PHARMACY:

An Introduction to the Profession

Notices

The author and publisher have made every effort to ensure the accuracy and completeness of the information presented in this book. However, the author and publisher cannot be held responsible for the continued currency of the information, any inadvertent errors or omissions, or the application of this information. Therefore, the author and publisher shall have no liability to any person or entity with regard to claims, loss, or damage caused or alleged to be caused, directly or indirectly, by the use of information contained herein.

PHARMACY:

An Introduction to the Profession
Second Edition

L. Michael Posey, BPharm
Editorial Director, Periodicals
American Pharmacists Association

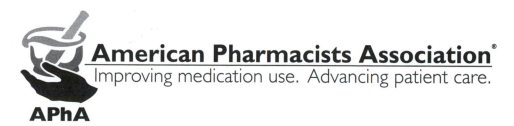

Washington, D.C.

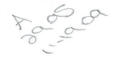
Acquiring Editor: Sandra J. Cannon
Production Editor: Paula Novash
Cover Design: Richard Muringer, APhA Creative Services
Layout and Graphics: Michele A. Danoff, Graphics by Design
Proofreader: Amy Morgante
Indexer: Mary Coe

© 2009 by the American Pharmacists Association
APhA was founded in 1852 as the American Pharmaceutical Association.

Published by the American Pharmacists Association
1100 15th Street, NW, Suite 400
Washington, DC 20005-1707
www.pharmacist.com

This textbook was published from 1992 through 2002 as an annually updated serial titled
Pharmacy Cadence by Pharmacy Editorial & News Services, Inc., Athens, Georgia.

To comment on this book via e-mail, send your message to the publisher at aphabooks@
aphanet.org

Library of Congress Cataloging-in-Publication Data

Posey, L. Michael.
  Pharmacy : an introduction to the profession / L. Michael Posey. –
2nd ed.
     p. ; cm.
  Includes bibliographical references and index.
  ISBN 978-1-58212-127-7
  1. Pharmacy. I. Title.
  [DNLM: 1. Pharmacy. 2. Career Choice. 3. Education, Pharmacy. QV
21 P856p 2009]

  RS91.P67 2009
  615'.1–dc22

                                                        2008045916

How to Order This Book
Online: www.pharmacist.com
By phone: 800-878-0729 (from the United States and Canada)
VISA®, MasterCard®, and American Express® cards accepted

Dedication

To the pharmacists of tomorrow

Contents

Preface | to the Second Edition

As students pass through the years of undergraduate education in America's colleges of pharmacy, they are presented with the opinions and viewpoints of dozens of faculty members, the perspectives and outlooks of hundreds of journal articles and textbooks, and the intricacies of thousands—some would say millions—of facts. Sometimes, amidst the cadence of all this information, the student never understands the bigger picture of how all the pieces fit together.

Since it was first published in 2003, the purpose of this textbook has been to provide a simple framework, in advance, so that the student will know better what a certain term means or what an issue is all about. This updated Second Edition contains the latest information on the state of pharmacy today, including how implementing MTM services has enhanced the practice of our profession.

During pharmacy school, the student is expected to undergo a process known as professionalization. This can begin only when the student has developed an accurate view of the profession he or she is entering and has come to understand the basic tenets of the profession and the critical issues it is now facing.

Pharmacy: An Introduction to the Profession provides that basis for the budding pharmacy student. Written for orientation to pharmacy courses (both preprofessional and professional level), this book has concise chapters focusing on the core knowledge needed to put information from other courses into perspective. The text is best supplemented with lectures from pharmacy faculty or administrators with expertise in the various subject areas. Also, practitioners from various areas of pharmacy practice should be invited to supplement the discussion of pharmacy career paths (Chapter 6) and post-graduate education (Chapter 10). When colleges of pharmacy do not have a standalone orientation course, this text can be used for supplemental reading in an appropriate preprofessional or early professional level course.

The new articles in Chapter 11 represent recent pharmacy literature that can help jump-start new student pharmacists. To keep this material current, a list of updated readings is available through the Publications page of APhA's Web site, www.pharmacist.com. Faculty members who wish to be notified of changes in these readings should request this in an e-mail message to aphabooks@aphanet.org.

Improvements in future editions of this textbook will be based on faculty and student feedback. Please contact me with ideas for expansion or improvement at the address shown below. Likewise, readers with suggested articles for inclusion in future editions are asked to bring those to my attention. Only through your efforts can this text gain more utility for tomorrow's students of pharmacy.

L. Michael Posey, BPharm (mposey@aphanet.org)
Washington, D.C.
May 2008

Acknowledgments

Development of this book would not have been possible without the advice and suggestions of the pharmacy deans and faculty who were surveyed during planning stages. The following individuals reviewed portions of the material before publication:

- Edward P. Armstrong
- Maude A. Babington
- Sandy Hunt Bentley
- Valerie Briggs
- Carmen A. Catizone
- Laura Cranston
- George Francisco
- Caroline Gaither
- John A. Gans
- Gregory J. Higby
- Randy P. Juhl
- Kenneth W. Kirk
- Kathryn Kuhn
- Ronald W. Maddox
- Lucinda Maine
- Michael L. Manolakis
- Vicki Meade
- Arthur A. Nelson
- Joseph A. Oddis
- Robert W. Piepho
- Gary Van Riper
- John S. Ruggiero
- Ralph Saroyan
- David J. Slatkin
- Rebecca P. Snead
- Ellen Wilcox
- Linda M. Williams
- William A. Zellmer

Bruce A. Berger of Auburn University contributed Chapter 4, Communications in Pharmacy Practice, which summarizes concepts presented in his book *Communication Skills for Pharmacists,* 2nd edition, published by APhA. Lauren Angelo, PharmD, MBA, of the APhA staff in Washington, D.C., assisted with development of material related to the Medicare Part D prescription drug benefit and medication therapy management. This information appears in Chapter 3, Pharmacy Reborn: Pharmaceutical Care and Medication Therapy Management, and Chapter 7, Governmental and Voluntary Oversight of Pharmacy.

Chapter 1 | Pharmacy's Cadence: Drumbeat of a Profession

Over the past 20 years, pharmacy has made a number of important decisions, ones that were very controversial among members of the profession. As we move toward the end of the first decade of the 21st century, I'm happy to report to you that those difficult choices are reaping dividends for pharmacy and pharmacists.

As you will read in the pages of Chapters 2 and 3 of this textbook, the profession of pharmacy has a long and illustrious history, one filled with challenges that led pharmacists to adapt and innovate. In recent years, change required pharmacists to expand from a singular focus on the medication and an economic reliance on payments generated by the transfer of drugs and drug products to the patient. The profession, recognizing that new and more powerful medications were presenting challenges to physicians and patients alike, needed to expand from being a source of the medications to also providing patients with the information needed to safely and appropriately use those drugs.

With the passage of the Medicare Prescription Drug, Improvement, and Modernization Act of 2003, pharmacy is now recognized in both the product and information aspects needed for today's practice. In this chapter, I briefly explain the importance of this legislation and its implications for pharmacy and also cover two other general trends of concern to the profession: the need for a recognized cadre of paraprofessionals to support pharmacists in their expanding roles and the exploding demand for medications and health care in general because of the number of senior citizens in the United States and other developed countries.

Medication therapy management: Pharmacy's raison d'être

For centuries, pharmacists have been paid when they provided a medicinal agent or product to patients. This system served the profession well for millennia. When the responsibilities of medicine and pharmacy were demarcated a few centuries ago, pharmacists focused their practices on the art of preparing the medicinals prescribed by physicians using unique equipment available in their apothecaries and developed new ways of making medicinal agents palatable, effective, and safe.

Over a few decades in the late 19th and early 20th century, the pharmaceutical industry gradually subsumed many of the compounding responsibilities of pharmacists, making the dispensing part of pharmacy not much more than counting and pouring from big bottles into little bottles, and then preparing a label and sticking it on the prescription vial or bottle. Pharmacy responded to this change in many ways; these are described more completely in Chapter 3. A key component of this response was to increase the medication information activities of pharmacists. This meant that in some cases pharmacists needed to contact physicians to suggest changes in prescriptions, or even to decline to dispense a prescription that might harm the patient. The problem was that, in these cases, the

"Shallow men believe in luck, believe in circumstance. Strong men believe in cause and effect."

—Ralph Waldo Emerson

"Chance favors the prepared mind."

—Louis Pasteur

Paradigm:
As used here, paradigm is the typical or standard activities of a pharmacist on a day-to-day basis.

pharmacist was not being reimbursed for the extra work, and if the prescription was not dispensed, no payment at all would occur.

The profession, starting in the 1960s and 1970s, developed information services, first in hospitals and then for patients in nursing homes. The systems were quickly incorporated into the institutional structures, and governmental regulations were soon developed for these settings. But patients in community pharmacies did not see much change. Since the public's overall perception of pharmacy relies on what they see in the community independent and chain pharmacy, people began to think that pharmacists really didn't do anything but "count, pour, lick, and stick."

Beginning with a federally mandated requirement to offer medication counseling to patients in the Medicaid program in the 1990s, this situation began to change in community pharmacies, but at a hopelessly glacial rate. As you will read in Chapter 3, the American Pharmacists Association (APhA) Foundation and motivated pharmacists in Asheville, N.C., finally created some movement in community pharmacies when they created models for community pharmacists to use in providing a new kind of care to patients with chronic diseases such as diabetes and high serum cholesterol levels. The resulting practice, called medication therapy management (MTM),[1] was included in the 2003 legislation that created a prescription drug benefit for disabled and senior citizens who receive health care under the federal Medicare program. In addition, pharmacists such as John Grabenstein, PhD, then with the U.S. Army and working closely with APhA staff, began to advocate that pharmacies were an ideal place for patients to be vaccinated against influenza and other infectious diseases. These events began to change the perception of the corner drugstore from a mercantile outlet to one where patients could obtain health care services.

Pharmacy technician:
A paraprofessional assistant to the pharmacist who helps with the mechanical preparation of medications for dispensing to patients. This person may interpret prescription orders, prepare the medication (including some compounding of medications and preparation of intravenous solutions), and check the work of other technicians in specific situations.

As this book goes to print in mid-2008, the prospects for MTM making a tremendous difference are excellent. Independent pharmacies have implemented MTM programs, and some pharmacy chains are looking at ways to have at least one pharmacist with special training in MTM in every unit. For this effort to succeed, pharmacy practitioners will need to work under a new, emerging **paradigm** that integrates accurate dispensing of the medications with MTM services that focus on how pharmacotherapy can improve the health of each patient.[2] Because the number of pharmacists is limited and the number of prescriptions dispensed annually is growing, accurate dispensing will rely on automation and **pharmacy technicians**, and pharmacy will need to develop sound systems for managing this process even as they meet with patients to discuss their use of medications.

As I wrote recently in APhA's MTM magazine, *Pharmacy Today,*[3] this new mode of pharmacy practice works,[4-10] employers whose budgets are being strained by health care costs ought to pay attention to the results afforded by pharmacist care of chronic diseases,[5,7,8] the model for pharmacist provision of such services has been tested and shown to work in a variety of pharmacy and geographic settings,[11] and pharmacists who have the knowledge, skills, and tools for delivering this type of care are available.[12,13] There's nothing else to wait for—we need only now to get to work providing MTM! Whether we do will have a lot to do with how—or perhaps whether—pharmacy is practiced a decade or two from now.

Health care: Economics of aging for the baby boomers

The world is changing. As a result of advances in medical science, people are living longer, especially in the developed countries of the world. Combined with a decreasing birth rate in many countries, the world's population is becoming older. As shown graphically in Figure 1.1 (see page 6), by 2030 the number of people in the retired age groups is predicted to be far larger than it has been in the past, both in numbers and as a percentage of the population. All in all, the percentage of Americans who are 65 years of age or older will increase from 12.4% in 2000 to 19.6% in 2030.[14-16] Older people have more diseases, especially degenerative conditions such as arthritis and Alzheimer's disease, that interfere with one's ability to walk, bathe, dress, feed oneself, or use the bathroom without assistance. Older patients generally also take many more medications than do younger people.

The implications of this demographic shift are far reaching. In the United States, the Social Security and Medicare programs are relied upon by millions of older Americans for basic social and medical care. These programs depend on continued contributions from current workers to pay benefits for recipients, and the number of workers per retired person is falling. As the 76 million baby boomers—those Americans born between 1946 and 1964—begin reaching retirement age in 2011, the existing system for social and health care of senior citizens will be increasingly stressed. Combine that fact with America's already burgeoning national debt, and the question of how America will pay for care of its senior citizens in the coming half century becomes even more challenging. Can fewer and fewer workers pay enough in taxes to provide support for an increasing number of senior citizens and service the national debt at the same time? If not, what then?

For pharmacists, will these changes translate into a population whose chronic diseases are a natural fit for the kind of MTM services described above? Or will the continually increasing cost of medications simply mean that fewer and fewer resources are left over to pay for the professional expertise needed to use those medications properly?

While no one knows the answers to such questions, the indicators for pharmacy are positive. First, drug-related problems (DRPs) are undoubtedly one of the big challenges facing the medical system in general and pharmacists in particular. Studies show that the cost of DRPs among ambulatory Americans (not counting those in hospitals and nursing homes) was $177 billion nearly a decade ago. This means that for every $1 spent on medications, another $1 is spent paying for problems associated with use of the medications.[17] Experts who have analyzed DRPs conclude that, while a lot of DRPs are unexpected and cannot be foreseen, pharmacists could have prevented or minimized many DRPs through timely interventions.

In addition to payment for such services under the Medicare Part D MTM program, the possibility that patients might pay pharmacists directly for help with managing medications is a positive sign.[18,19] As a sufficient number of patients experience MTM services and conclude that they are valuable, a tipping point may be reached that will lead to widespread patient demand for pharmacists' services. If and when that occurs, then coverage by **pharmacy benefits managers** and other third-party payers will be common.

Pharmacy benefits managers (PBMs): Companies that contract with managed-care organizations, insurance companies, or employers to provide prescriptions and pharmaceutical care to a covered population. PBMs often contract with networks of independent or chain pharmacies to provide this care in accordance with guidelines and rules that can reduce the cost of prescriptions.

If pharmacists are preoccupied with detecting and preventing DRPs, who will be responsible for getting the right drug to the right patient at the right time? Fortunately, several trends have converged to provide pharmacists with a lot of assistance in the process of drug preparation.

Pharmacists getting out of drug preparation

Pharmacists have for years had helpers who assisted with various tasks in the pharmacy and have used tools to make the job easier or faster. Advances in technology are producing sophisticated dispensing machines and robotic devices that, using bar-code scanners, are virtually replacing pharmacists in their dispensing roles. Likewise, pharmacy technicians have emerged as an identifiable group of competent assistants who can perform many of the tasks formerly handled by pharmacists.

As applied in pharmacy practice, automated devices include systems for dispensing tablets and capsules. These systems generally combine a computer, bar-code scanner, and counting device. Some systems produce strip packs of medications sealed into individual pouches, while others put all the medications for a certain time of administration into a single pouch.

Automated dispensing systems are now being linked to computerized physician order entry systems in both hospitals and the ambulatory settings. Medication errors caused by poor handwriting and other types of ineffective communication are driving physicians to write prescriptions on computers and personal digital assistants,[20] and Medicare Part D is expected to mandate an increased level of computerized physician order entry.

Robotic devices are more common in hospitals. Some robots deliver medications to nursing stations located around the building, while others are used to fill patient cassettes in unit-dose dispensing systems.[21]

Many exciting changes have been made with respect to the training, recognition, and legal status of pharmacy technicians. These paraprofessionals assist with the process of filling prescriptions. While the tasks that technicians may legally perform vary from state to state, they generally include reading the physician's order, computer entry of the information, placing the drugs into a container for the patient, affixing the label, and giving the completed materials to a pharmacist for checking.

Pharmacies that rely on technicians heavily—such as chain pharmacies, mail-service operations, and hospitals—often have formal training programs that combine classroom work with on-the-job experiences. Additionally, community colleges and technical schools are implementing more and more technician-training programs, which usually require one or two years of schooling. The U.S. military has an excellent training program for technicians.

In response to the advancing level of importance of pharmacy technicians within practice, a national certification examination was established for pharmacy technicians. Housed physically within the headquarters of the American Pharmacists Association, the Pharmacy Technician Certification Board is an independent organization responsible for administering the examination, which tests the knowledge of pharmacy technicians. First administered in 1995, the examination has a high rate of passage—usually above 80%.

The number of Certified Pharmacy Technicians (CPhTs) exceeded 300,000 by mid-2008. In comparison, the number of licensed pharmacists in the United States is about 200,000.

Planning for change

As the quotations at the beginning of this chapter indicate, pharmacy has two choices in dealing with the break-neck pattern of change sweeping through health care: plan and prepare for it, or hope for the best. On the assumption than the former option is preferred, *Pharmacy: An Introduction to the Profession* will present the history, forces, trends, and concepts that influence pharmacy in its present state. You—the new student pharmacist in the early decades of a new millennium—can use this information in planning for the future of your new profession, pharmacy.

REFERENCES

1. American Pharmacists Association and National Association of Chain Drug Stores Foundation. Medication therapy management in pharmacy practice: core elements of an MTM service model. Version 2.0. *J Am Pharm Assoc.* 2008; 48: 341-53.
2. Posey LM. Proving that pharmaceutical care makes a difference in community pharmacy [editorial]. *J Am Pharm Assoc.* 2003; 43: 136-8.
3. Posey LM. MTM: The pieces fit together. *Pharm Today.* 2008(Mar); 14(3).
4. Cranor CW, Christensen DB. The Asheville Project: short-term outcomes of a community pharmacy diabetes care program. *J Am Pharm Assoc.* 2003;43:149-59.
5. Cranor CW, Bunting BA, Christensen DB. The Asheville Project: long-term clinical and economic outcomes in a community pharmacy diabetes care program. *J Am Pharm Assoc.* 2003;43:173-84.
6. Garrett DG, Martin LA. The Asheville Project: participants' perceptions of factors contributing to the success of a Patient Self-Management Program for Diabetes. *J Am Pharm Assoc.* 2003;43:185-90.
7. Bunting BA, Cranor CW. The Asheville Project: long-term clinical, humanistic, and economic outcomes of a community-based medication therapy management program for asthma. *J Am Pharm Assoc.* 2006;46:133-47.
8. Bunting BA, Smith BH, Sutherland SE. The Asheville Project: Clinical and economic outcomes of a community-based long-term medication therapy management program for hypertension and dyslipidemia. *J Am Pharm Assoc.* 2008;48:23-31.
9. Bluml BM, McKenney JM, Cziraky MJ. Pharmaceutical care services and results in Project ImPACT: Hyperlipidemia. *J Am Pharm Assoc.* 2000;40:157-65.
10. Bluml BM, Garrett DG. Patient self-management program for diabetes: first-year clinical, humanistic, and economic outcomes. *J Am Pharm Assoc.* 2005;45:130-7.
11. Fera T, Bluml BM, Ellis WM, Schaller CW, Garrett DG. The Diabetes Ten City Challenge: Interim clinical and humanistic outcomes of a multisite community pharmacy diabetes care program. *J Am Pharm Assoc.* 2008;48:181-90.
12. Schommer JC, Planas LG, Johnson KA, Doucette WR. Pharmacist-provided medication therapy management (part 1): provider perspectives in 2007. *J Am Pharm Assoc.* 2008;48:354-63.
13. Schommer JC, Planas LG, Johnson KA, Doucette WR. Pharmacist-provided medication therapy management (part 2): payer perspectives in 2007. *J Am Pharm Assoc.* 2008;48:e46-e54.
14. Institute of Medicine. Retooling for an Aging America: Building the Health Care Workforce. Washington, D.C.: Institute of Medicine; 2008. Accessed at www.iom.edu/?ID=53452, May 10, 2008.
15. Centers for Disease Control and Prevention. Public health and aging: trends in aging—United States and worldwide. *MMWR.* 2003;52:101-6.
16. Posey LM. America ages, pharmacy prepares. *Pharm Today.* 2003(May): 1, 11, 13.
17. Ernst FR, Grizzle AJ. Drug-related morbidity and mortality: updating the cost-of-illness model. *J Am Pharm Assoc.* 2001;41:156-7.
18. Ganther JM. Third party reimbursement for pharmacist services: why has it been so difficult to obtain and is it really the answer for pharmacy? *J Am Pharm Assoc.* 2002; 42: 875-9.

19. Winckler SC. Pharmacist services: insurance need not be the only answer [editorial]. *J Am Pharm Assoc*. 2002; 42: 826.

20. Posey LM. Electronic physician order entry: segue to a fully automated medication system. *Pharm Today*. 2001(Sept):1, 9, 10.

21. Posey LM. Medication errors: the pain, the problems, the process. *Pharm Today*. 2001(Feb): 1, 21.

Figure 1.1 | Population age distribution for developing and developed countries, by age group and sex—worldwide, 1950, 1990, and 2030.

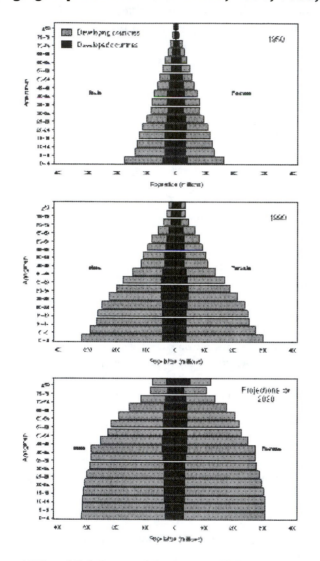

Source: United Nations, 1999, and U.S. Bureau of the Census, 2000.

Chapter 2 | Development of Pharmacy in History as a Healing Profession

For as long as the human species has encountered disease, injury, and illness, people have sought relief. Several detailed accounts of pharmacy history are available for the interested reader[1-3]; presented here is a brief overview of the roots of this profession. Noteworthy are the 40 original oil paintings commissioned by Parke–Davis, now a part of Pfizer, and recently donated to the American Pharmacists Association (APhA).[3] The development of this Robert Thom series has been reviewed by George Griffenhagen, APhA historian.[4] Reproductions of this series hang in many schools of pharmacy across the United States. Griffenhagen has also compiled the history of pharmacy as recorded on stamps and postal imprints.[5] An excellent illustrated history of pharmacy has been published, written by respected historians David L. Cowen and William H. Helfland.[6] Tables 2.1 through 2.6 provide interested students with detailed listings of key dates in pharmacy and world history.

In this chapter, we will study the history of pharmacy from its origins in ancient Babylonia through the middle of the twentieth century, when pharmacy's status as a profession was questioned by medicine and other parts of society. Chapter 3 details the more recent history of pharmacy as a process of reprofessionalization took hold.

"... if the preparation of medicines is taken from the apothecary and he becomes merely the dispenser of them, his business is shorn of half its dignity and importance, and he relapses into a simple shopkeeper."

—William Procter, 1858

Pharmacy in ancient times

Pharmacy was undoubtedly "practiced" in prehistoric times as people instinctively used the water, plants, and earth around them for soothing compresses on wounds and ailments. As civilization dawned in ancient Mesopotamia (2600 B.C.), Babylonian healing practitioners combined the responsibilities of priest, physician, and pharmacist,[3] and some of the oldest pharmacy records are found in Sumerian (Babylonian) clay cuneiform tablets that date to about 2000 B.C. Retailers of drugs were concentrated on a certain street in Babylon by 2111 B.C.[1,3,7]

In Ancient China (circa 2000 B.C.), legend tells that Emperor Shen Nung investigated the medicinal properties of hundreds of herbs, and he recorded 365 native herbal drugs in the first Pen T'sao.[3]

Egyptian priests, as part of their duties, prepared medicines. The Ebers papyrus, which dates from 1900 to 1100 B.C., is the best known and most important pharmaceutical record from ancient history. It contains 800 prescriptions using 700 drugs. Of particular note in the papyrus is inclusion of quantities of substances, which were largely missing in the Babylonian clay tablets. Many modern dosage forms are also referred to in the Ebers papyrus—gargles, snuffs, inhalations, suppositories, fumigations, enemas, poultices, decoctions, infusions, pills, troches, lotions, ointments, and plasters.[1]

Table 2.1 | Selected World & Pharmacy Events Before the Middle Ages[a]

YEAR	EVENT	YEAR	EVENT
50,000 B.C.	Neanderthal man existed on earth.	429–347 B.C.	Plato.
35,000 B.C.	Cro-Magnon man existed (late Palaeolithic Age).	384–322 B.C.	Aristotle.
7000-2000 B.C.	Neolithic Age in Europe.	338–323 B.C.	Alexander the Great.
5000-4500 B.C.	Dawn of Sumerian, Egyptian, and Minoan cultures.	44 B.C.	Julius Caesar assassinated.
2500 B.C.	Surgical operations depicted in Egyptian pyramids.	4 B.C.	Jesus Christ born.
2000-1000 B.C.	Bronze Age in Europe.	79	Plague following eruption of Vesuvius. Pompeii destroyed.
1500 B.C.	Ebers papyrus.	130-201	Galen.
1237 B.C.	Death of Asclepius.	220	Han Dynasty ends in China.
1000-500 B.C.	Earlier Iron Age in Europe.	303	Martyrdom of Saints Cosmas and Damian (patron saints of medicine and pharmacy).
950 B.C.	Homer.		
753 B.C.	Founding of Rome.	369	Hospital of St. Basil erected at Caesarea by Justinian.
600 B.C.	Massage and acupuncture practiced by Japanese.	395–1453	Byzantine Empire.
580-489 B.C.	Pythagoras.	400	First hospital established in western Europe.
550 B.C.	Buddha and Confucius lived.	476	Fall of Roman Empire.
525 B.C.	Asclepius raised to rank of God of Medicine in Greece.		
522 B.C.	Medical school founded at Athens.		
500 B.C.	Later Iron Age.		
460–361 B.C.	Hippocrates.		

[a] Adapted from reference 3.

In ancient Greece lived the Father of Botany, Theophrastus (about 300 B.C.). In addition to studying plants in general, his observations about the medicinal qualities of herbs have proven uncannily accurate.[3] Hippocrates of Cos formulated the theory of the four humors that parallel the four elements (air—blood, water—phlegm, earth—black bile, fire—yellow bile); he surmised that disease was caused by an imbalance of these bad humors. This led to centuries of medicine aimed at expelling from the ill person of the offending, excess bad humors.[1]

Galenicals:
Historically used to refer to a class of pharmaceutical products that were compounded through mechanical means.

Galen (A.D. 130–200) practiced and taught medicine and pharmacy in ancient Rome. He developed principles of preparing and compounding medicinal agents that were followed for 1500 years, and the word **galenicals**, derived from his name, is still used to refer to medicinal agents derived from natural sources that are prepared mechanically.[3] Galen and his followers sought to restore humoral balance within a patient by the use of medicines of opposing qualities (for example, inflammation would be treated with cucumber, a cool drug). He also drew from many available sources and attempted to organize and systematize the work begun by Hippocrates.[1]

Also from the Roman era come the patron saints of pharmacy and medicine, the twin brothers Damian and Cosmas. These devout Christians of Arab descent offered religious and medicinal solaces to those who came to them, until their twin careers were cut short in 303 by martyrdom. Damian, the apothecary, and Cosmas, the physician, became the patron saints of their closely allied professions.[3]

Table 2.2 | World & Pharmacy Events During the Middle Ages[a]

YEAR	EVENT	YEAR	EVENT
571–632	Mohammed.	1345	First apothecary shop in London.
711	Moslems invaded Spain.	1348–1350	Black Death.
768–814	Charlemagne.	1368	Ming Dynasty in China.
871–901	Alfred the Great.	1376	Board of Medical Examiners founded in London.
980–1036	Avicenna.	1440–1450	Invention of printing.
1066	Battle of Hastings.	1452–1519	Leonardo da Vinci.
1096–1272	Crusades.	1454	Gutenberg Bible printed.
1198	Hospital movement inaugurated by Innocent III.	1457	First medical publication (Gutenberg Purgation-Calendar).
1215	Magna Carta signed in Britain.	1478	Spanish Inquisition.
1227–1274	Thomas Aquinas.	1479	First edition of Avicenna printed.
1231	Medical school at Salerno.		
1271	Marco Polo began travels.	[a] Adapted from reference 3.	
1330	Gunpowder used in warfare.		
1336–1453	Hundred Years' War.		

Pharmacy differentiates during the middle ages

Pharmaceutical knowledge—and the number of drugs available—grew considerably during the Middle Ages, thanks primarily to the Arabic world. Pharmacy as a separate activity began to develop, and privately owned pharmacies were established in Islamic lands. Medicine and pharmacy were for the first time separated.[1] The first known apothecary shop was opened in Baghdad in the eighth century, and the Moslems carried this concept into Europe during wars and other excursions into Africa, Spain, and southern France. The "Persian Galen," Ibn Sina (circa 980–1037), is known as Avicenna by the Western world. An intellectual giant, he was a physician, poet, philosopher, diplomat, and companion of Persian princes and rulers.[3] His Canon Medicinae brought together the best knowledge of the Greeks and Arabs into a single medical text.

Priests were also important in advancing the use of plants and other substances as medicines for patients during the Middle Ages.[1]

German Emperor Frederick II issued an edict in about 1240 that legally separated pharmacy from medicine in southern Italy and Sicily. Known as the Magna Carta of pharmacy, the edict contained three decrees[1]:
1. The pharmaceutical profession was to be separated from the medical profession.
2. The pharmaceutical profession should be supervised officially.
3. Pharmacists should take an oath to prepare drugs reliably, according to skilled art, and in a uniform suitable quality.

Each of these three requirements was critical in pharmacy's recognition by society and in later developments in the history of pharmacy.

Table 2.3 | World & Pharmacy Events During the Renaissance[a]

YEAR	EVENT
1492	Columbus discovers America.
1493–1541	Paracelsus.
1498	First official pharmacopeia (Florentine Receptario).
1509–1547	Reign of Henry VIII in England.
1517	Luther propounded his theses at Wittenberg.
1518	Royal College of Physicians founded in England.
1524	Cortes erected hospital in Mexico.
1526	Paracelsus founded chemotherapy.
1540	English barbers and surgeons united as "Commonalty of the Barbers and Surgeons."
1543	Copernicus described revolution of earth around sun.
1543	English apothecaries legalized by Act of Parliament.
1558–1603	Reign of Elizabeth I.
1561–1626	Francis Bacon.
1564–1616	Shakespeare.
1564–1642	Galileo.
1578–1657	William Harvey.
1584	Sir Walter Raleigh brought curare from Guiana.
1590	Compound microscope invented.
1604–1609	Galileo elucidated law of falling bodies.
1606–1669	Rembrandt.
1607	Settlement of Jamestown, Virginia.
1609	Galileo turns telescope on the night sky.
1609–1618	Kepler stated laws of planetary motion.
1615–1616	Harvey lectured on circulation of blood.
1617	Guild of Apothecaries of the City of London founded.
1618	First edition of London Pharmacopoeia.
1618–1648	Thirty Years' War.
1620	Pilgrims landed at Plymouth, Massachusetts.
1620	Van Helmont stressed chemical role of gastric juice in digestion.
1622–1673	Molière.
1628	Harvey published *De Motu Cordis*.
1630–1638	Treatment of malarial fever with cinchona bark known in Peru.
1632–1723	Antony van Leeuwenhoek (inventor of microscope).
1636	Harvard College founded.
1639	First hospital in Canada.
1639–1650	Juan del Vigo introduced cinchona into Spain and Italy.
1643	Sir Edward Greaves described typhus fever as a "new disease" in England.
1648	Francesco Redi disproved theory of spontaneous generation.
1654–1715	Reign of Louis XIV.
1660	Willis described puerperal fever.
1661	Malpighi published first account of capillary system (*De pulmonibus*).
1661	Robert Boyle defined chemical elements and isolated acetone.
1661	Descartes published first treatise on physiology (*De homine*).
1665	Newton discovered binomial theorem and law of gravitation.
1665	Great Plague of London.
1666	Great Fire of London.
1669	Lower showed that venous blood takes up air in the lungs.
1670	Malpighi discovered malpighian bodies in spleen and kidneys.
1670	Willis discovered sweet taste of diabetic urine.
1672	De Graaf described the graafian follicles in ovary.
1673	Leeuwenhoek began making microscopes.
1675	Leeuwenhoek discovered protozoa.
1682–1725	Peter the Great rules Russia.
1683	Sydenham's treatise on gout published.
1683	Leeuwenhoek described and sketched bacteria.
1685–1750	Johann Sebastian Bach.
1690	Locke's "Essay Concerning Human Understanding" published.

[a] Adapted from reference 3.

The Renaissance: Pharmacists flourished too

Following the Middle Ages, many parts of European society re-examined the Greek and Roman tenets that they had held as fact. Thus, just as Copernicus challenged the Roman Catholic Church with his conclusion that the earth revolved around the sun, pharmacists stood ready to consider new approaches to the prevention and treatment of disease.

Among the ideas that failed to stand up to closer scrutiny were the humoral pathology concepts of Hippocrates and their systemization by Galen and Avicenna.[1] The Swiss physician Parcelsus (1493-1541) was particularly important in that he introduced two ideas: (1) Disease might be localized in a specific organ (rather than the entire body being affected), and such conditions could be treated internally using the chemical properties of medicinal agents, and (2) some plants and other substances contained minute quantities of active chemicals, which could be removed by making tinctures, extracts, and essences.[1]

Professional associations of pharmacists emerged during the Renaissance, although some date back to the 1200s. In England, pharmacists had been under the jurisdiction of the Guild of Grocers, which monopolized the drug and spice trade. In 1617, King James I granted a charter recognizing the Society of Apothecaries of London.[3]

Other contemporaries in the sixteenth and seventeenth centuries believed that disease was produced through an imbalance of acid and alkaline substances in the body. The theory of iatrochemistry held that food was transformed by saliva and by a ferment secreted by the pancreas and that blood was made life-giving through ferments from the gall bladder and lymph glands. These ideas provided convenient ways to categorize chemicals and drugs based on observed effects. Homeopathy, or treatment of disease with substances that produced similar symptoms as did the disease, also has its origins in the Renaissance period.[1]

Pharmacy in the United States: The early days

With the increased recognition and application of the scientific method in the 1700s and 1800s, modern pharmacy emerged. Progress in inorganic and organic chemistry, immunology, and chemotherapy began to change pharmacy from an empirically-based profession to a knowledge-based one.[7]

Medicine and pharmacy in the New World was necessarily based on practices from Europe, but the Americas also adapted European practices to meet new needs and take advantage of new opportunities. Many new medicinal plants were exported from the New to the Old World, including guaicum, sassafras, copaiba, and balsam of Peru. Four distinct types of pharmacies could be found in the Americas by the 18th Century: the dispensing physician, the apothecary shop, the general store, and the **wholesale druggist**. Dispensing physicians became less and less common, dying out around the end of the nineteenth century (they made a comeback recently, however, with some physicians establishing dispensing rooms in their offices as an additional profit center). Also of interest was that wholesale druggists of this period generally would have a dispensing operation that operated like the apothecary shops.[1]

Wholesale druggists: Intermediaries in the mercantile chain between manufacturers and retail outlets such as pharmacies.

Table 2.4 | World & Pharmacy Events in the Eighteenth Century[a]

YEAR	EVENT
1702	Stahl stated phlogiston theory.
1718	Geoffroy published table of chemical relationships.
1719	Neumann reported thymol.
1721	Zabdiel Boylston inoculated for smallpox.
1730	Frobenius described preparation of sulfuric ether.
1740	Thomas Dover developed "Dover's Powder."
1740–1786	Reign of Frederick the Great.
1743	Red Cross arrangement at Battle of Dettingen.
1743–1794	Antoine Laurent Lavoisier.
1749–1823	Edward Jenner.
1750	Griffith Hughes gave classic account of yellow fever of 1715 (Barbados).
1751	Pennsylvania Hospital established in Philadelphia with Jonathan Roberts as apothecary.
1752	Medical Society founded in London.
1754–1757	Black discovered carbon dioxide.
1755	John Morgan appointed as second apothecary at Pennsylvania Hospital.
1767	Kay and Hargreaves invented spinning jenny (beginning of Industrial Revolution in England).
1768	Baumé created the hydrometer.
1768	Margraaf discovered hydrogen fluoride.
1769–1821	Napoleon Bonaparte.
1769	Scheele discovered tartaric acid.
1770	First medical degree in United States conferred.
1770–1827	Beethoven.
1771–1774	Priestley and Scheele isolated oxygen ("dephlogisticated air").
1772	Priestley discovered nitrogen and nitrous oxide.
1773	Medical Society of London founded.
1773	Rouelle discovered urea.
1774	Scheele discovered chlorine.
1774	Wiegleb discovered myristic acid.
1774	Rouelle defined chemical nature of a salt.
1775	Lavoisier isolated and defined oxygen and defined an acid.
1775	Andrew Craigie became first Apothecary General of the United States.
1775–1783	American Revolution.
1777	Lavoisier described exchange of gases in respiration.
1777	Scheele's experiments with silver chloride laid groundwork for photography.
1778	William Brown published first American pharmacopeia, called the Lititz pharmacopeia.
1780	Benjamin Franklin invented bifocal lenses.
1781–1826	René Théophile-Hyacinthe Laennec.
1783	Scheele discovered glycerin.
1783	First balloon ascension.
1783–1785	Lavoisier decomposed water and overthrew phlogiston theory.
1784	Scheele discovered citric acid.
1785	Minkelers first used illuminating gas in balloons.
1785	Withering's treatise on the foxglove (digitalis) published.
1785	Scheele discovered malic acid.
1789	Klaproth discovered uranium and zirconium.
1789–1799	French Revolution.
1792	Cotton gin invented by Eli Whitney.
1793	Benjamin Bell differentiated between gonorrhea and syphilis.
1793	Lowitz discovered mono- and tri-chloroacetic acids.
1793–1794	Reign of Terror in France.
1794	Lavoisier beheaded.
1794	Thomas Percival's code of medical ethics privately printed.
1795	Joseph B. Caventou, French pharmacist and scientist, born.
1795–1796	Société de Médecine de Paris founded.
1796	Jenner vaccinated James Phipps.
1796	Lowitz prepared absolute alcohol and pure ether.
1796–1815	Napoleonic Wars.
1797	Vauqueline discovered chromium.
1798	Jenner's Inquiry published.
1799	Davy discovered anesthetic properties of laughing gas (nitrous oxide).
1800	Royal College of Surgeons of London chartered.

[a] Adapted from references 1–3 and 9–11.

Among the well-known pharmacists of the period were Christopher Marshall of Philadelphia, Hugh Mercer of Fredericksburg, Virginia, and Andrew Craigie, the Apothecary General during the Revolutionary War.[1]

Pharmacy in the United States: The nineteenth century

Wholesale druggists and individual apothecaries began manufacturing and selling chemicals in the late 1700s; this was the basis for the later establishment of pharmaceutical companies. The world was changing from an agriculturally-based economy to an industrial-based one, and pharmacy found itself caught in this shift. Some drugs could be manufactured using the newly discovered principles of chemistry. The smallpox vaccine of Jenner was proving that one could be made immune to the ravages of infectious diseases. By the end of the nineteenth century, Koch's postulates had clearly proven the microbial basis of many diseases. A German chemist, Friedrich Wilhelm Adam SertÅrner, first isolated the drug morphine from opium and thereby created recognition of the alkaloids as a distinct class of medicinal agents.[3]

In January 1820, an important meeting took place in the Senate chambers of the U.S. Capitol in Washington. There, delegates met to begin work on a national **pharmacopeia**. Thanks largely to the impetus provided by physician Lyman Spalding, the first *Pharmacopeia of the United States* was published that year, and it was the precursor to today's *United States Pharmacopeia*. The phrase "USP" at the end of drug names today denotes that the product complies with the standards set by the United States Pharmacopeial Convention, which continues to meet every five years to revise standards for the nation's drugs.[1]

> **Pharmacopeia:**
> Books listing drugs and other medical devices, including standards for their preparation and analysis, that are recognized by a governmental authority.

By the early 1800s, states were issuing licenses to apothecaries, often based on examination provided by the medical examining board; South Carolina the first state do so. In 1821, the Philadelphia College of Pharmacy (PCP) was founded, the first pharmacy organization in the United States. PCP soon provided classes for apprentices to learn pharmacy. The Philadelphia pharmacists were responding to two major threats: Deterioration of the practice of pharmacy and discriminatory classification by the University of Pennsylvania medical faculty. Other schools followed quickly, often with help from PCP[1]:

- Massachusetts College of Pharmacy (1823)
- College of Pharmacy of the City (and County) of New York (1829)
- Maryland College of Pharmacy (1840)
- Cincinnati College of Pharmacy (1850)
- Chicago College of Pharmacy (1859)
- St. Louis College of Pharmacy (1864)

The school at Philadelphia became the heart of American pharmacy in the 1800s. In addition to setting the tone and direction for pharmacy education, its faculty and alumni were instrumental in the formation of APhA, founded as the American Pharmaceutical Association, during a convention of 20 delegates at PCP in 1852.

Indeed, in the rotunda of the APhA building in Washington today sits a statue of William Procter, Jr., of PCP, known as "The Father of American Pharmacy." Procter was an 1837 PCP graduate who served on the faculty for 20 years and for 30 years on the United States Pharmacopeial Convention's Committee on Revision. The first secretary of APhA, he was editor of the *American Journal of Pharmacy* for 22 years.

Table 2.5 | World & Pharmacy Events of the Nineteenth Century[a]

YEAR	EVENT	YEAR	EVENT
1801–1820	Discoveries and/or isolation of cerium, morphine, mannitol, cinchonic acid, iodine, lecithin, daphnin, narcotine, strychnine, brucine, colchicine, quinine, and cinchonine.	1841	Pharmaceutical Society of Great Britain founded.
		1842	Long introduced ether anesthesia.
		1843	O. W. Holmes pointed out contagiousness of puerperal fever.
1803–1808	Lewis and Clark expedition.	1845–1923	Wilhelm Conrad Röentgen.
1806	End of Holy Roman Empire.	1846	Morton introduced ether anesthesia.
1809	McDowell performed ovariotomy.	1846	J. Marion Sims devised a vaginal speculum.
1810	Figuier published qualities of animal charcoal.	1847	American Medical Association organized.
1811	Valentine Seaman published the first civilian American pharmacopeia at the New York Hospital.	1847	Helmholtz published treatise on Conservation of Energy.
		1847	Sir J. Y. Simpson introduced chloroform anesthesia.
1815–1878	Crawford W. Long.	1847	Semmelwise discovered pathogenesis of puerperal fever.
1816	Laennec invented stethoscope.	1848	Fehling introduced test for sugar in urine.
1818	Meissner coined name "alkaloid."	1848	Claude Bernard demonstrated that glycogen is synthesized in the liver.
1819	Braconnet obtained grape sugar, treating sawdust with sulfuric acid.	1849	J. Marion Sims successfully operated for vesico-vaginal fistula.
1819–1868	William Thomas Green Morton.	1850	Claude Bernard published studies on arrow poisons.
1820	First *U. S. Pharmacopeia* published.	1850	Fehling developed solution for detection of sugar.
1820–1910	Florence Nightingale.	1851	Helmholtz invented ophthalmoscope.
1821–1840	Discovery and/or isolation of caffeine, iodoform, pectin, pectic acid, bromine, ethyl bromide, aluminum, santonin, chloroform, coniine, codeine, narceine, thebaine, dextrin, carbolic acid, aniline, and pure chloroform.	1851–1902	Walter Reed.
		1851–1853	Pravaz introduced the hypodermic needle.
		1852	American Pharmaceutical Association founded (now American Pharmacists Association).
1821	Döbereiner discovered the process of catalysis.	1853–1856	Crimean War, during which Florence Nightingale founded the modern nursing profession.
1821	Philadelphia College of Pharmacy founded.	1854–1915	Paul Ehrlich.
1822–1895	Louis Pasteur.	1859	Darwin's *Origin of Species* published.
1825	Publication of the *American Journal of Pharmacy,* first professional pharmacy periodical in English.	1860	Pasteur demonstrated presence of bacteria in air.
		1861–1865	Civil War in the United States.
1827–1912	Lord Joseph Lister.	1865	Lister introduced antiseptic treatment of wounds.
1829	Dagueree introduced photography.	1865	Gregor Mendel published memoirs about plant hybridity.
1829	Tuéry demonstrated antidotal properties of charcoal.		
1830–1848	Reign of Louis Philippe.	1865	First International Pharmaceutical Congress convened in Brunswick, Germany.
1832	British Medical Association founded.		
1832–1905	Albert B. Prescott.	1866	A. J. Ångström introduced Ångström units.
1833	Johannes MÅller's treatise on physiology published.	1867	Lister introduced antiseptic surgery.
1833	William Beaumont published experiments on gastric digestion.	1868	Clinical thermometer introduced.
		1869	Virchow urged medical inspection of schools.
1835	Berzelius coined term "catalysis."	1870	Fritsch and Hitzig investigated the localization of function of brain.
1837	Gerhard differentiated between typhus and typhoid fevers.		
1837	Victoria became Queen of England.	1870–1871	Franco-Prussian War (test of vaccination).
1839	Schwann published treatise on cell theory.	1871	Lister noted antibiotic phenomena.
1840	Henle published statement of germ theory of communicable diseases.	1876	Koch obtained pure cultures of anthrax bacilli on artificial media.
1841–1860	Discovery/isolation of niobium, cocaine from coca leaves, aniline dyes, and pure cocaine.	1876	Bell telephone introduced.

continued on page 15

Table 2.5 | World & Pharmacy Events of the Nineteenth Century,[a] continued

YEAR	EVENT	YEAR	EVENT
1878	Von Basch measured blood pressure with sphygmomanometer.	1895	Marconi introduced wireless telegraph.
1878	Edison invented platinum-wire (incandescent) electric light bulb.	1897	Emil Fischer synthesized caffeine, theobromine, xanthine, guanine, and adenine.
1879	Billings and Fletcher started *Index Medicus.*	1897	Ehrlich stated the side chain theory of immunity.
1881	Pasteur produced anthrax vaccine.	1898	P. and M. Curie discovered radium.
1883	Susan Hayhurst was first woman graduate of the Philadelphia College of Pharmacy. She was in charge of the pharmacy of the Woman's Hospital of Philadelphia for three decades.	1898	Dreser introduced heroin.
		1898	National Association of Retail Druggists (now National Community Pharmacists Association) founded.
1885	Pasteur introduced rabies vaccine.	1899	Walter Reed and others demonstrated mosquito transmission of yellow fever.
1886	Limousin developed glass ampuls for storage of hypodermic solutions.	1899	H. Dreser introduced aspirin.
1889	Behring introduced antitoxins.	1900	Conference of Pharmaceutical Faculties founded (now American Association of Colleges of Pharmacy).
1895	Röentgen discovered x-rays.		

[a] Adapted from reference 3.

During the latter half of the nineteenth century, pharmacy schools operated primarily as finishing schools; pharmacy apprentices with several years' experience in apothecary shops would attend school for a limited amount of time before becoming licensed pharmacists. A physician-chemist at the University of Michigan changed that. Albert B. Prescott believed that the scientific foundation of pharmacy should be laid first through didactic educational programs and only then should the student attempt to learn the practical side of the trade through an apprenticeship. Prescott, dean of pharmacy at the University of Michigan, went up against organized pharmacy with his beliefs, and for it he was rejected as a delegate at the 1871 APhA convention in St. Louis. But time proved him right, and by the turn of the century, most schools began adopting his model. He served as president of APhA in 1899–1900 and of the predecessor organization of the American Association of Colleges of Pharmacy in 1900.[8]

Twentieth century pharmacy: A business or a profession?

William Procter, the influential PCP faculty member, was prescient when he identified what would become a chief problem for twentieth century pharmacists. As quoted by Hepler,[7] Procter wrote in 1858:

"... if the preparation of medicines is taken from the apothecary and he becomes merely the dispenser of them, his business is shorn of half its dignity and importance, and he relapses into a simple shopkeeper."

By the beginning of the twentieth century, the pharmaceutical industry had begun to make an impact on the daily lives of pharmacists. More and more products were produced ready to dispense, and problems with adulteration and quackery caused the United States Congress to pass the Pure Food and Drug Act in 1906 (see Chapter 7, Governmental and Voluntary Oversight of Pharmacy). In Germany, new discoveries in organic chemistry

Table 2.6 | World & Pharmacy Events, 1901–1950[a]

YEAR	EVENT
1901	Landsteiner discovered blood groups (isoagglutination).
1901	Awarding of Nobel prizes began.
1902–1903	Jensen propagated cancer through several generations of mice.
1903	Wright brothers make successful flight with airplane.
1904–1914	Panama Canal built.
1906	Pure Food and Drugs Act passed in the United States.
1910	Abraham Flexner published survey of medical schools and education.
Early 1900s	Several hormones and vitamins identified.
1914–1918	World War I.
1914	Flexner stated that pharmacy was not a profession.
1915	Twort reported on bacteriophages.
1916	Bull introduced antitoxin for gas gangrene.
1918	Surgeon General rules that pharmacy was not a profession.
1918–1919	Spanish influenza pandemic.
1921	Banting and Best isolated insulin.
1925	First state association of hospital pharmacists formed, in California.
1926	E. L. Kennaway extracted the first known cancer-causing chemical, 3,4–benzpyrene.
1926	Förster developed the brain-function chart.
1927	Lindbergh crossed the Atlantic in airplane alone.
1928	Alexander Fleming discovered penicillin.
1928	Forssmann performed the first heart catheterization.
1929	Worldwide stock market crash; beginning of Great Depression.
1931	Development of electron microscope.
1932	Chadwick, Joliot-Curie, and Urey discovered, respectively, the neutron, positron, and heavy hydrogen.
1932	Zernike developed the phase-contrast microscope.
1933	Hitler rose to power in Germany.
1935	Trefouel, Nitti, and Bovet discovered prontosil's action to be caused by sulfanilamide.
1935	Kendall and Reichstein isolated cortisone.
1935	Stanley discovered the virus agent of tobacco mosaic, a "living" molecule.
1935	Nucleic acids found to be the principal components of viruses and genes.
1936	Hospital pharmacy section of APhA formed.
1937	Sulfonamide therapy for gonorrhea introduced.
1938	Federal Food, Drug and Cosmetic Act passed, increasing federal oversight of drugs.
1938	Hess discovered the regulatory function of the midbrain.
1938	Hahn developed a device for nuclear fission.
1939–1945	World War II.
1939	Florey and Chain developed penicillin to stage of therapeutic use.
1939	More than 150 different kinds of synthetic materials were known.
1940	Karl Link discovered dicumarol.
1940	Landsteiner and Wiener discovered the Rhesus factor in blood.
1940	American College of Apothecaries founded.
1942	Atomic energy released and controlled in first nuclear chain reaction.
1942	First jet aircraft tested.
1942	American Society of Hospital (now Health-System) Pharmacists founded.
1943	Penicillin production gets underway.
1944	Waksman announced discovery of streptomycin.
1944	Synthesis of quinine.
1945	Worldwide antimalarial campaign using DDT.
1945	United Nations formed.
1946	Penicillin produced synthetically.
1947	Chloramphenicol discovered.
1948	Farber found that antagonists to folic acid alleviated leukemia.
1948	World Health Organization founded.
1948	Kinsey report on Sexual Behavior of the Human Male.
1948	200-inch telescope installed at Mount Palomar Observatory.
1950–1953	Korean Conflict.

[a] Adapted from reference 3.

were making possible the increased rational design of drugs (as well as creating the additional horrors during World War I because of the use of lethal nerve gases).

As the century progressed, the pharmaceutical industry became stronger. The dramatic acceleration came during and following World War II. The military had an urgent need for penicillin, which had lain dormant in Fleming's laboratory for 10 years. The technology, scientific knowledge, and need were present all at once, and the post-World War II pharmaceutical industry began producing drugs that were much more powerful and specific than those available previously.

The effect of this on pharmacists was twofold: (1) The art of **compounding** rapidly became less important, as most prescriptions could be filled with manufactured dosage forms, and (2) the knowledge about the drugs, their mechanisms of action, and their side effects became much more complicated.

> **Compounding:**
> The preparation of prescriptions specifically for a patient based on an individualized drug order from a prescriber.

Pharmacy had already encountered problems during the first half of the twentieth century in maintaining or gaining recognition as a profession. In 1918, the Surgeon General refused to recognize pharmacy as such, which meant that pharmacists could not be commissionable officers in the Armed Forces as were professionals such as physicians and engineers. Pharmacy had responded in 1932 by standardizing pharmacy school curricula as four-year programs leading to attainment of the bachelor of science degree in pharmacy.[7] This was not enough, however, and pharmacists remained enlisted personnel during World War II.

Consequently, the end of World War II found a pharmacy profession in an emaciated state. As Brushwood wrote during the celebration of APhA's sesquicentennial, "By 1952 pharmacists had become what they sought to be: respected custodians of the nation's drug supply, at the tail end of the chain of distribution. This is an important role, but not a fulfillment of the promise of the profession in 1902, when an expansive patient-oriented practice appeared to be developing."[12] Because pharmacists were not recognized as professionals by the military,[13] schools had been decimated by conscription during the war, and much of pharmacists' knowledge and skills were being rendered useless by the new technologies of pharmaceutical industry. A major challenge for the leaders of pharmacy lay in store during the latter half of the twentieth century.

REFERENCES

1. Sonnedecker G. Kremers and Urdang's history of pharmacy. 4th ed. Philadelphia, PA: J. B. Lippincott Company; 1976. (Copies of this book are available from the American Institute of the History of Pharmacy, Pharmacy Building, Madison, WI 53706.)
2. LaWall CH. Four thousand years of pharmacy: an outline history of pharmacy and the allied sciences. Philadelphia, PA: J. B. Lippincott Company; 1927.
3. Bender GA. Great moments in pharmacy. Detroit: Northwood Institute Press; 1967. (Note: This book contains reprints of the Parke-Davis History of Pharmacy oil paintings; however, it is not the best source of specific historical information.)
4. Griffenhagen GB. Great moments in pharmacy: development of the Robert Thom series depicting pharmacy's history. *J Am Pharm Assoc.* 2002;42:170–82.
5. Griffenhagen G. Pharmaceutical philately. Johnstown, PA: American Topical Association; 1990.
6. Cowen DL, Helfand WH. Pharmacy: an illustrated history. New York: Harry N. Abrams, Inc.; 1990.

7. Hepler CD. The third wave in pharmaceutical education: the clinical movement. *Am J Pharm Ed.* 1987;51:369-85.

8. Manasse HR Jr. Albert B. Prescott's legacy to pharmaceutical education in America. *Pharm Hist.* 1973; 15:22-8.

9. Schmidt JE. Medical discoveries: who and when. Springfield, IL: Charles C Thomas; 1959.

10. Morton LT. A medical bibliography (Garrison and Morton). London: Gower Publishing Company;1983.

11. The new encyclopedia britannica. 15th ed. Chicago: Encyclopedia Britannica; 1991.

12. Brushwood DB. Governance of pharmacy, 1902-52. *J Am Pharm Assoc.* 2001;41:376-7.

13. Worthen D. Carl Thomas Durham (1892-1974): pharmacy's representative. *J Am Pharm Assoc.* 2005;45:295-8.

Chapter 3 | Pharmacy Reborn: Pharmaceutical Care and Medication Therapy Management

As reflected in the history presented in Chapter 2, societies have for centuries devised systems to provide solutions to people's problems. In the caves of thousands of years ago, our predecessors probably had job descriptions very similar to one another: find food, prepare it, protect themselves and their family from harm, and reproduce. Life was difficult, but the jobs were all about the same.

As the human species evolved, specialized tasks became more the norm. Some people were farmers, while others worked with newly discovered metals. Curing the affirms of the ill became the main activity of some people, and discovering grand schemes of making war was the motivation for others.

For centuries, people continued to develop more and more specialized roles, and a person in need would seek the materials, services, advice, or expertise of his neighbors in a community of people. Little need existed for any formal recognition of specialized expertise, since most people knew each other and knew for what each could be relied upon. Travel was difficult, leaving most people restricted to a small geographic area throughout their disease- and war-shortened lives.

However, as the Middle Ages began to wane, people became more mobile, and cities began to grow. People no longer knew all of their neighbors. Jobs became more specialized. In response, a variety of alliances and organizations began to develop of merchants and businessmen involved in similar activities. These organizations were often formed with self-serving interests in mind, such as to limit competition by requiring all parties to abide by certain standards. But they also served a useful purpose in that standards began to develop by which various trades began to practice. Some of these sponsoring organizations evolved into professional associations, others into labor unions, and some into trade groups.

By the eighteenth century, many of these standards or restrictions had been adopted by governmental bodies, giving the force of law to the previously voluntary requirements. The Industrial Revolution, generally considered to be from the late 1700s until the mid-twentieth century, accelerated this change, as did the rapid pace of scientific discoveries. Jobs became highly specialized, and the tasks performed by a given group of workers are not easily completed by those not in that field.

Occupations vs. professions

As society recognized the increasing complexity of some jobs, people began to differentiate further between a work activity that was a job, a lifelong or long-term devotion to an occupation, and the specialized knowledge and unique requirements of a profession.

"Pharmaceutical care gives us hope that our profession can restore its past greatness, not by our becoming chemists again, but rather by our making a commitment to outcomes that are valuable beyond price to our patients, in a health care environment that is being stood on its head by rapid change."

— Charles D. Hepler, in "Four Virtues for the Future," 1997 Remington Lecture

Differentiating between an occupation and a profession has occupied many sociologists' minds for decades. Charles D. Hepler, a pharmacist and pharmacy professor at the University of Florida, wrote extensively about pharmacy and its professional status in the1980s and 1990s. Let's look at some of his conclusions.

Hepler[1] relies on the basic observations of Larsen[2] in characterizing a profession. Three basic characteristics have become the hallmarks of professions[1]:

- The services offered are closely linked to major human values, such as health, property, or religion.
- The services require a degree of knowledge, skill, and understanding beyond those possessed by ordinary people of the day and beyond a layman's ability to evaluate (for example, the accuracy of a diagnosis or the purity of a prescription).
- The services are inherently personal or individualized in nature, meaning that they cannot be readily standardized or mass-produced.

These three requirements surely prove that pharmacy of the nineteenth century was a profession, Hepler concluded. Pharmacy has always concerned itself with health. One has to have special training—indeed, special tools—to determine what ingredients are present in a tablet or tincture. And a brief review of the prescription files crumbling from age in an old pharmacy will show that few patients received the same medications; medicaments were highly individualized, and the pharmacist compounded many prescriptions specifically for a patient immediately before dispensing.[1,3]

However, what about pharmacy of the twentieth century? Amendments to the Federal Food, Drug and Cosmetic Act required pharmaceutical manufacturers to spend millions of dollars in premarket testing of drugs, and advances in technology allowed mass production of ready-to-dispense tablets, capsules, suppositories, liquids, and injectables. Prescriptions became so standardized that some pharmaceutical companies gave physicians preprinted prescription pads complete with drug name, quantity to dispense, and directions. As Hepler noted, the only individualization was the patient's name and the prescription number, and "the complexity of most pharmaceutical service was reduced in the public mind, and often in reality, to the infamous sequence of counting, pouring, licking, and sticking."[3]

Pharmacy, always plagued by the image of the merchant interested primarily in moving the drug products, thus had come perilously close to losing any valid status as a profession.

Pharmaceutical care as reprofessionalization

Luckily, the same development that threatened pharmacy—the industrialization of the pharmaceutical industry in the first half of the twentieth century—also provided the profession with a valuable opportunity.

Any cursory review of pharmacology or medical books from just a few decades ago quickly demonstrates that efficacious drugs were few and far between. While the explosion in knowledge of chemicals described in Chapter 2 had provided some powerful agents, many of the drugs were merely palliative. Antibiotics were not yet available, the pathophysiologies of many disease states were not well understood, and the best many patients could hope for was relief from suffering until the disease took its course.

Efficacy:
The ability of a drug to produce desired therapeutic effects.

Safety:
The ability of a drug not to produce harmful or deleterious side effects or adverse reactions.

Table 3.1 | Pharmacy & World Events, 1951–Present[a]

YEAR	EVENT
1951	Durham-Humphrey Amendments to Food, Drug and Cosmetic Act passed by U.S. Congress, more clearly identifying drugs that required prescribing by a licensed medical practitioner.
1951	Ludwig Gross showed virus transmission of leukemia in mice.
1951	André–Thomas developed the heart-lung machine.
1951	International Pharmacopoeia published by World Health Organization.
1951	Effect of fluoride on dental caries discovered.
1952	Reserpine discovered.
1952	First open-heart operation by Baily.
1952	First hydrogen bomb explosion.
1955	Jonas Salk developed polio vaccine.
1957	First space satellite launched.
1959	Polonski described the function of DNA.
1960	Introduction of the laser.
1961	First manned space travel.
1962	Drug Amendments passed, requiring efficacy of new drugs (in addition to a previous requirement of safety).
1963	ASHP begins accreditation of hospital pharmacy residencies.
1963	Lasers used in medicine.
1963	Oxytocic drugs used in obstetrics.
1963	John F. Kennedy assassinated.
1964	Pharmacist Hubert H. Humphrey elected Vice President of the United States.
1964–73	Americans involved in combat in Vietnam.
1966	Ninth Floor Project begins at University of California–San Francisco, leading to clinical pharmacy movement.
1967	First human heart transplant by Christiaan Barnard.
1969	American Society of Consultant Pharmacists founded.
1969	Americans land on moon.
1970	Bureau of Narcotics and Dangerous Drugs reorganized as Drug Enforcement Administration.
1972	United States postage stamp issued in honor of pharmacy.
1974	Richard Nixon resigned presidency as a result of Watergate scandal.
1974	Restriction endonucleases discovered, thus permitting genetic engineering and sparking the biotechnologic revolution.
1975	Supreme Court decision in Portland Retail Druggists Association v. Abbott Laboratories et al. limits distribution of specially priced pharmaceutical drugs by nonprofit entities.
1975	ASHP formed special-interest groups to meet the diverse needs of emerging practice areas.
1975	Millis Commission issues report on the future of pharmacy.
1979	American College of Clinical Pharmacy founded.
1980	FDA required mandatory patient package inserts for 10 major drugs and drug classes during waning days of Carter Administration (the regulations were rescinded in 1981 by the Reagan Administration).
1981	AACP rejected PharmD as entry-level degree.
1981	Michigan Pharmacists Association began certifying pharmacy technicians based on examination.
1983	APhA President William S. Apple died.
1984	First Pharmacy in the 21st Century conference held.
1985	Directions in Clinical Pharmacy Practice conference held at Hilton Head, S.C.
1989	ACPE proposed elimination of the B.S. Pharmacy degree, leading to establishment of PharmD as entry-level degree for pharmacy.
1989	Academy of Managed Care Pharmacy founded.
1989–90	Congress first passed but then repealed legislation covering outpatient prescription drugs for the elderly.
1990	Congress passes amendments to the Omnibus Budget Reconciliation Act requiring pharmacists to offer medication counseling to Medicaid prescriptions when they are dispensed the first time. Many state boards of pharmacy extended the requirement to include all patients.
1992	APhA, ASHP, and AACP conducted the Scope of Pharmacy Practice project, with a goal of redefining the typical activities of pharmacists and technicians.
1994	ASHP changes its name to the American Society of Health-System Pharmacists.
1995	First administration of a national pharmacy technician certification examination.
1997	Joseph A. Oddis retires after 37 years as chief executive officer at ASHP.
1997	Pharmacists in Asheville, N.C., begin providing pharmaceutical care to patients with diabetes in what would become known as the "Asheville Project."
1998	Pharmacists named most trusted professionals in U.S. for 10th year in a row.
1999	Internet pharmacies become common on the World Wide Web.
1999	FDA begins requiring patient package inserts with some prescription drugs.
2000	ACPE regulations for the new PharmD degree became effective.
2001	Robert R. Courtney, a Kansas City pharmacist, is arrested for providing to physicians for cancer patients intravenous solutions that contained little or no medication.
2001	September 11 terrorist attacks.
2001	Pharmacists fall to fourth in trust/ethics poll, tied with policemen and trailing firefighters, the U.S. military, and nurses.
2003	Iraqi War begins.
2003	APhA changes its name to American Pharmacists Association.
2003	Medicare Part D created by Congress covering outpatient prescription drugs.
2006	Number of Certified Pharmacy Technicians passes 250,000 mark, exceeding number of licensed pharmacists.
2008	Permanent CPT billing codes for medication therapy management services take effect.

[a] Adapted in part from reference 9.

In the 1950s, scientists began to make major strides in understanding biological systems; remember that it was not until 1953 that DNA was proven to be the genetic material of living organisms. Just as physics had been advanced in the 1600s and chemistry made great strides in the 1800s and early 1900s, the time for biology came in the 1900s. Finally, medical scientists understood specifically what underlying metabolic or genetic defect caused certain diseases, and with this knowledge powerful new drugs were identified or in some cases created to cure the conditions (see Table 3.1).

Additionally, literally thousands of compounds were tested for antibacterial, antifungal, and antiviral activity in the ensuing decades. Despite the current concern over antibiotic resistance, myriad commercially available antibiotics are available for treating diseases that regularly killed and debilitated people only half a century ago. Some people attribute the so-called sexual revolution of the 1960s not only to the availability of oral contraceptives ("birth control pills") but just as much to the marketing of antibiotics that could cure sexually transmitted bacterial infections. In short, new drugs were changing the world.

In the late 1950s and 1960s, astute pharmacists such as Donald C. Brodie of the University of California-San Francisco, Donald E. Francke of the University of Michigan, and Paul F. Parker of the University of Kentucky began to conceptualize a new role for pharmacists that would involve the specialized provision of information about these powerful new agents that were beginning to reach the market. As it came to be known, the clinical pharmacy movement sought to create a role for pharmacists in the provision of patient-specific drug information or advice to physicians and other members of the health care team.

Hepler has identified three simultaneous trends that served as the basis for the clinical pharmacy movement: (1) **drug information**, (2) **drug distribution**, especially **decentralized** programs in hospitals, and (3) teaching and research programs in **pharmacology** and **biopharmaceutics**.[3] These three currents combined for the first time in the famous 1966 "Ninth Floor Project" at the University of California-San Francisco, in which faculty sought to find a way to train students for a role that did not previously exist. The problem was stated this way[4]:

"[Although] the concept of the pharmacist as a drug consultant was stressed and attempts were made to instruct the student in how his pharmaceutical knowledge related to patient care ... the faculty had no opportunity to test their techniques of instruction for there was no laboratory at that time where the students could put their training into practice."

The project began in September 1966 with the following goals[4]:
- To develop a hospital floor-based pharmaceutical service that would provide maximal patient safety in the utilization of drugs.
- To charge the pharmacist with the responsibility for all phases of drug distribution, except the administration of medication to the patient.
- To provide an unbiased and easily available source of reliable drug information (the pharmacist) and to disseminate information according to the needs of professional personnel.
- To provide clinical experience for interns and residents and other qualified pharmacy students in hospital pharmacy.

Drug information:
A service provided by pharmacists to other health professionals or to the public in which basic or detailed information about drugs is provided.

Decentralized drug distribution:
Systems in hospitals of distributing drugs to patients in which pharmacy services are located in several locations near patient-care areas rather than in one central pharmacy.

Pharmacology:
The study of the action of drugs in biological systems.

Biopharmaceutics:
The study of a drug's physical and chemical properties as they relate to the effects of the drug on the body (absorption, distribution, and metabolism or elimination).

Table 3.2 | **Summary of the Concepts, Findings, and Recommendations of the Study Commission on Pharmacy[5]**

1. Among deficiencies in the health care system is the unavailability of adequate information for those who consume, prescribe, dispense, and administer drugs. Pharmacists are health professionals who could make an important contribution to the health care system of the future by providing information about drugs to consumers and health professionals. Education and training of pharmacists must be developed to meet these important responsibilities.

2. Pharmacy should be conceived basically as a knowledge system that renders a health service by concerning itself with understanding drugs and their effects upon people and animals.

3. A pharmacist must be defined as an individual who is engaged in one of the steps of a system called pharmacy.... A pharmacist is characterized by the common denominator of drug knowledge and the differentiated additional knowledge and skill required by his particular role.

4. The system of pharmacy must be described as being both effective and efficient in developing, manufacturing, and distributing drug products. However, it cannot be described at present as either effective or efficient in developing, organizing, and distributing knowledge and information about drugs.

5. Major attention should be given to the problems of drug information—specifically in defining who needs to know, what he needs to know, and how these needs can best be met with speed and economy.

6. Despite the real and multifaceted differentiation in the practice roles of pharmacists, there is a common body of knowledge, skill, attitudes, and behavior all pharmacists must possess. The objectives of pharmacy education must be stated in terms of both the common knowledge and skill and of the differentiated and/or additional knowledge and skill required for specific practice roles.

7. The Study Commission recommends the following three component educational objectives for pharmacy education:
   a. The mastery of the knowledge and the acquisition of the skills common to all of the roles of pharmacy practice.
   b. The mastery of the additional knowledge and the acquisition of the additional skills needed for those differentiated roles that require additional pharmacy knowledge and experience.
   c. The mastery of the additional knowledge and the acquisition of the additional skills needed for those differentiated roles that require additional knowledge and skill other than pharmacy.

8. Every school of pharmacy should promptly find the ways and means to provide appropriate practice opportunities for its faculty members having clinical teaching responsibilities so that they may serve as effective role models for their students.

9. The curricula of the schools of pharmacy should be based on the competencies desired for their graduates rather than upon the basis of knowledge available in the several relevant sciences.

10. The greatest weakness of the schools of pharmacy is a lack of an adequate number of clinical scientists who can relate their specialized scientific knowledge to the development of practice skills.

11. Pharmacy is a knowledge system in which chemical substances and people called patients interact. Needed and optimally effective drug therapy results only when drugs and those who consume them are fully understood. One of the first steps in reviewing the educational program of a college of pharmacy should be weighing the relative emphasis given to the physical and biological sciences in the curriculum for the first professional pharmacy degree.

12. Those schools of pharmacy with adequate resources should develop, in addition to the first professional degree, programs of instruction at the graduate and advanced professional level for more differentiated roles of pharmacy practice.

13. The optimal environment for pharmacy education is the university health science center, for the full range of knowledge, skill, and practice can be found there. However, the Commission does not believe that it is practical or in the public interest to recommend that all colleges of pharmacy must be so located. Alternative arrangements, if effectively used, can provide an acceptable environment for the education of students at the baccalaureate level.

14. All aspects of the credentialling of pharmacists and pharmacy education would be enhanced by the services of a National Board of Pharmacy Examiners, created by joint action of the National Association of Boards of Pharmacy, the American Council on Pharmaceutical Education, and the American Association of Colleges of Pharmacy.

Drug-regimen review:
A clinical pharmacy service provided to residents of nursing homes in which pharmacists review the drug therapy of residents and provide suggestions to physicians about drug selection, duplication, necessity, adverse effects, or monitoring.

Nursing homes:
Facilities that provide residential care and health care to residents who live in them. Residents are typically deficient in one or more activities of daily living: ambulating, feeding, bathing, or toileting.

- To design and conduct studies in cooperation with the physician and nurse so that a full evaluation may be obtained of institutional pharmacy service within the framework of the team approach to patient care.

All of these roles were radical departures from prior functions of pharmacists. But gradually, the worth of such services took hold, and schools of pharmacy across the country began to create a demand for clinical pharmacy services by placing pharmacy faculty in acute-care institutions and giving medical residents and interns a taste of what highly motivated and competent pharmacists could accomplish.

The publication of *Drug Intelligence and Clinical Pharmacy* (now *Annals of Pharmacotherapy*) began in 1967, and two pharmacy therapeutics textbooks came out of San Francisco in 1972. By 1974, the federal government recognized a clinical role for pharmacists when it began requiring the pharmacist to conduct monthly **drug-regimen reviews** of residents in skilled-care **nursing homes**, thanks to the efforts of pharmacists such as George F. Archambault, Richard S. Berrman, and other leaders of the fledgling American Society of Consultant Pharmacists.

Thus, the clinical pharmacy movement created the opportunity for pharmacy to continue as a profession worthy of the respect and trust of its patients: Clinical pharmacy was involved in the health care of patients, it required specialized knowledge and skills, and it was individualized.

Affirmation of the trend: The Millis Report

In 1975, the American Association of Colleges of Pharmacy commissioned a study of pharmacy by a 12-member group headed by Dr. John Millis, a nonpharmacist educator who had recently completed a study of physician education. Known commonly as the Millis Commission, the group issued its findings in a 161-page report called *Pharmacists for the Future: The Report of the Study Commission on Pharmacy*.

The Commission made 14 recommendations, which are paraphrased or summarized in Table 3.2. Among the changes in pharmacy and pharmacy education as a direct result of the Millis Commission were the following:
- Acceleration of development of clinical sites for pharmacy school faculty
- Development of a national examination for licensure of pharmacists, now called the NAPLEX® (North American Pharmacist Licensure Examination®)
- Increased movement toward making pharmacy a knowledge-based clinical profession
- Creation of a small number of clinical scientists programs in schools of pharmacy at the doctor of philosophy level
- Creation of a Board of Pharmaceutical Specialties within APhA to recognize specialty practices in pharmacy and certify individuals in those specialties

However, as Hepler has noted,[3] the Millis Report failed to produce a real spark in shifting pharmacy dramatically and irreversibly toward its desired goals. Unlike some previous similar reports in pharmacy or medicine, the Millis Report did not outline specific changes in pharmacy school curricula or give a blueprint for the future. It provided only external recognition for the advances made by pharmacy as a clinical profession.

Hepler raises the stakes with pharmaceutical care

The clinical pharmacy movement continued in the 1980s. Two new journals were published: *Pharmacotherapy* was founded in 1981 by the late Russell R. Miller, a clinical scientist of the ilk envisioned by the Millis Commission, and *Clinical Pharmacy*, by the American Society of Hospital Pharmacists from 1982 through 1993. A third textbook in the clinical pharmacy field, *Pharmacotherapy: A Pathophysiologic Approach*, was first published in 1989.

The term pharmacotherapist was chosen to designate specialists in clinical pharmacy when the Board of Pharmaceutical Specialties recognized this part of practice in 1988. Certified Pharmacotherapy Specialists carry the initials "BCPS" following their names.

But Hepler began to conclude that the clinical pharmacy and pharmacotherapy movement was not the sole answer to pharmacy's problems. Beginning at the 1985 Directions for Clinical Practice in Pharmacy (called commonly the Hilton Head conference because of its South Carolina meeting site), Hepler expounded on the notion that pharmacists had to do more than just try to control the use of drugs. Hepler preached that they had to take responsibility for the care provided to patients through the clinical use of drugs. In 1987, he first applied the term pharmaceutical care[3] in describing what he and colleague Linda Strand called these new self-actualizing roles for pharmacists.[6]

Table 3.3 provides the definition of pharmaceutical care, as proposed by Hepler and Strand. Several trends are reflected in the concept. For many years, healthcare institutions and organizations had relied on process criteria in judging various systems. If a pharmacist used the correct process for filling and dispensing a prescription, then the results of that process were assumed to be of adequate quality. In the pharmaceutical care definition, contemporary outcomes-oriented language is presented in the first paragraph. Thus, where a hospital in the past might have been required to have a certain type of drug-distribution system, now the hospital would be checked for medication error rates. Instead of trying to define the process, only the outcomes were of interest.

For pharmaceutical care, the four outcomes as shown should be related to the purposes for which a medication is being administered to a patient, as defined in the first paragraph.

The team approach is endorsed in the second paragraph, reflecting pharmacy's shared purpose with other health care professions. Also identified in that paragraph are the kinds of functions a pharmacist would be expected to provide.

The third paragraph is the key to the concept of pharmaceutical care. The pharmacist has a direct relationship with the patient and a direct responsibility to that patient to provide competent pharmaceutical care (as defined in the first two paragraphs). If the pharmacist was not providing services appropriate to those of a profession (value, complexity, and specificity), then Hepler argued that the pharmacist had broken his or her professional **covenant** with that patient.[3]

Finally, the fourth paragraph stated that the provision of pharmaceutical care should occur anytime and anywhere a pharmacist encountered a patient. Thus, the same prin-

Covenant:
A promise or an agreement between two parties in which each provides something of value to the other. In pharmacy, the patient gives money to the pharmacist, who provides a patient-specific pharmaceutical product along with information on the proper use and adverse effects of that product.

Table 3.3 | Definition of Pharmaceutical Care[6]

Pharmaceutical care is the responsible provision of drug therapy for the purpose of achieving definite outcomes that improve a patient's quality of life. These outcomes are (1) cure of a disease; (2) elimination or reduction of a patient's symptomatology; (3) arresting or slowing of a disease process; and (4) preventing a disease or symptomatology.

Pharmaceutical care involves the process through which a pharmacist cooperates with a patient and other professionals in designing, implementing, and monitoring a therapeutic plan that will produce specific therapeutic outcomes for the patient. This in turn involves three major functions: (1) identifying potential and actual drug-related problems; (2) resolving actual drug-related problems; and (3) preventing potential drug-related problems.

Pharmaceutical care is a necessary element of health care, and should be integrated with other elements. Pharmaceutical care is, however, provided for the direct benefit of the patient, and the pharmacist is responsible directly to the patient for the quality of that care. The fundamental relationship in pharmaceutical care is a mutually beneficial exchange in which the patient grants authority to the provider, and the provider gives competence and commitment (accepts responsibility) to the patient.

The fundamental goals, processes, and relationships of pharmaceutical care exist regardless of practice setting.

Deep discounter:
A type of mercantile outlet that reduces prices far below those of normal retail outlets and relies on volume to make a profit.

ciples applied whether the patient was in an intensive-care unit at a major medical center or was asking about a skin rash in a busy, **deep-discounting** chain or mass-merchandise pharmacy.

The concept of pharmaceutical care struck a responsive chord with many practitioners. It was termed pharmacy's mission for the 1990s,[7] and links between pharmaceutical care and the quality of care to patients were made.[8]

By 1990, the contributions that pharmacists could make clinically had been recognized by society through two key federal laws. In 1974 and again in 1987, the federal government ruled that consultant pharmacists must check the dose regimens of nursing home patients each month. In 1990, Congress passed a law that pharmacists must offer counsel to ambulatory Medicaid patients about these medications, and many state legislatures and boards of pharmacy extended this requirement to all patients through changes in pharmacy statutes and regulations.

Making a decision about the entry-level degree

The pharmacy profession struggled and debated for 40 years as to what the appropriate entry-level degree for pharmacy should be. Finally, in the early 1990s, the profession settled on the Doctor of Pharmacy. But the battle took its toll on pharmacists and their national associations.

An increasing number of student pharmacists had been voluntarily seeking the PharmD degree during the 1980s, but many of them did so after first obtaining their baccalaureate degrees and, in many cases, working for a few years. Most pharmacy graduates (6,000 of 7,000 graduates in 1990), however, finished with B.S. degrees in pharmacy. By 1995, the enrollment in PharmD programs would total 9,346 individuals, compared with 24,069 in B.S. degree programs.

In 1989, the American Council on Pharmaceutical Education (now the Accreditation Council on Pharmacy Education), which accredits schools of pharmacy, announced plans to consider revising its accreditation standards such that the B.S. Pharmacy degree would be eliminated by 2000. Since many state boards require pharmacists to be graduates of ACPE-approved programs, this ACPE action essentially eliminated the B.S. Pharmacy as an entry-level degree for pharmacy practice, replacing it with the PharmD credential.

By 1992, all major pharmacy practitioner organizations had endorsed a "new PharmD" as the entry-level degree. The course was affirmed that summer, when the House of Delegates of the American Association of Colleges of Pharmacy supported the PharmD as pharmacy's entry-level degree.

ACPE in 1997 finalized the standards for the PharmD programs of the twenty-first century, marking completion of nearly 10 years of hearings, confrontations, and oppositions about the profession's entry-level degree. Today, all U.S. pharmacy schools offer only the PharmD degree as an entry credential for pharmacy practice.

MTM: Pharmaceutical care in community pharmacies

Until the mid-1990s, pharmaceutical care was provided primarily in hospitals with clinical pharmacy services and long-term care facilities where consultant pharmacists reviewed medication therapy on a monthly basis. In community pharmacy, practice remained primarily as Hepler had described it: Count, pour, lick, and stick.

In 1997, in the North Carolina mountain town of Asheville, that began to change. What became known as the Asheville Project was implemented when the city of Asheville tried to figure out how to contain its rapidly rising employee health costs. The result was a system in which pharmacists developed thriving pharmaceutical care practices in their local community pharmacies; employees, retirees, and dependents with diabetes had lower overall health costs, missed fewer days of work or school, and required less intensive health care interventions; and the city found its health care dollars being spent to keep people well instead of dealing with their illnesses after they had worsened.[9-11] This positive experience with diabetes would be replicated in patients with asthma,[12] cardiovascular disease,[13] and depression (unpublished data).

As the Asheville Project got off the ground, William M. Ellis joined the APhA Foundation, and he brought a new level of energy to this venerable organization. The Foundation's Quality Center initiated the Pinnacle Awards, given annually to recognize an individual, a group practice, health system, or corporation; and a government agency, nonprofit organization, or association to recognize pioneering, innovative ways to improve medication-use processes that increase medication adherence, reduce drug misadventures, improve patient outcomes, and increase communication among all members of the health care team. The Foundation sponsored Project ImPACT: Hyperlipidemia, a research study in which 26 pharmacies significantly improved serum cholesterol levels in 397 patients with dyslipidemias through education and adherence initiatives.[14] The Foundation also became involved in the Asheville Project including an effort to demonstrate the importance of patient self-management in diabetes,[15] a project that proved this local effort could be replicated in communities across the country in the Diabetes Ten City Challenge.[16]

As described further in Chapter 5, pharmacy achieved a ringing endorsement for the concept of pharmaceutical care in 2003 when the U.S. Congress created a medication therapy management (MTM) benefit as part of newly established prescription drug coverage ("Part D") for the Medicare program, which covers elderly and the disabled citizens. The Medicare Prescription Drug, Improvement, and Modernization Act of 2003 required that MTM services be provided to high-risk patients with the goals of enhancing patients' understanding of appropriate drug use, increasing adherence to medication therapy, and improving the detection of adverse drug events.[17]

In keeping with the spirit and precepts of pharmaceutical care, MTM services go far beyond the brief counseling encounters required under OBRA '90. A document presenting the consensus of national pharmacy organizations notes, "MTM services encompass the assessment and evaluation of the patient's complete medication therapy regimen, rather than focusing on an individual medication product. This model framework describes baseline core elements of MTM service delivery in pharmacy practice and does not represent all services that could be delivered by pharmacists."

As presented in the second version of a "core elements" document, the MTM service model in pharmacy practice includes the following five core elements[17]:
- Medication therapy review
- Personal medication record
- Medication-related action plan
- Intervention and/or referral
- Documentation and follow-up

Pharmacy: The future belongs to you

If they choose to be part of the solution to America's health care crisis, pharmacists are now positioned well to be the drug-therapy experts on the health care team. The biotechnology and pharmacogenomics revolutions are producing complicated new drugs that defy categorization based on past schemes, and drugs are more important than ever in therapeutics. The bold decisions made about the appropriate role for pharmacists and the entry-level degree have produced formal recognition of pharmacists' clinical services, and through MTM, many believe that pharmacists in coming years will spend most of their time in this mode of practice rather than in the drug preparation duties that dominated in the past.

REFERENCES

1. Hepler CD. Pharmacy as a clinical profession. *Am J Hosp Pharm.* 1985; 42:1298-306.
2. Larsen MS. The rise of professionalism. Berkeley, CA: University of California Press; 1977.
3. Hepler CD. The third wave in pharmaceutical education: the clinical movement. *Am J Pharm Educ.* 1987; 51:369-85.
4. Day RL, Goyan JE, Herfindal ET, Sorby DL. The origins of the clinical pharmacy program at the University of California, San Francisco. DICP *Ann Pharmacother.* 1991; 25:308-14.
5. Study Commission on Pharmacy. Pharmacists for the future. Ann Arbor, Michigan: Health Administration Press; 1975: 139-43.
6. Hepler CD, Strand LM. Opportunities and responsibilities in pharmaceutical care. *Am J Pharm Educ.* 1989; 53(suppl):7S-15S.

7. Penna RP. Pharmaceutical care: pharmacy's mission for the 1990s. *Am J Hosp Pharm.* 1990; 47:543-9.

8. Angaran DM. Quality assurance to quality improvement: measuring and monitoring pharmaceutical care. *Am J Hosp Pharm.* 1991; 48:1901-7.

9. Cranor CW, Christensen DB. The Asheville Project: short-term outcomes of a community pharmacy diabetes care program. *J Am Pharm Assoc.* 2003;43:149-59.

10. Cranor CW, Bunting BA, Christensen DB. The Asheville Project: long-term clinical and economic outcomes in a community pharmacy diabetes care program. *J Am Pharm Assoc.* 2003;43:173-84.

11. Garrett DG, Martin LA. The Asheville Project: participants' perceptions of factors contributing to the success of a Patient Self-Management Program for Diabetes. *J Am Pharm Assoc.* 2003;43:185-90.

12. Bunting BA, Cranor CW. The Asheville Project: long-term clinical, humanistic, and economic outcomes of a community-based medication therapy management program for asthma. *J Am Pharm Assoc.* 2006;46:133-47.

13. Bunting BA, Smith BH, Sutherland SE. The Asheville Project: Clinical and economic outcomes of a community-based long-term medication therapy management program for hypertension and dyslipidemia. *J Am Pharm Assoc.* 2008;48:23-31.

14. Bluml BM, McKenney JM, Cziraky MJ. Pharmaceutical care services and results in Project ImPACT: Hyperlipidemia. *J Am Pharm Assoc.* 2000;40:157-65.

15. Bluml BM, Garrett DG. Patient self-management program for diabetes: first-year clinical, humanistic, and economic outcomes. *J Am Pharm Assoc.* 2005;45:130-7.

16. Fera T, Bluml BM, Ellis WM, Schaller CW, Garrett DG. The Diabetes Ten City Challenge: Interim clinical and humanistic outcomes of a multisite community pharmacy diabetes care program. *J Am Pharm Assoc.* 2008;48:181-90.

17. American Pharmacists Association and National Association of Chain Drug Stores Foundation. Medication therapy management in pharmacy practice: core elements of an MTM service model. Version 2.0. *J Am Pharm Assoc.* 2008; 48: 341-53.

Chapter 4

Communications in Pharmacy Practice

Bruce A. Berger, PhD, RPh
Professor and Head of Pharmacy Care Systems
Auburn University Harrison School of Pharmacy
Auburn University, Alabama

Successful communication of information, ideas, and concepts is an important part of modern life, and it is an integral skill that must be learned, developed, and used by competent pharmacists. Medications are complicated technologies that must be used properly. Pharmacists can help patients make the best use of pharmacotherapy by making sure that they understand the need for each drug, when and how to take it, and what benefits and adverse effects to expect.

For you, the new pharmacist in training, communication skills must be developed early in your studies. Direct patient contact is a component of early experiential programs in curricula of schools of pharmacy, and pharmacy students must be ready to talk with patients about their health and feelings. In addition, communication skills are important in group discussions and interdisciplinary projects used for teaching purposes within the school itself.

In this chapter, proven techniques that you can use to build relationships and improve patient care are described. This material is based on the second edition of a book published by APhA, *Communication Skills for Pharmacists: Building Relationships, Improving Patient Care*, by Bruce A Berger of the Auburn University Harrison School of Pharmacy, and further information about each topic is available in that text along with more complete lists of references.

Developing the relationship

As described in Chapter 3, the concept of pharmaceutical care is based on a covenantal relationship between pharmacists and patients, and like all relationships, this one must be established and maintained. Without a patient-pharmacist relationship, pharmaceutical care and medication therapy management cannot be provided.

Relationships between patients and pharmacists are important for many reasons, but the key aspect for purposes of this chapter is that relationships provide the basis for effective and valued communications. Unless the pharmacist and patient know each other and recognize that the other is a living, breathing, feeling person—that is, unless they have a relationship—then it is all too easy to simply view the other party as an impediment or nuisance who keeps us from doing what we really want to do.

"Can I permit myself to enter into the private world of my patients, explore their feelings without judging them, and in some significant and honest way, respond in a manner that lets them know that I have listened and I want to provide whatever assistance or comfort that I can? Can I see this person as unique in his/her reaction to illness? Can I see what is different and the same about this person so that any insight or assistance I may give is the most useful to this patient?"

—Bruce A. Berger

Acknowledgment: Content of this chapter is based on *Communication Skills for Pharmacists: Building Relationships, Improving Patient Care*, second edition, authored by Bruce A. Berger and published by the American Pharmacists Association. Many of its ideas, examples, and concepts appeared originally in *U.S. Pharmacist* and were adapted with permission of Jobson Publishing, LLC, publisher of that journal.

Chapter 4

The viewing of other people in a self-centered way, such as obstacles to one's own goals or a vehicle through which one's own goals can be realized without regard for the feelings of the other person.

In books published by the Arbinger Institute, two ways of responding to people are described: the responsive way and the resistant way.[1,2] When we recognize that other people are complex human beings with feelings, wants, and dreams, we treat them *responsively*. We appreciate their successes and their joys, and we respond to those feelings. But when we deal with other people in the *resistant way*, we treat them as vehicles, obstacles, or irrelevant (**objectification**), and our own self-centeredness prevents us from recognizing their human qualities. Such an attitude impairs or impedes the proper provision of information needed as part of the process of pharmaceutical care.[3,4]

The term "mental health" means "happiness" for many people, but a more correct definition for it is the adjustment of one's internal tensions rather than attempts to change the external environment to fit our own selfish wants. As pointed out by Peck in his classic 1978 book, *The Road Less Traveled*,[5] the first great realization of the Buddha was that life is suffering, resulting in disease and old age, and that in fact these are inevitable outcomes of life as we know it. As people recognize that they daily face a certain degree of suffering and learn ways of coping with it, they achieve mental health in the sense I have described here.

In pharmacy, we often encounter our patients at times when they have just learned that they have an acute or chronic disease, or after they have found out that they have cancer or some other terminal condition. During the course of a busy day in the pharmacy or a frustrating time in our own lives, we must remember the nature of the covenant we have with our patients. As patients struggle to balance their own feelings with the realities of their lives, we as pharmacists should remember a few basic tenets that underlie healthy responses in such situations.

First, people behave in certain ways to get their needs met. In the pharmacy, patients may complain because it is the only way they know to get attention. They may be dealing with stress and have only dysfunctional strategies for dealing with change, loss, or disappointment. But somewhere underlying behaviors are feelings, and the pharmacists' recognition of those emotional needs may provide much information about how to best help patients with their medications and diseases.

Second, feelings are real. Feelings provide us with feedback—be they physical sensations such as heat or pain or the emotional feelings of joy, happiness, or loss. Feelings come from within one's self; they are not caused by other people. Feelings are caused by those meanings we assign others' communications in a given context. As health professionals, we are expected to appropriately manage our own feelings even as we acknowledge and validate the feelings of our patients. This can be difficult. We must remember that we can be aware of our own feelings and our rights to feel that way, but we should not inappropriately express those feelings to our patients.

Third, patients ultimately have responsibility for their own medication-taking behaviors, but we can have substantial influence over those behaviors. As pharmacists, we promise to provide patients with the medications they need, the information necessary for proper use of those medications, and the monitoring needed to safeguard patients' health during the medication-use process. Patients pay us for these services. While we cannot be held responsible for solving patients' problems, we can provide them with the best tools available for addressing those concerns and create an environment in which effective communication can occur. While ultimately patients must take responsibility for taking medicines when and how they should, we play a major role in assisting them with this by providing thorough and accurate information and taking time to answer their questions and address their concerns.

Fourth, communication can be evaluated as appropriate or inappropriate only in relation to the objectives of the communicator. As pharmacists, we are in control of our own communication goals, and we should strive to keep those professional and appropriate to the mission of improving patient's health.

Finally, unrealistic expectations can drive you crazy. Pharmacists are quite familiar with the patient who constantly complains about medication prices. But yet, since these individuals return month after month to make purchases, and they apparently feel the need to complain, they obviously are more than willing to buy the pharmacy's products and services at the fair price offered. Remember, life is suffering, and the fact that patients complain may be more related to that than to any of their specific complaints.

Listening and empathic responding

To demonstrate the depth and meaning of the professional relationship with a patient, the pharmacist must hear, understand, and respond effectively to the concerns expressed by the patient. To do so requires a great deal of active effort and, in a sense, courage. Let me explain.

Listening begins with an act of will; we must choose to listen—really listen—to someone else (Figure 4.1). Active listening requires our complete and undivided attention. By giving our patients our attention and focusing our energies upon them, we show each patient that we have a trusting, caring relationship, one embodied in the concept of pharmaceutical care.

Figure 4.1 | The process of listening and empathic response.

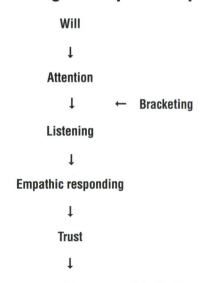

Will
↓
Attention
↓ ← Bracketing
Listening
↓
Empathic responding
↓
Trust
↓
Further exploration of thoughts and feelings

True listening requires the listener to temporarily suspend his or her own beliefs, opinions, and ideas, a process called bracketing by psychologists.[5] The greatest barrier to this type of listening is our tendency to judge or evaluate the information using our own ideals. When we do so, we have not listened, and we simply lump the patient into a stereotyped category and fail to truly understand the unique emotions the patient has about a newly diagnosed chronic or terminal disease, the fear of being pregnant after a birth control method failed, or an unexpected adverse effect of a medication. Great courage is required to truly listen, because when we suspend our values, we open ourselves to the chance that we may need to change our own ideas or beliefs.

After we truly listen to patients, our next responsibility as pharmacists is to respond empathically. Empathy is different from sympathy, which is one's own emotional response to the problems of another. Empathy is the feeling or experiencing of another's affective response to a problem or situation. As with true listening, this experiencing is done without the interference of one's own values or judgments. While many people think they can be more empathic if they have personally experienced a similar loss or tragedy, that is not necessarily the case, as one's own emotional perspective about the situation may get in the way of seeing the patient's unique perspective.

When pharmacists respond with empathy to our patients, we show courage, as the process requires the opening up of one's self to the pain and other affective responses that people have to the problems in their lives. Thus, empathy is often not all soothing—in fact, it can be quite painful and unsettling.

In many situations we find ourselves in as pharmacists, we must remember that empathy does not mean that we have to give up our own values, ideals, opinions, or positions. We can express our understanding of others' situations without unauthorized (and illegal) dispensing of prescription drugs or controlled substances, loaning money to employees or patients, or placing orders from sales representatives for goods we do not need.

Finally, remember that we must respond empathically for patients to know that we care about them and their health problems. The best way to do this is to reflect back what patients are saying to us. We should not minimize the problem, try to claim that the patient has nothing to worry about, or maintain that the patient should not be so depressed. Whatever emotions or difficulties the patient expresses as we truly listen, those should be reflected back to demonstrate an empathic response.

Supportive communication

Many of the patient–pharmacist interactions described in this chapter have involved situations in which patients were upset or concerned about their health status. Pharmacists commonly encounter patients with such apprehensions, and as a result, they often need to engage in supportive communication.

Supportive communication allows people to feel understood and less alone.[6] When patients express their concerns openly and physicians respond to them, studies have shown that patient **adherence** to therapy is greater, health professionals are more satisfied with the relationship, and patients perceive their physicians to be more understanding and

Adherence:
The rate at which patients actually take a prescribed treatment. Known formerly as "compliance." A related term, persistence, describes the rate at which patients continue to take their medications over time.

caring.[7] A study of physician interactions with patients showed that supportive communication had physical and health benefits, improved resistance to infection and disease, and even extended life.[8]

Pharmacists can be supportive in their communications by legitimizing the patient's feelings, acknowledging the importance and permanence of the loss to the patient, and encouraging the patient to accept the loss.[7] These losses can involve loss of mobility or independence, or of habits the patient considers good, desirable, or pleasurable, such as certain foods or smoking.

In validating the patient's feelings, we as pharmacists can use the processes and techniques described above under listening and empathic responses. When we do, we must remember that our goal is to demonstrate caring and concern for the patient so that they are better prepared to deal with the anger and fear they may be feeling, accept their situation, and be more likely to adhere to treatments.

The goal of supportive communication is not to solve the patient's problems, to cheer the patient up, or make everything better. No matter what we say or do, the patient may remain upset or agitated. Consider this situation: a patient storms into the pharmacy, demanding that a prescription be filled immediately because the person has a flight to catch. You are busy, with several patients who have waited 20 minutes or more for their medications. In this situation, you must communicate supportively with the patient, but you should not accept responsibility for the patient's failure to plan ahead. It will take a certain amount of uninterrupted time to convey to this patient that you understand his problem but that you also have responsibilities to other patients. But the alternative is more costly.

When patients have diseases or conditions that evoke shame or feelings of guilt, they often convert these emotions to anger, and pharmacists may sometimes bear the brunt of their frustration. The stigma society attaches to conditions such as depression or HIV infection make patients' feelings understandable, and pharmacists should make every effort to communicate with these patients in a supportive manner and to avoid responding to their anger with attacks or avoidance. More than most, these patients need support and confirmation.

In dealing with patients who are upset, we should avoid conveying unhelpful or unsupportive messages, including ones that show that we are trying to fix the problem. We must learn to simply listen and legitimize feelings, for that is what will alleviate some of these people's stress.

Patient counseling

As you advance in pharmacy school, you will increasingly be called upon to provide information to patients about their medications and the diseases being treated. This will happen initially in your early pharmacy practice experiences, but you may also find that, in social situations or at family reunions, people will ask you questions about their own experiences with medications. Later, during advanced pharmacy practice experiences and courses in which you deal directly with patients, you—as the emerging drug therapy expert on the health care team—will apply your unique knowledge and skills in helping patients understand how to best use their medications in the prevention and treatment of disease.

Patient counseling is the general term for provision of information to patients in such settings. Required by law (see Chapter 7), patient counseling should accompany the dispensing of every prescription. However, here we refer to patient counseling as an *exchange* of information. We give information about the patient's medicines and condition, but we also get information about what the patient already knows and what concerns may exist (see Table 4.1) It is not enough to coerce patients into signing away their right to counseling as part of the transfer of medications by pharmacy staff, as is done far too often in many of the nation's community pharmacies. The pharmacist is a professional with responsibilities to the patient that are required under law, regulation, and the profession's own code of ethics (see Chapter 5), and the privilege of being a pharmacist can be revoked if the person does not comply with these requirements. Along with getting the right drug to the right patient at the right time, the provision of adequate information about the medication is a basic responsibility that we have as pharmacists.

The scope and nature of patient counseling will become clearer as you advance in the curriculum of your school of pharmacy. For now, consider the steps in the checklist shown in Table 4.1, and begin thinking about how you will convey in simple terms the information you are beginning to learn about medications.

Interacting with physicians

Another situation you may soon experience is interacting on a professional level with physicians. While pharmacists often contact physicians about potential errors made in the prescribing process, a collaborative relationship must be established between these members of the health care team. Out of mutual concern over the best interests of the patient, pharmacists and physicians must develop mutual respect for one another.

As a pharmacist in training, you will mostly be in situations where you are a temporary member of a health care unit. But as you enter practice, you will be in more permanent situations, and in these it is important to begin building rapport with your physician colleagues before you need to contact them about a specific patient. A pharmacy's innovative services can be presented in one-on-one meetings with physicians or through lectures to local medical societies. Volunteering to work on public health or disaster-preparedness committees in your community is another forum within which to interact with physicians and other health care professionals. In each of these efforts, one goal is to establish oneself as a professional with a unique set of knowledge and skills that are of value to the other members of the health care team and to the community.

Drug interactions:
Detrimental (or occasionally positive) effects produced when two or more drugs are used at the same time. By checking the patient profile for interacting drugs, the computer can alert the pharmacist to consider whether both drugs can be safely used together in a patient.

When situations arise in which the pharmacist needs to call a physician, the focus of that communication should be on the patient and drug-related problems that need to be solved or averted. These may involve **drug interactions**, diseases that have not been recognized or treated, suboptimal medication choice, or incorrect dosages. Whatever the problem, the pharmacist should be prepared before contacting the physician, including having a recommendation and a rationale for that solution to the problem.

During a face-to-face encounter or a telephone call, follow this process for communicating with the physician and his or her staff:

Table 4.1 | Patient Counseling Checklist[a]

1. Pharmacist introduces self.
2. Identifies patient or patient's agent.
3. Asks if patient has time to discuss medication.
4. Explains purpose and importance of counseling session.
5. Asks patient what physician told him or her about medication and what it is treating. Asks what patient knows or understands about the disease. Uses any available patient profile information (including possible allergies).
6. Asks patient if he or she has any concerns prior to information provision.
7. Responds with appropriate empathy, listening, and attention to concerns. Uses these skills throughout counseling session.
8. Tells patient name, indication, and route of administration of the medication.
9. Tells patient the dosage regimen.
10. Asks patient if he or she will have a problem taking the medication as prescribed.
11. Tailors medication regimen to patient's daily routine.
12. Tells patient how long it will take for the medication to show an effect.
13. Tells patient how long he or she might be on the medication.
14. Tells patient when he or she is due back for a refill (and number of refills).
15. Emphasizes the benefits of the medication and supports its use before talking about side effects and barriers.
16. Discusses major side effects of the drug and whether they will go away in time.
17. Points out that additional rare (emphasizes this to patient) side effects are listed in the information sheet (to be given to patient at the end of counseling session). Encourages patient to call if he or she has any concerns about these.
18. Uses written information to support counseling where appropriate.
19. Discusses precautions (e.g., activities to avoid).
20. Discusses beneficial activities (e.g., exercise, decreased salt intake, diet, self-monitoring).
21. Discusses drug–drug, drug–food, and drug–disease interactions.
22. Discusses storage recommendations and ancillary instructions (e.g., shake well, refrigerate).
23. Explains to patient in precise terms what to do if he or she misses a dose.
24. Checks for understanding by asking patient to repeat back key information (e.g., drug name, side effects, what to do about missed doses).
25. Rechecks for any additional concerns or questions.
26. Advises patients to always check their medicines before they leave the pharmacy.
27. Uses appropriate language throughout counseling session.
28. Maintains control of counseling session.
29. Organizes information in an appropriate manner.
30. Follows up to determine how patient is doing.

[a] Developed by the author of this chapter and Bill G. Felkey, MS, a faculty colleague at the Auburn University Harrison School of Pharmacy. Reprinted from *Communication Skills for Pharmacists: Building Relationships, Improving Patient Care,* second edition, by Bruce A. Berger and published by the American Pharmacists Association.

---

1. State who you are and the purpose of the call. Be pleasant: "Hello, Dr. Jones. I am Joe Smith from Smith's Pharmacy. I need to talk with you about Carla Brown's prescription for (name of medication). Is this a good time?"
2. State the problem and recommended solution: "You prescribed (name of prescribed medication) for Carla. She does not have any third-party coverage and would have to pay for this medication out of her own pocket. She says she cannot afford it. I would like to recommend (name of alternative medication) if you are treating (indication). This would be affordable to her and would be equally or nearly as effective."
3. If you meet resistance: Stay focused on the problem. Make good eye contact (if in person), and repeat back your understanding of what the physician's resistance is about. "So, if I understand you correctly, you simply don't like (name of alternative medication) because you have had better success with (name of prescribed medication)." The physician confirms this, and you state, "Given that you are treating (indication), I have found (give citation of study), and it shows that (name of alternative medication)

is very effective. I'm very concerned that Ms. Brown won't take the (name of prescribed medication) because it is too expensive for her. I have tried to convince her that it might prevent future visits, but she insists that she won't take it. Can we try (name of alternative medication) instead?"

Professional communications of this nature do much to establish, maintain, and strengthen the collegial relationship between pharmacists and physicians who work together in caring for patients. By focusing on the problem, relying on facts, and staying away from interpersonal conflicts, these health care professionals provide the best possible care for their patients.

Immediacy: Word choice and nonverbal cues

Much of the discussion in this chapter has focused on the central messages that you as a pharmacist in training should convey to patients and colleagues in various situations. But those messages are only a small part of the communication process—7% in some studies. The message received is influenced more by how you say something and what your body does while you are saying it. About 55% of the meaning attached to communications comes from nonverbal clues, and the other 38% comes from vocal cues.[9]

The choice of words used in a communication is important. For instance, the difference between saying "you and I should discuss this matter" and "we should discuss this matter" is great. The sentences technically mean the same thing, but use of "we" implies much greater verbal immediacy and greater sense of unity in solving a problem.

What is nonimmediate language? Consider the differences in perceived meaning by the following statements that all convey the same information:
• Remember, we said that you should come in for a checkup. (most immediate)
• Remember, you said that you would come in for a checkup.
• Remember, it was said that you should come in for a checkup. (least immediate)

Nonimmediate language is used by both patients and professionals to discuss topics with which they are uncomfortable, including death, dying, and serious conditions such as AIDS. Such distancing behavior is a normal means of coping with uncomfortable subjects or possibilities, but it fails to help patients address and accept their situations.

A three-step process can be used to increase the amount of immediate language in your communications:
1. Identify topics and issues that make you uncomfortable, and identify groups and persons with whom you feel uncomfortable.
2. Identify nonimmediate language when it is spoken.
3. Identify when and with whom you use nonimmediate language.

By recognizing when and how we are switching from open, direct language to words that create distance and discomfort, we are taking the first step toward improving our ability to convey empathy and provide truly supportive communications.

Nonverbal cues in communications come from a variety of indicators:

- How far away we stand while talking with others (proxemics)
- Use of time in our communications (chronemics)
- Amount of eye contact or gaze (oculesics)
- Use of touch (haptics)
- Body movements (kinesics)
- Use and choice of objects in communications, such as clothing and symbols (objectics)
- Use and quality of the voice, such as changes in tone and pitch (vocalics)

Nonverbal means of communications are very important in our discussions with patients. If we show boredom or disregard in our facial expressions, patients will believe those messages and ignore noncongruent words and messages. Windows and counters in prescription departments and elevation of pharmacists above the patients create barriers to effective communication. Americans are resentful when they are made to wait for more than 5 minutes in most situations.[10] Eye contact is very important in communicating understanding and caring. Touching a patient's arm can be an effective means of conveying empathy if the health professional does so in a comfortable and appropriate manner. All of these elements must be incorporated into the pharmacist's professional demeanor so that patients comprehend conveyed communications correctly and perceive that their pharmacist is a trusting, caring professional with whom a strong relationship is paramount.

Conclusion

The ability to communicate is important for every pharmacist. By beginning to develop the skills described in this chapter, you will be ready when the time comes for you to convey important information about medications with your family, your friends, and your patients.

REFERENCES

1. Arbinger Institute. Leadership and Self-Deception: Getting Out of the Box. San Francisco: Barrett-Koehler Publishers; 2002.
2. Warner CT. Bonds That Make Us Free: Healing Our Relationships, Coming to Ourselves. Salt Lake City: Deseret Book Company; 2001.
3. Berger BA, Smith RE. Patient interaction. Part 1. The right choice. *US Pharm.* 2003(Apr).
4. Smith RE, Berger BA. The right choice: a pharmacy fable. Part 2. *US Pharm.* 2003(May).
5. Peck MS. The Road Less Traveled. New York: Simon & Schuster; 1978.
6. Basch MF. Empathic understanding: a review of the concept and some theoretical considerations. *J Am Psychoanal Assoc.* 1983;31:101-6.
7. Squier RW. A model of empathic understanding and adherence to treatment regimens in practitioner patient relationships. *Soc Sci Med.* 1990;30:325-39.
8. Albrecht TL, Burleson BR, Goldsmith D. Supportive communication. In: Knapp ML, Miller GR, eds. Handbook of Interpersonal Communication. 2nd ed. Thousand Oaks, Calif.: Sage Publications; 1994.
9. Mehrabian A. Silent Messages. Belmont, Calif.: Wadsworth Publishing; 1971.
10. McCroskey JC. An Introduction to Rhetorical Communication. Englewood Cliffs, N.J.: Prentice Hall; 1982.

Chapter 5 | Ethics in Pharmacy Practice

In Chapters 3 and 4, reference was made to the idea of a "covenant," or promise, between the pharmacist and the patient. This professional covenant is similar to a legal contract, in which each party makes certain promises. In this case, the pharmacist agrees to provide pharmaceutical care to the patient, and the patient agrees to provide payment and any needed information to the pharmacist.

Implicit in this covenant is the idea that the pharmacist has certain moral obligations to the patient, specifically to provide quality pharmaceutical care. A component of pharmaceutical care is the provision of drug therapy that will improve the patient's health or well-being. What happens if the patient doesn't want to take the drug, even though the pharmacist knows the patient may suffer or even die as a result? What if the patient needs the drug but has no money to pay the pharmacist for it? What if the pharmacist knows that the patient is an alcoholic, and an alternative drug is available that doesn't interact with alcohol? What if the drug is for AIDS and the pharmacist knows that the patient's wife is unaware of her husband's condition?

Each of these situations represents an ethical dilemma requiring choices that the pharmacist must make. Because of their professional roles, pharmacists have access to, or knowledge of, confidential information. Patients turn to pharmacists as knowledgeable, competent advisors about drug therapy and health care in general, and they expect to deal with an ethical, competent practitioner.

While much has been written about some of the major controversial ethical issues of our day—decisions about death and dying (assisted suicides, abortion), about rationing of health care resources, about who should make health care decisions (payers, patients, or health care providers)—pharmacists often encounter the simplest but most irreconcilable problems. A prominent citizen may ask for an unauthorized but medically needed refill on a Saturday when the prescribing physician is unavailable. A local physician may be overprescribing diet pills, but the pharmacy may be making a lot of money filling these questionable prescriptions. A physician may prescribe a **placebo** or nonprescription drug for a **hypochondriac** and ask the pharmacist to counsel the patient as if the medicine were a powerful analgesic. In social settings, pharmacists and student pharmacists are often asked about the usual use of certain medicines, whether a medication can cause a certain effect, and whether a given dose "is a lot."

In these and many other situations, pharmacists must make ethical decisions every day. Health professionals have struggled with some of these situations since the days when the Hippocratic Oath was first written; other dilemmas are the result of modern technologies that can preserve people as legally alive but mentally deceased. But what is ethics? What are the ethical principles that pharmacists can use as guides in making these difficult decisions?

"As to disease, make a habit of two things — to help, or at least to do no harm."

—Hippocratic Oath

Placebo:
A preparation with no known pharmacologic or medicinal properties. Placebos can sometimes "work" by making the patient believe that a real drug is being given, and placebos are used in some research as a way of identifying the beneficial properties of drugs.

Hypochondriac:
A patient with a psychologic disorder in which he or she complains of imagined medical problems.

The moralistic basis of biomedical ethics

In all human societies in the world, various behaviors are deemed to be right or wrong based on moralistic codes; these behaviors can be very different from culture to culture. In one of the best textbooks on biomedical ethics, Beauchamp and Childress differentiate between general moral codes, which apply to all members of a society, and professional moral codes, which apply to groups of people engaged in a certain profession or occupation.[1]

Beauchamp and Childress use the following logic sequence to illustrate four hierarchies of moral reasoning:

4. **Ethical theories** are derived from
3. **Principles**, which are derived from
2. **Rules**, which are derived from
1. **Particular judgments and actions**

As these levels suggest, people first learn about moral reasoning as small children by observing their own and others' actions and developing opinions about right and wrong. These opinions are codified into rules, which kindergarten and elementary school children use in a strict "good versus bad" view of the world. As the child matures, he or she develops principles of behavior that can be used as guides in the moralistic dilemmas of adolescence. And finally, ethical theories are developed by an individual, a group of individuals, or society as a whole (through the laws and court systems) to guide behavior when rules and principles may conflict with one another.

Within pharmacy, moralistic reasoning is embodied in various professional codes of conduct. The most universal in the profession is that of the American Pharmacists Association (Table 5.1). Of the two major schools of thought in Western ethics, the APhA Code tends to take the position of the nonconsequentialists, which is based on the following principles[2]:

1. Autonomy: An action is right if it respects the autonomy, or independent choice, of others.
2. Veracity: Telling the truth is right.
3. Fidelity: Keeping promises, commitments, contracts, and covenants is right.
4. Avoiding killing: Taking of human life is wrong.
5. Justice: Fair distribution of goods and harms is right.

The other major school of thought, consequentialism, generally considers actions to be right when they have beneficial outcomes for the people involved and wrong if they have detrimental consequences. This line of reasoning is embodied in the principle of beneficence, which is a person's moral obligation to help others—to contribute to the welfare of others. Beneficence may be thought of as the Good Samaritan, a person who interrupts his or her own life so that a person in need can be assisted. The principle of nonmaleficence is somewhat different from this concept: The health professional should above all keep the patient from harm.[2] These two principles are embodied in this quote from the Hippocratic Oath: "As to disease, make a habit of two things—to help, or at least to do no harm."

When discussing ethical issues in a chapter as brief as this one, it is difficult to maintain a separation between beneficence and nonmaleficence. In medicine, as in the world in general, no action or procedure is completely safe or completely effective. Thus, the line

Table 5.1. | Code of Ethics of the American Pharmacists Association[a]

Preamble: Pharmacists are health professionals who assist individuals in making the best use of medications. This Code, prepared and supported by pharmacists, is intended to state publicly the principles that form the fundamental basis of the roles and responsibilities of pharmacists. These principles, based on moral obligations and virtues, are established to guide pharmacists in relationships with patients, health professionals, and society.

I. A pharmacist respects the covenantal relationship between the patient and pharmacist.

Considering the patient–pharmacist relationship as a covenant means that a pharmacist has moral obligations in response to the gift of trust received from society. In return for this gift, a pharmacist promises to help individuals achieve optimum benefit from their medications, to be committed to their welfare, and to maintain their trust.

II. A pharmacist promotes the good of every patient in a caring, compassionate, and confidential manner.

A pharmacist places concern for the well-being of the patient at the center of professional practice. In doing so, a pharmacist considers needs stated by the patient as well as those defined by health science. A pharmacist is dedicated to protecting the dignity of the patient. With a caring attitude and a compassionate spirit, a pharmacist focuses on serving the patient in a private and confidential manner.

III. A pharmacist respects the autonomy and dignity of each patient.

A pharmacist promotes the right of self-determination and recognizes individual self-worth by encouraging patients to participate in decisions about their health. A pharmacist communicates with patients in terms that are understandable. In all cases, a pharmacist respects personal and cultural differences among patients.

IV. A pharmacist acts with honesty and integrity in professional relationships.

A pharmacist has a duty to tell the truth and to act with conviction of conscience. A pharmacist avoids discriminatory practices, behavior or work conditions that impair professional judgment, and actions that compromise dedication to the best interests of patients.

V. A pharmacist maintains professional competence.

A pharmacist has a duty to maintain knowledge and abilities as new medications, devices, and technologies become available and as health information advances.

VI. A pharmacist respects the values and abilities of colleagues and other health professionals.

When appropriate, a pharmacist asks for the consultation of colleagues or other health professionals or refers the patient. A pharmacist acknowledges that colleagues and other health professionals may differ in the beliefs and values they apply to the care of the patient.

VII. A pharmacist serves individual, community, and societal needs.

The primary obligation of a pharmacist is to individual patients. However, the obligations of a pharmacist may at times extend beyond the individual to the community and society. In these situations, the pharmacist recognizes the responsibilities that accompany these obligations and acts accordingly.

VIII. A pharmacist seeks justice in the distribution of health resources.

When health resources are allocated, a pharmacist is fair and equitable, balancing the needs of patients and society.

[a] Adopted by the membership of the American Pharmaceutical (now Pharmacists) Association, October 27, 1994.
Copyright © 1994, American Pharmacists Association, Inc.
Reprinted with permission.

can blur between doing good and not doing harm, for in doing good one can inadvertently do harm. However, it is important to differentiate between the two concepts so that ethical dilemmas may be properly analyzed.

Medical ethics is derived from a combination of the above elements, but the subject can be discussed by looking at four principles that embody all of the above concepts:

- Respect for patient autonomy
- Nonmaleficence
- Beneficence
- Justice

From these four principles come the obligations of the professional to be truthful with patients (veracity), to respect a patient's wishes to be left alone (privacy), not to disclose without permission information about the patient's medical condition (confidentiality), and to keep promises made to the patient (fidelity). Let's look at each of these underlying principles in more detail.

Respect for autonomy

In medicine, the principle of respect for autonomy is manifest in various types of informed consents to treatment and medical research. Medicine at one time operated under a paternalistic system in which the physician was considered the best decision-maker, since he or she had the range of knowledge about the disease state, the available alternatives, and the patient's condition. However, people have now realized that the risk–benefit ratio for a medical intervention is often quite different when considered by a patient whose life might be endangered by the procedure and a physician who stands to gain materially if the procedure is performed. This conflict has now been largely resolved by acceptance of the principle of respect for autonomy into medical practice: It is the patient who makes the final decision about whether a procedure will be performed on his or her body.

Five elements of informed consent must be met for the patient to make a proper decision about whether to submit to certain medical treatments[1]:

I. Threshold element
   A. Competence
II. Information elements
   A. Disclosure of information
   B. Understanding of information
III. Consent elements
   A. Voluntariness
   B. Authorization

Competence refers to the ability of the patient to understand the decision at hand. Comatose patients cannot communicate, and therefore are unable to provide informed consent. Other types of physical incompetence may also prevent informed decisions, as can cases of psychological incompetence (for example, patients with Alzheimer's disease or memory impairment).

In such cases, the next of kin or legal guardian of the patient must make an informed decision about therapy. Many life-or-death decisions end up in court when the decision of the legal guardian or relatives conflicts with institutional policies, governmental laws, or other people's opinions. People are increasingly preparing documents known as living wills, or advance directives, that attempt to spell out in advance what decisions they would make in certain clinical situations. Or patients may sign a durable power of attorney for health care, which allows spouses or other persons who know the patients well to make such decisions in cases of incompetence.

Whatever the situation, informed consent or refusal of treatment cannot occur without a competent patient or legal guardian involved.

The informational elements include both disclosure and understanding. Disclosure must be appropriate based on contemporary professional standards or appropriate for what a "reasonable person" would expect to be told in a similar situation. Exceptions to the disclosure element have been recognized in cases of emergency or when "sound medical judgment" would lead the health professional not to disclose certain information to, for example, a depressed or unstable patient.[1]

Assuring that the patient understands the decision being made is quite problematic, since the means to measure understanding are often unavailable. Some patients are capable of understanding one day but not the next. Others may be in a stage of denial of their diseases and thereby be incapable of understanding the relevance of a medical procedure. Patients' definitions of medical terms may vary substantially, thus impeding understanding. Or a procedure may be explained only minutes before it is to occur, giving the patient insufficient time to process the information before a decision is required.[1]

Because of the wide variability of problems with understanding as an element of informed consent, no clearly established models or definitions exist. But health professionals continue to have an ethical obligation to assure that patients truly understand the options they have when making informed decisions about their medical care.

Finally, the patient must give consent voluntarily and authorize the procedure through a legally valid document. Voluntariness, as used here, is defined this way: "A person acts voluntarily to the degree he or she wills the action without being under the control of another agent's influence."[1] Thus, voluntariness can be affected by coercion or manipulation by health professionals or relatives and by drugs or psychological disorders. Manipulation is the presentation of information in such a way that the patient's view of the situation is altered so that the patient does what the manipulator wants.

Thus, the patient has the right under currently held ethical principles to make autonomous decisions, and health professionals should respect them. This should be not confused with autonomy itself, but rather it is restricted to a respect for autonomous decision-making. However, this is but one element underlying biomedical ethical principles, and it must be considered along with the other three elements: Nonmaleficence, beneficence, and justice.[1]

Nonmaleficence

Nonmaleficence is best summarized in the most famous sentence in physicians' Hippocratic Oath: "At least, do no harm." It is differentiated from beneficence in that nonmaleficence refers to not taking actions that would inflict harm, while beneficence refers to taking actions that will do good. Conflict between the two principles is inevitable, since no medical or drug treatment is completely effective or completely safe; there are always cases of therapeutic failure and adverse unintended consequences.

Negligence:
Failure of a professional to provide the standard of due care to patients who seek that care.

The principle of nonmaleficence is integrated into a professional standard of due care, which is the basis used by courts in trying professional misconduct or **negligence** cases. The moralistic due care standard, comprising the following elements, is similar to the legalistic standard of due care[1]:

1. The professional must have a duty to the affected party.
2. The professional must breach that duty.
3. The affected party must experience a harm or injury.
4. This harm must be caused by the breach of duty.

All four elements must be met; if the professional is not recognized by society or by the courts as having a duty to a specific patient, then no breach has occurred. Similarly, if the patient does not experience harm or if the harm does not result from the breach of duty, then no breach is recognized.

Over the past two decades, several widely publicized court cases have involved conflicts over the principle of nonmaleficence, often in situations that require a distinction between allowing a patient to die versus killing a patient. Generally recognized is that health care professionals should provide due care to patients but are not obligated to provide care, especially "heroic" means, when biological death is imminent in a person with serious or severe illnesses or conditions. The range of pertinent distinctions is as follows[1]:

I. Obligatory care
II. Optional care (may be neutral or heroic care)
III. Wrong care (obligatory not to provide)

Living will:
A legal document that provides guidance to healthcare professionals about what actions a patient would like taken if he or she is unable to provide an informed decision because of illness or injury. Also known as an advance directive.

How does a medical professional decide what care should be provided to a given patient? Three factors are involved: the patient's clinical condition, the patient's prior wishes as expressed informally or in a **living will**, and laws and societal rules.

Courts have generally supported the withholding of care—including such basic needs as nutrition and respiratory support—to patients whose mental function is minimal or nonexistent and whose conditions are considered irreversible. In cases where no living will is available, the next-of-kin, legal guardian, or designated proxy is consulted about the possible courses of action. Thus, even obligatory care may not be necessary in every patient-care situation.

Heroic measures are a result of modern scientific and technologic developments that provide people with ways of prolonging life even though a person is clinically nonfunctional. The acceptability of failing to provide heroic measures is reflected in "do not resuscitate" orders in nursing homes for elderly patients who do not wish to be revived if cardiopulmonary failure occurs.

46 | **PHARMACY:** *An Introduction to the Profession*

Failure to provide care to incompetent patients or to those who do not wish to be resuscitated conjures up thoughts that there is such a thing as a life not worth living.[1] The ethical principle being espoused is that to provide care in these situations would in effect harm that patient, but to not provide care means that the patient will die. The idea that death is better than life conflicts with many people's own moral principles; this conflict is at the heart of many of the deepest, most emotional issues of our day. To some degree, even parts of the abortion controversy fall under this heading, since people argue that the life of an unwanted baby would be worse than not living at all.

Because of the conflicts and differences of opinion, the obligation of the health care professional to do no harm is becoming more and more complicated in today's world. Only through a proper understanding of the patient's wishes (as defined through respect for autonomy) and through evaluation of what is in the patient's best interests (nonmaleficence versus beneficence) can ethical decisions be reached.[1]

Beneficence

While the lessons learned by studying nonmaleficence are important, the obligations of a healthcare professional go far beyond this concept. No one would ever seek medical care if the only promise was that no harm would be done. The APhA Code of Ethics exemplifies practice beyond nonmaleficence in that it requires pharmacists to render unto patients "the full measure of professional ability."

This is the concept of beneficence—to do good, to remove harms, to promote welfare. A corollary to the principle is that benefits and risks of therapy must be balanced. How are these concepts being applied in pharmacy today?

All members of society are expected to render aid to those in need, but the obligations of a health care professional become larger because of the specialized knowledge possessed and because of the authority that society has given the individual. The professional is expected to render aid even when some degree of personal risk is involved. Just as a lifeguard is expected to rescue drowning swimmers at personal risk, the physician is expected to provide care to patients with infectious diseases such as AIDS or hepatitis at personal risk of acquiring those diseases.[1]

However, the professional covenant cannot be activated unless both parties agree to its terms, and health care professionals do have some legal and ethical rights to select whom they will serve. Just because a patient has a need does not mean that the provider must care for that patient in nonemergency situations. Of course, legal restrictions would prevent physicians from discriminating on the basis of race, creed, color, nationality, or handicap. Diseases, including AIDS, have often been recognized as "handicaps," thus preventing health care professionals from refusing to care for patients with certain conditions.

The application of the principle of beneficence in healthcare often leads to conflict with respect of patient autonomy. As was discussed earlier in the chapter, the practice of paternalism in healthcare was the result of the provider unilaterally deciding what was in the best interest of the patient. This practice has now largely been replaced by the concept of respect for autonomy—that an informed patient is best able to choose from several potential therapies.

But this does not mean that the conflict between autonomy and beneficence has ended. Paternalism conflicts with respect for autonomy when a mentally unstable patient is not told that he or she has a terminal disease; here the patient is never given the information necessary to make an informed decision because the provider (the "father") believes that the patient would be incapable of rational thought or of making the best decision. Debates continue about how far health care professionals should be allowed to go in applying the principle of beneficence when it is in conflict with the patient's expressed or potential wishes.

The other key component of beneficence is the development of risk–benefit models that can be used to help with ethical decisions. In recent years, cost has been added to this model as the price of health care—and especially medications—has risen dramatically in comparison with the costs of other goods in American society.

The evaluation of relative costs, benefits, and risks is based on the ethical theory of utilitarianism. It states that, given a choice between equally effective therapies, healthcare providers should seek to maximize benefits and minimize costs and risks. To analyze these three variables, various formal models of cost-effectiveness and cost-benefit analysis have been developed. Risk assessment is another technique used to focus on the amount of risk a patient must encounter in a given procedure.[1]

As students of algebra will recall, one cannot solve a single equation with two variables. Either one variable must be held constant, or more information (another equation, in the algebraic problems) must be available. A similar line of thinking involves the ethical dilemmas of modern medicine: How can one select ethically from among different therapies that are equally effective but with different costs and risks? Or what processes can be used to choose between alternatives that are equally safe but with different costs and efficacies? In the final analysis, who will live and who will die? If the decision turns on costs and the relative wealth of the individual, has justice been done? That is the next element in ethical reasoning.

Justice

On first blush, the application of the principle of justice to health care makes one think of equal opportunity to obtain treatment for all people, regardless of wealth or social status. Despite its ethical appeal, this is probably not a realistic position, as some 40 million Americans have no health insurance, those with insurance must meet all kinds of conditions and copayments that they may not be able to afford, and only a few of America's super-wealthy citizens could afford to pay their own health care bills throughout a lifetime.

So, what is justice when it comes to health care?

Aristotle noted that justice was the equal treatment of equals and the unequal treatment of unequals. But America purports to be a society of equals. Several major theories of justice are debated in America today[1]:

- *Utilitarian theories of justice:* Justice is merely a form of the most paramount and stringent form of utility, so the system for evaluating risks, benefits, and costs must balance the private and public benefits, risks, and costs.

Table 5.2 | Six Stages of Moral Reasoning About Unauthorized Refills in Pharmacy Practice[a]

Classes of Morality	Stage No.	Example of Stage
Preconventional	1	Obedience: A pharmacist dispensing an unauthorized refill to avoid reprimands by owners of a pharmacy.
	2	Instrumental egoism and simple exchange: A pharmacist dispensing an unauthorized refill to do what he was being paid for and to give the patient what he wanted.
Conventional	3	Interpersonal concordance: A pharmacist dispensing an unauthorized refill because of a belief that the physician would be happy, the patient would be happy, and the pharmacy owner would be happy.
	4	Law and duty to the social order: A pharmacist dispensing an unauthorized refill only after calling the physician, or not dispensing it, because to do otherwise would be illegal.
Postconventional	5	Societal consensus: A pharmacist working with the pharmacy owner or nearby physicians to set up a system for handling unauthorized refills.
	6	Nonarbitrary social cooperation: Presented with a request for an unauthorized refill, a pharmacist dispensing it or refusing to dispense it based on the ultimate welfare of the patient.

[a] Adapted from reference 3.

- *Libertarian theories of justice*: Individual liberty is the most important factor in libertarian thinking, so a free-market basis for health care is considered the most just. Perhaps even if people elect to buy and sell babies or organs for transplant, the libertarian would be happy so long as the government does not interfere with this expression of individual freedom.
- *Egalitarian theories of justice*: While not every person is entitled to an equal share of available goods and services, egalitarians believe that certain distributions of burdens and benefits should be equally available. This line of thinking serves to create basic rights for all citizens, some of which are stated (the right to vote) and some of which are implied (health care).

As the United States struggles to fix its ailing but very expensive health care system, the central problems will lie in the application of the principle of justice and the irreconcilable differences contained in the above three theories. So long as the financial resources of all citizens are not equal, it is certain that wealthier people will be able to seek medical interventions not available to other citizens. Perhaps a basic right to a certain minimum level of health care services will be identified, or perhaps a system of resource allocation or rationing on some other basis will be devised. Whatever the final decision, the application of the principle of justice along with respect for autonomy, nonmaleficence, and beneficence will keep medical ethicists busy for many years.

Ethical considerations in pharmacy practice

How do all these ethical principles translate into actual pharmacy practice? Like many theories, the information is more easily stated than applied. While the scope of this text does not allow detailed discussions of ethical dilemmas in pharmacy, many excellent analyses have been published in the medical and pharmacy literature. The *American Journal of Health-System Pharmacy* and *U.S. Pharmacist* have published much material on ethics in pharmacy over the years. Interested readers and classes should consult these for group discussions.

One article can assist in analyzing and categorizing pharmacy-related ethical principles. Dolinsky and Gottlieb[3] applied the model shown in Table 5.2 to pharmacy situations. The authors attribute actions taken in stages 1–3 as being primarily from self-interest, while stage 4 is legalistic. Stages 5 and 6 are based on principles and are more likely to be ethically proper—even though they may be illegal. As a practice exercise, describe ethical dilemmas that you have encountered while working in or visiting a pharmacy, and try to describe the stages of moral reasoning and the principles of ethics involved in the decision the pharmacist made.

Balancing the demands of society

As the healthcare professional with responsibility for the proper use of drugs in society, pharmacists are faced daily with ethical quandaries. Some of these are addressed in a minute-by-minute fashion, as patients and prescriptions come and go. Others develop over time, such as the physician who prescribes increasing amounts of narcotics for members of his or her family. Still others occur for pharmacists when they are fulfilling their roles as responsible members of the healthcare team or of the community (for example, offering advice to local governments about controlling illegal drugs). Without a moral and ethical framework within which to focus rational thought, pharmacists are at a loss in fulfilling their professional covenant with patients.

REFERENCES

1. Beauchamp TL, Childress JF. Principles of biomedical ethics. 5th ed. New York: Oxford University Press; 2001.
2. Veatch RM. Hospital pharmacy: what is ethical? *Am J Hosp Pharm.* 1989; 46:109-15.
3. Dolinsky D, Gottlieb J. Moral dilemmas in pharmacy practice. *Am J Pharm Educ.* 1986; 50:56-9.

Chapter 6 | Career Planning: Practice Areas in Pharmacy

One of the great benefits of having a degree in pharmacy is the wide variety of career options that it opens to the individual. From going back to the corner drugstore in one's hometown to rising through the ranks of multinational corporate conglomerates, the possibilities are endless for the new pharmacy graduate.

In this chapter, the major areas of practice in pharmacy are presented along with some general concepts of career planning and obtaining a job. In many pharmacy orientation courses, these brief oversights of practice areas are supplemented with presentations by guest lecturers who work in various practice settings. But don't let your investigation stop there—if an area of practice appeals to you, contact alumni from your school or local practitioners who work in that part of pharmacy. If you decide on a path for your career, begin planning now so that you can take the elective courses that will give you a jump-start after you graduate.

One caveat is in order at this point in pharmacy history: Times are changing. As you learned in Chapter 3, medication therapy management (MTM) is becoming more common in community pharmacy, and no one knows now what practice will be like in a few years. Likewise, the availability of increasingly sophisticated robotic equipment and computerized systems along with a growing number of Certified Pharmacy Technicians are affecting the practice of pharmacy in all settings. If pharmacists "play their cards right," MTM could be a dominant mode of practice by the time this edition of this textbook goes out of print. At a minimum, pharmacists' daily activities should be greatly different in a few years, and I discuss this possibility at appropriate places in this chapter.

"In youth my wings were strong and tireless,
But I did not know the mountains.
In age I knew the mountains
But my weary wings could not follow my vision—
Genius is wisdom and youth."

—Epitaph of Alexander Throckmorton, from *Spoon River Anthology*, by Edgar Lee Masters

Identifying a career option in pharmacy

A successful career is built on two things: good planning and good luck. And one of my favorite quotes is that I'd rather be lucky than good.

However, that does not mean that good planning counts for nothing in charting a career. While one never knows precisely when certain unique opportunities may be available, the wide variety of pharmacy positions available in many different settings can accommodate many plans for advancement throughout a career. And, without planning, one will not be ready to seize the opportunities when they do arise.

While every aspect in career planning could not be presented in any one book, the best advice to the student pharmacist is to find a good mentor. Identify the pharmacy faculty in your school who seem knowledgeable about the parts of pharmacy that interest you, and ask them to give you advice on what courses and experiences will best prepare you for that career. Ask about personality inventory tests or other assessment tools that

Figure 6.1 | **Critical job factors for pharmacy careers. Use this chart to ask yourself what you feel is important in your future pharmacy career.[a]**

Glaxo Pathway Evaluation Program for Pharmacy Professionals *Self-assessment Decision-Making Chart*		
Critical Job Factors	**Present Position**	**Optimal Position**
Counseling Spend time with patients, public		
Continuity of Relationships Maintain ongoing, long-term patient, consumer contact		
Helping People Directly or indirectly add to well-being of individuals, society		
Professional Interaction Involvement with other health care professionals		
Educating Other Professionals Time devoted to educating other health care professionals		
Repetition Very repetitive daily activities, tasks		
Multiple Task Handling Juggle many tasks at a time with interruptions		
Problem-solving Solve problems with tried, true solutions; or by exploring untested solutions		
Focus of Expertise Specialist or generalist		
Innovative Thinking Generate new ideas about pharmacy, pharmaceuticals		
Applying Scientific Knowledge Applying scientific or medical knowledge		
Business Management Organize, manage, assume risks of business		
Pressure Deal with crisis, quickly interpret medical, technical information		
Work Schedule Regular vs. irregular, long hours		
Leisure/Family Time Little vs. ample time for family, leisure activities		
Job Security Secure position and income		
Opportunity for Advancement Limited vs. many advancement opportunities		
Community Prestige Opportunity to gain recognition in the community		
Professional Prestige Opportunity to gain recognition in the profession		
Income Income level to meet lifestyle expectations		

[a]Adapted with permission from reference 1.

Figure 6.2 | **Pharmacy, people, and big picture skills needed in various levels of management of pharmacies.**[a]

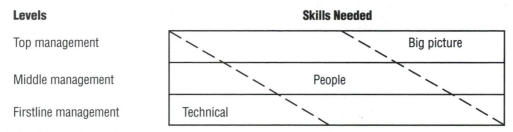

Levels	Skills Needed		
Top management			Big picture
Middle management		People	
Firstline management	Technical		

[a]*Reprinted with permission from reference 2.*

may be available for identifying your strengths and interests. Find out whether advanced study beyond your entry-level degree will be needed, and ask yourself whether you are willing or able to devote the extra time, money, and energy for more studies. Learn whether you would be required to relocate for that career, and talk with your spouse, significant other, or family about what that might mean. With proper advice, input, and thought, your career choices should become obvious.

An important tool available to student pharmacists for career planning is the Pathways Evaluation Program for Pharmacy Professionals. Originally developed by Glaxo (now GlaxoSmithKline) in the 1980s, this program was transferred to the American Pharmacists Association in 2001. It helps student pharmacists as well as pharmacists considering a career switch to evaluate the importance to the individual of several factors that vary among pharmacy practice settings (Figure 6.1)[1]:

- Applying scientific knowledge
- Business management
- Pressure
- Work schedule
- Leisure/family time
- Job security
- Opportunity for advancement
- Community prestige
- Professional prestige
- Income

Pathways materials can be accessed in the Careers center on www.pharmacist.com, the APhA Web site. The online version of the Pathway evaluation allows you to rate 48 different factors that are similar to those shown in Fig. 6.1 on a 1–10 scale. Based on these responses, the specific positions and work settings most likely to fit your responses are identified, along with detailed information about each. The system also includes results of a 2007 survey of people in each type of position along with salary and other relevant information.

For further information about APhA's services that can enhance your career choices, contact the Association at 800/237-APhA (2742).

Descriptions of various pharmacy practice settings are also available on the Web site of the American Association of Colleges of Pharmacy (www.aacp.org; click on "Career Options" in the Student section of the site).

Table 6.1 | Contact Persons for Internship Programs

Pharmaceutical industry
Contact your Dean or the Advisor of your Academy of Students of Pharmacy Chapter for an application.
Deadline for applications: November 30 of each year

Federal pharmacy
COSTEP
Public Health Service Recruitment
5600 Fishers Lane, Room 7A-07
Rockville, MD 20852
301/443-5740
www.fda.gov
Deadline for summer applications: December 31 of each year

Drug information
United States Pharmacopeial Convention
12601 Twinbrook Parkway
Rockville, MD 20852
301/816-8390
www.usp.org
Deadline for summer applications: February 1 of each year

National Council on Patient Information and Education
4915 Saint Elmo Avenue, Suite 505
Bethesda, MD 20814-6082
301/656-8565
www.talkaboutrx.org
Deadline for summer applications: March 1 of each year

Association management
American Pharmacists Association[a]
2215 Constitution Ave., NW
Washington, DC 20037
800/237-APhA (2742)
www.pharmacist.com
Deadline for summer application: February 1 of each year

National Community Pharmacists Association
205 Daingerfield Road
Alexandria, VA 22314
703/683-8200
www.ncpanet.org
Deadline for summer applications: April 15 of each year

American Society of Health-System Pharmacists
7272 Wisconsin Avenue
Bethesda, MD 20814
301/657-3000
www.ashp.org
Deadline for summer applications: February 1 of each year

Paul G. Cano Legislative Internship
American Society of Consultant Pharmacists
1321 Duke Street
Alexandria, VA 22314-3563
703/739-1300, Ext 126
www.ascp.com
(call to determine availability and schedule)

Pharmacy fraternities
Phi Delta Chi (www.phideltachi.org) and
Lambda Kappa Sigma (www.lks.org)
have periodically offered summer internships.

[a]Until early to mid-2009, APhA is temporarily located at 1100 15th St., NW, Washington, DC 20005; telephone numbers will remain the same.

Getting ready to pursue a career

One of the best ways to determine if you like a certain part of pharmacy is to work in that setting. Luckily, many possible options are available for doing that if you will look around and be willing to go where the job is.

Gaining this work experience is important in three ways: (1) It provides you with the chance to see what your daily activities would be like in that setting, (2) your experience there makes your school work more relevant by showing you why you need to know "all this stuff," and (3) your commitment to that career option will appear stronger to potential employers when you are graduating. You should also remember that the time you spend searching for a job after you graduate is money lost—and your postgraduate salary will be many times greater than what you can make during school! Taking a lower-paying job during school to aid your career planning could be an important investment in your future.

If you are considering a career in pharmacy practice in community, hospital, or consultant pharmacy, positions should be available in your area. Talking with faculty members who deal a lot with alumni, looking in the newspaper, or visiting local pharmacies (or hospital pharmacies) can all be productive. To identify consultant pharmacists, you may need to contact the American Society of Consultant Pharmacists at the address shown in Table 6.1 and Chapter 8, since these are often **"closed-shop" pharmacies** located in industrial parks or office complexes.

For jobs in alternative pharmacy career paths, investigate the possibility of summer internships (Table 6.1). For instance, the APhA–ASP sponsors a summer internship program in the pharmaceutical industry. Student pharmacists from all over the United States work at various major research-oriented pharmaceutical companies for the summer. There, the students rotate through all the major parts of the company, learning about research and development of new drugs, marketing, sales, drug information, and professional relations.

Likewise, the Public Health Service has COSTEP (Commissioned Officer Student Training and Extern Program). This three-month experience is available for student pharmacists to learn more about the role pharmacists can play in the federal government, including the Food and Drug Administration, the Indian Health Service, the Public Health Service, and the National Institutes of Health.

For student pharmacists who are intrigued by a career working in pharmacy associations, summer internships are available from APhA, the National Community Pharmacists Association (NCPA), the American Society of Health-System Pharmacists (ASHP), and periodically the pharmacy fraternities Lambda Kappa Sigma and Phi Delta Chi. All these are approximately three-month stints at the headquarters of these groups that involve rotations in various aspects of association work: membership, financial, conference planning, legal, executive support, editorial, and marketing. The NCPA and ASHP rotations are open to all student pharmacists; the fraternity groups generally choose from among their own members.

Experiences focused more on the provision of drug information as a career are also available at the United States Pharmacopeial Convention and the National Council on Patient Information and Education.

In addition to the nationally oriented experiences shown in Table 6.1, many state pharmaceutical associations have part-time, temporary, and summer positions available. Ask your pharmacy school faculty about those possibilities.

These experiences can be critical in knowing beforehand whether certain areas of pharmacy are for you. Valuable postgraduate time can be saved by experiencing a part of pharmacy before entering the workplace, even if you learn that your expectations were not met and that another segment of the profession is more appealing.

Closed-shop pharmacies:
A pharmacy not open to the public. It usually provides services to nursing homes or other types of long-term care facilities. These services may be drug dispensing, consulting on patients' drug therapy, or both.

One final point about career planning. Figure 6.2 on page 53 shows the kinds of skills that will be needed in various parts of a pharmacy career, pretty much regardless of where you practice. Pharmacy school is designed to teach you much of the technical aspects of the profession; it touches only slightly on people and big-picture skills. Throughout your career, people skills will be very important; you must learn how to live, work, and communicate with others. And, as you are promoted throughout your career, what you learned in school will become less important than keeping the big picture in mind. This all means that you can never stop learning, and that you should take advantage now of opportunities to advance your people skills. The best place to do that in pharmacy school is through involvement in student organizations, where you can learn about small-group decision-making, conflict resolution, communication, teamwork, and goal setting.

With that background, let's look at the major areas of practice within pharmacy:
- Community independent pharmacy
- Community chain pharmacy
- Institutional pharmacy
- Consultant pharmacy
- Managed care or home care
- Pharmaceutical industry, government, and associations

For each of the above areas of pharmacy practice, the following components will be addressed during each synopsis:
- Definition and scope of practice
- Position availability
- Salary
- Typical day
- Common rewards and frustrations
- Prospects of growth and advancement

Community independent pharmacy

As related in Chapter 2 on the history of pharmacy, the independent pharmacy is where the profession began, and it is still in many ways the heart and soul of pharmacy. Many of today's pharmacists came into the profession because of the respect they had for "doc" at the corner drugstore; in fact, for a sizable fraction of pharmacists, "doc" was their father or some other close relative. The spirit of entrepreneurship and the American dream of owning one's own business lives on in our country's 25,000 independent pharmacies, which have endured through decades of increasing competition from larger, better financed chain stores and decreasing reimbursement levels that have led to lower profit margins.

For independent pharmacists, the key word is "independent." Pharmacists who choose to practice in independent community pharmacy are uniquely able to practice their profession in the way they choose, and this means they can more quickly transition their practices into MTM if they choose to do so. They are able to respond quickly to changing consumer needs and have a real and lasting impact in their community. Through independent pharmacy, each practitioner has the opportunity to succeed or to fail. Each practitioner has the privilege—and the risk that comes with it—of setting the rules and determining the policies for the pharmacy.

According to the *2007 NCPA–Pfizer Digest,* the typical independent pharmacy dispenses 196 prescriptions per day, assuming a six-day workweek for the independent pharmacy. Nationally, independent pharmacies dispense 1.4 billion prescriptions annually, which is 41% of all prescriptions dispensed in the community pharmacies. Just under 60% of prescriptions are dispensed using generics. The average pharmacy has total gross sales of $3.9 million, with 90% of sales coming through prescriptions. An average of 13.4 full-time equivalent employees work in the independent pharmacy, including 3.2 FTE pharmacists (counting the owner) and 4.6 FTE technicians. Overall, 91% of pharmacies offer nutrition services, 86% deliver prescriptions, 86% offer charge accounts, 79% have compounding services, and 75% carry herbal medicines.[4]

About 37% of independent pharmacies are located in downtown areas, 24% in non-business residential areas, 12% in hospitals or medical professional centers, and 9% in shopping malls.

A survey conducted by NCPA showed that 98% of independent pharmacists counsel their patients and that the independent pharmacist, in a typical day, talks with physicians 23 times, and spends nearly 2 hours counseling patients.

Pharmacist positions are available in independent stores, and the country is filled with success stories for those who want to compete in this environment. Profiles of successful community pharmacists are published regularly in the NCPA magazine, *America's Pharmacist* (www.americaspharmacist.net; membership required), and APhA's *Pharmacy Today* (www.pharmacytoday.org; open access) profiles a successful MTM practitioner—including many in independent pharmacy practice—in each issue. While starting salaries in independent pharmacies are often a little lower than in chain pharmacies, the prospects for advancement are different, especially if there is a chance to buy the pharmacy or start one's own pharmacy at some point.

All industries tend to go through three stages of development: Sales growth, multiple locations, and diversification. Independent community pharmacy is no different. Most successful community pharmacies today have either several locations (30% of independent owners owned two or more locations in the 2007 data[4]), which increases the company's sales and buying power, and/or diverse services, such as compounding, veterinary pharmacy, home care, **durable medical equipment**, long-term care (nursing homes or residential care facilities), or intravenous therapy. The growth possibilities in these emerging areas of MTM and health care are limitless.

For pharmacists in entry-level positions in independent community pharmacy, much of the day is spent in drug-dispensing and patient-counseling activities. Many community pharmacies have pharmacy technicians who assist the pharmacist with the filling of prescriptions for checking and dispensing by the pharmacist. Computers are tremendously important in today's community pharmacy, as they have enabled pharmacies to provide advanced services, such as keeping **patient profiles**, checking for drug interactions, and providing patient-specific information for counseling, billing, drug-use review, or insurance purposes. MTM services are facilitated in some computer software packages, including conducting and documenting medication therapy reviews, providing patients with a personal medication record, and generating medication-related action plans that are shared

Durable medical equipment:
Items such as wheelchairs, walkers, and bedside toilets that patients buy when their health fails or rent during rehabilitative periods after surgery or injury. The term can also include various types of intravenous (also called parenteral) or enteral services that require special catheters or pumps to deliver fluids or nutrition through the patient's veins or the gastrointestinal tract safely.

Patient profiles:
A record, usually computerized, of all medications a patient has received at a given pharmacy. Ideally, the profiles should include both prescription and nonprescription medicines.

with physicians and other primary care providers.[4] The community pharmacist may compound special prescriptions for patients or prepare drugs for intravenous administration. As pharmaceutical care and MTM have become the norm and patient counseling is provided more universally in pharmacy, the pharmacist is spending increasing fractions of his or her time in direct patient contact. This trend is making the pharmacist a source of primary care, making communication skills, patient-assessment techniques, and clinical knowledge all the more important.[5-8]

For managers or owners of community pharmacies, time is spent ordering merchandise and drugs, dealing with cash flow and accounts receivable or payable, handling personnel problems, marketing MTM and consulting services offered by the pharmacy, and planning for the future. Of course, since most independent pharmacies are small businesses, any employee may be called on to do almost anything—from managing the store while the owner is out of town to mopping the floors.

Practice in independent community pharmacies can be very rewarding for pharmacists who like to really know their patients, are attracted by the excitement of entrepreneurship that small businesses provide, or want the flexibility of finding a job in their hometown or virtually any other city or hamlet in the country. Independent pharmacists deal directly with the public, and they sometimes complain about some of those interactions, especially patients' criticisms about the skyrocketing prices of prescription drugs and problems with third-party payers. The pharmacist here feels caught in the middle, since the prices are dictated by the pharmaceutical manufacturer and the policies set by insurance companies and pharmacy benefits managers. The situation has been compounded further by pharmaceutical companies that have become "whipping boys" in the public discourse for their pricing and marketing practices. Combined with the long hours of standing on one's feet with few breaks to even go to the rest room—much less sit down to eat—some pharmacists have experienced frustration in community independent pharmacy.

The entrepreneurial spirit definitely lives on for the pharmacy owner. In addition to a salary, the owner may also benefit financially from the profits of the business, and he or she can sell the store when the time comes to retire or move on to some other situation.

All in all, independent community pharmacy provides a nice home for thousands of American pharmacists. Because of the nature of owning one's own business, many of these pharmacists are leaders in the profession, and they face today's challenges with just as much resolve, grit, and determination as did their predecessors who fought back intrusions by the merchants and grocers in Renaissance England.

Community chain pharmacy

Community chain pharmacists practice in cities and towns of all sizes and shapes and in a variety of settings, including the traditional chain pharmacy (such as CVS/pharmacy and Rite Aid), supermarkets, and mass merchants (such as Target and Wal-Mart). Chain pharmacies often have a large selection of merchandise in the front of the store; the pharmacy is often placed in back of the store to encourage consumers to pick up other items while they are getting their prescriptions filled.

While the day-to-day operations of a prescription department are similar to those in independent pharmacies, a chain pharmacist is part of a larger corporate structure that provides numerous personal growth and career-development opportunities. Chain pharmacies operated in 2006 nearly 40,000 units, as shown in Table 6.2. As you can see, the number of traditional chain pharmacies has increased slightly since 1996, while the number of supermarket and mass merchant outlets has ballooned by 60% or more over this 11-year period.[9]

A total of 188 corporate chains are members of the National Association of Chain Drug Stores (NACDS). Even though the perception of a chain drug store typically is that of a large retail outlet carrying a wide variety of merchandise, about two of every three NACDS members are small chains, meaning they operate at least four but no more than 50 stores. Many of these small chains operate like a typical independent pharmacy by carrying limited merchandise and focusing almost entirely on providing health-related products and services.[9]

The NACDS Web site (www.nacds.org) contains basic information and contact information for its member companies. If you're looking for a job or a career in community chain practice, this is a great place to start. The largest members of NACDS include Rite Aid, CVS/pharmacy, Walgreen, Wal-Mart, Albertson's, K-Mart, Medicine Shoppe International, Safeway, TrueCare Pharmacies, Ahold USA, and Target. Nationally, sales in all chain pharmacies totaled $198.9 billion in 2007, a 5.0% increase over 2006. Prescription drugs accounted for about three-quarters of this amount, $159.01 billion, including $104.8 billion in traditional chains, $25.66 billion in mass merchants, and $28.54 billion in supermarkets.[10]

More than one half of new pharmacy graduates enter chain practice each year. Reasons for this high proportion include job availability in nearly any part of the country, excellent salary and fringe benefit packages, store locations in areas of high population density, and the opportunity to interact with the public in a health care environment. New chain pharmacies are opening every day as they battle for market share in a competitive field. Chain pharmacists can expect to dispense an average of about 180 prescriptions per day in the typical chain pharmacy, based on national data available on the NACDS Web site.[10]

The "front-line" or staff pharmacist practicing in a chain pharmacy, no matter what the size, is afforded one of the greatest opportunities for patient interaction, if they can extract themselves from the prescription-filling process and find time for patient counseling and MTM. High prescription volume pharmacies heavily use trained technicians and automation to provide pharmacists with the time to counsel patients on their drug therapy and answer their questions.

Table 6.2 | NACDS Chain Member Pharmacies

	1990	1995	2006
Traditional	16,970	17,004	19,535
Supermarket	1,336	3,148	9,552
Mass Market	2,451	4,286	7,144
Total	20,757	24,438	36,231

Source: National Association of Chain Drug Stores

Community chain pharmacies have led the pharmacy profession in developing the computer technology needed to keep up with the growing number of medications being used by patients each year. Sophisticated software programs have been developed by chains to maintain each patient's complete medication profile record and detect any potential drug interactions that could occur when a new drug is added to that profile. Online verification of a patient's eligibility under a specific insurance plan results in significantly reduced paperwork and handling of claims. Inventory control and pricing accuracy also are greatly enhanced by this heavy reliance upon computers.

A primary key to a satisfying career as a chain pharmacist is the continual contact with patients. As one chain pharmacist stated, "I've found that the key to good pharmacist–patient rapport lies in never losing sight of the patient's needs and perspective. To make sure this happens, it's important to be sympathetic to their conditions. With many of my older customers, the communication between us is just as important as the medications they use."

Numerous chain pharmacists become active in local, state, and national pharmacy associations, and typically chain employers are highly supportive when their pharmacists have opportunities to serve in leadership positions in these organizations or on state boards of pharmacy. Countless chain pharmacists actively support the educational programs of nearby pharmacy schools by serving as preceptors of student externs. Some chain pharmacists even serve as practitioner members of various schools' curriculum committees.

Many chains are expanding their scope of services into other health-related areas such as MTM, immunizations, nutrition and weight loss programs (including some in which supermarket pharmacists take patients on shopping tours of the grocery store and teach them how to read food labels and plan their diets), home health care, nursing home consulting, and home infusion therapy. This further increases the professional opportunities that await pharmacists who choose to practice in a corporate chain setting. Most chains have established pilot programs in MTM, and some have had hundreds of their pharmacists become certified in MTM delivery and/or immunizations. If these initial efforts take hold and the payment for services becomes routine, the face of pharmacy practice will be changed in the coming years.

A growing area in most corporate chain pharmacy organizations is the managed care department. Here, pharmacists negotiate contracts with health-maintenance organizations, employer groups, and pharmacy benefit managers. In a chain pharmacy's purchasing department, pharmacists work with vendors and with generic and research-based pharmaceutical manufacturers in making drug-product-selection decisions.

Some pharmacists become so interested and involved in corporate management that they leave the pharmacy and health service division of their company and are promoted into positions in general merchandising, store layout and design, and even site selection and real estate negotiations. For those pharmacists who want to combine their professional talents with the challenge of the fast-paced retail business, numerous middle- and upper-level management positions are available. Many chains offer management training programs and specialized educational support that can help pharmacists chart a path that leads from the prescription department to one of several career tracks in management at the store, district, regional, and corporate levels.

Pharmacists in chain practice are satisfied by the level of job security, the provision of continuing education directly by the employer, and the predictability that a corporate environment gives their careers and their personal lives. Practice can be just as rewarding in terms of patient contact if the pharmacist is allowed to practice professionally based on corporate policies and workload. The frustrations of patients complaining about prescription prices is worse in chains, since the patients there are more often bargain shoppers who are looking to save money. At the local level, pharmacists are sometimes frustrated by nonpharmacist managers of a store, who may interfere with the pharmacist's professional obligations to the patient. And, there can be the frustration of reaching a **"terminal" position** early in one's career but being frozen into that position by the high salaries offered by chains.

The largest group of pharmacy graduates, year in and year out, goes directly into community chain pharmacy. Many of these people find a satisfying career there that gives them a lifetime of professional growth and opportunity.

Institutional pharmacy

Institutional pharmacy, traditionally practiced in hospitals and other "organized" health care settings, offers a diverse realm of possibilities to the new pharmacy graduate. Within today's disparate corporate hospital-based structures, an entire spectrum of pharmacist positions can be found in institutional pharmacy. Dispensing-only jobs require little contact with patients or other professionals outside the pharmacy, other than via telephone. Clinical pharmacy (analogous to MTM in community pharmacies) was born in hospitals, and positions with full-time clinical responsibilities are available on patient-care units where interactions with physicians, nurses, and the rest of the **health care team** go on continuously. And there is management, dealing with multimillion-dollar personnel and drug budgets that can make or break the sales goals of pharmaceutical industry representatives in the area. If that is not enough, there are separate divisions and corporations for home care, outpatient pharmacies, drug information, drug research, and nutritional therapy.

A definition of hospital or institutional pharmacy is therefore difficult. The primary commonality is that all the segments are part of a corporate structure that has grown since the 1950s, when the federal government funded the Hill-Burton Act for building new hospitals, and since 1966, when Medicare and Medicaid reimbursement began under Lyndon Johnson's Great Society program.

Jobs in hospital pharmacy are easy to find, but one needs to consider carefully what terminal position is desired. In 1963, hospital pharmacy began accrediting residencies (see Chapters 7 and 10), and today many jobs—especially management positions in the pharmacy—require that applicants have completed such a residency. If one wants to leap from the pharmacy into hospital administration, an appropriate masters degree (e.g., in business or hospital administration) would likely be needed. Large hospitals are often affiliated with schools of medicine or pharmacy, and most clinical positions require a PharmD degree plus postgraduate residencies and/or fellowships. One's career in hospital pharmacy, particularly larger institutions, can thus be greatly affected by decisions made as a student or young practitioner.

Terminal position:
A position in a corporate hierarchy from which one has little hope for advancement because of an individual's education and corporate policies.

Health care team:
A group of professionals with various skills who work together in providing patient care.

Chapter 6

Pharmacokinetic monitoring:
A part of pharmaceutical care required by patients on certain medications. For some drugs, the difference between a therapeutic blood level and a toxic blood level is very small, and the doses of those drugs need to be calculated carefully and blood levels checked to assure optimal therapy.

Nutrition support:
For patients whose medical conditions do not permit them to take a normal diet, nutrition support is provided. This may entail oral feedings using liquid foods or intravenous feedings using specialized solutions. The pharmacist is an important member of the nutrition support team because of special expertise in both product-preparation and clinical areas.

Controlled substances:
Any of several dangerous drugs, such as morphine, cocaine, codeine, diazepam (Valium), and amphetamines, that are handled, dispensed, and recorded specially under federal law. Some controlled substances, such as marijuana and heroin, are completely illegal, since they have no accepted medical use in the United States.

Rounding:
Once or more often each day in a teaching hospital, members of the healthcare team gather to conduct "rounds," which usually involve walking to the room of each patient that the team is currently caring for. During rounds, each member of the team has an opportunity to share with the others important information about the patient. Since these are teaching institutions, rounds also serve an important role in imparting knowledge among the members of the team.

Salaries in hospital pharmacy have historically been somewhat lower than in community pharmacy, especially in chain pharmacies. That may be true to some degree still, but the gap has been largely closed as a result of pharmacist shortages in the late 1990s and early 2000s. The possibilities for advancement are strong in this field, and more than a few hospital pharmacy directors have been promoted into hospital executive positions. In these, they are administratively responsible for numerous departments that can range from the clinical laboratory to material management or housekeeping. For an employee who is not at financial risk (as would be an independent pharmacy owner), the salaries of hospital pharmacy director and executive positions are high. However, because of the pyramid shape of hospital pharmacy staffs, the competition for the management positions can be keen.

Benefits in hospitals tend to be very favorable, compared with other parts of pharmacy. This results from the large number of employees in hospitals, including some unionized groups that have demanded and received favorable benefits packages over the years.

For the pharmacist whose responsibilities are centered around drug distribution, the daily mission is to get the right drugs to the right patient at the right time. Most hospitals employ pharmacy technicians who assist greatly with this task. These technicians are quite capable, many of them having weeks or months of training, years of experience, and certification from the Pharmacy Technician Certification Board. In some hospitals, technicians are responsible for providing the **controlled substances** to nursing units and for making intravenous solutions for patient administration.

Clinical pharmacists in the hospital are involved in more patient care and drug information activities. Some pharmacists **"round"** with the healthcare team, which comprises physicians, nurses, respiratory therapists, social workers, and physical or occupational therapists. Other pharmacists provide care to patients who need specialized pharmacy services, such as **pharmacokinetic monitoring** or **nutrition support**. Some larger institutions have drug information centers, where pharmacists answer questions from health care professionals or the public about drugs, poisonings, and medication use.

Institutional pharmacy administrators in midsize and larger facilities have a life similar to that of midlevel managers in many corporations. Little time is spent in direct pharmacy practice; life instead is personnel schedules and problems, budgeting, purchasing, and dealing with situations ranging from medication errors to pharmacists or technicians stealing controlled substances for personal use or street sale. As mentioned above, a fair number of pharmacist managers are able to rise into hospital administration after they have obtained masters degrees in either business administration or hospital administration.

Most pharmacists seem to either love or hate hospital practice. In pharmacy school, hospital pharmacy is sometimes glorified because of the important role it has played in creating the clinical pharmacy and pharmaceutical care movements, which led to the establishment of MTM in community pharmacies. But the hospital is threatening to some— it is a large building with hundreds or thousands of employees and patients. Introductory and advance pharmacy practice experiences may consist of helping pharmacy technicians fill **patient carts** with **unit dose packages** of drugs in a windowless basement pharmacy.

The preceptor, often the director of pharmacy, may never be around, as he or she attends a seemingly endless string of committee meetings in other parts of the hospital. Thus, many student pharmacists or young pharmacists become turned off by hospital practice, based on a short but not necessarily representative experience.

But for those who love the institutional environment, the hospital is great. Many patients are quite ill, so the rewards are immediately apparent when the pharmacist attends a successful **"code blue."** In larger hospitals, dozens of other pharmacists interact daily, and it is easy to trade schedules or get vacation time. The hours are very predictable, usually one of three shifts: 7 a.m. to 3 p.m., 3 p.m. to 11 p.m., or 11 p.m. to 7 a.m. However, many hospital pharmacies are open 24 hours a day each day of the year, and staffing requirements can lead to conflicts with pharmacists' personal lives.

The possibilities for professional growth in hospital pharmacy have been very good, and the largest pharmacy convention in the world is the American Society of Health-System Pharmacists' Midyear Clinical Meeting, which is held the first week of December each year. Up to 20,000 people regularly attend that meeting. With such a concentration of well-trained health care professionals, the hospital provides an intellectually stimulating atmosphere devoid of many of the frustrations one finds in community practice.

Disappointments in hospital pharmacy are similar to those alluded to above: Feelings of isolation if confined to a basement pharmacy for drug distribution; difficulties with bureaucratic tendencies; and a lack of face-to-face patient contact for those without clinical responsibilities. Salaries are not overly aggressive, as many people are willing to trade some of the advantages of hospital work for a slightly lower salary.

Institutional pharmacy practice continues to be a very exciting, dynamic area of practice. Virtually every kind of pharmacy practice can be found in hospitals somewhere: Outpatient (ambulatory) pharmacy, acute care, emergency care, nuclear pharmacy (handling of radioactive drugs), long-term care, and home care. About 5,000–6,000 hospitals provide care in virtually all areas of the United States except the most rural or least populated. Hospital pharmacy has provided much of pharmacy's reprofessionalization over the past seven decades (see Chapter 3), and practice there can be very rewarding for those who prefer its environment.

Long-term care pharmacy

Another area of pharmacy practice with rich clinical opportunities is the provision of services to patients who are institutionalized in long-term care facilities. While nursing homes commonly provide this institutional care, a number of factors are leading to the establishment of many other kinds of facilities collectively known as community-based long-term care. In nursing homes, patients (or residents as they are called in this setting) are deficient in one or more of the normal activities of daily living: Ambulating, eating, bathing and dressing, or toileting. In community-based long-term care, the resident may simply need assistance with taking their medications at the right time or with preparing meals. In fact, the resident may be living at home, and the long-term care service may be a nurse or personal assistant who comes by once a day to help with such activities.

Patient carts:
Hospital pharmacies often use carts with small drawers, one for each patient on a nursing station, to deliver medications from a central or decentral pharmacy to the patient-care floors. Each nursing station cart is exchanged periodically, usually once a day, with a new supply of medications for each patient.

Unit dose packages:
In hospitals and some nursing homes, medications are packaged in strips, with each dose labeled with the brand name, strength, and generic name of the drug. Even though this packaging costs more, it speeds the pharmacy operation and permits return of unused medication to the pharmacy.

Code blue:
This term refers to the hospital's response when a patient is in cardiopulmonary arrest (the heart and/or lungs have stopped). Various healthcare professionals respond to the Code Blue, and the pharmacist attends to help calculate doses and draw up drugs to be administered in this emergency situation. Hospitals differ in what they call the situation; Code Blue is a common term derived from the fact that the patient is turning blue from a lack of oxygen. Other names are Code Red or Code 99.

This is the world of the long-term care pharmacist, who is also called a consultant pharmacist because the relationship between the facility or agency and the pharmacist is most often contractual (that is, the pharmacist consults to the facility under contract, rather than working as an employee of the nursing home). Consultant pharmacists work from a variety of settings, most of them remote from the nursing home or facility:

- Community independent or chain pharmacies that provide a limited amount of long-term care services
- Stand-alone long-term care pharmacies, owned either independently or by a chain pharmacy or large long-term care corporation
- Pharmacies that provide no drugs but only consult on the proper procedures and therapies in a facility
- Hospital pharmacies
- Pharmacies located in nursing homes (where the pharmacist may very well be an employee of the facility)

Consultant pharmacist services to nursing homes are mandated under federal law. To qualify for Medicaid reimbursement, a nursing home must have the drug regimens of all residents reviewed by a pharmacist each month. This clinical pharmacy service, first mandated in 1974, was the only one recognized in federal statutes until Congress began requiring pharmacists to counsel all Medicaid patients in 1990.

Salaries for consultant pharmacists usually start out between the independent/hospital range and the chain range. Some consultant pharmacists who own their own businesses have done extremely well; a survey of consultant pharmacists noted that one practitioner earned nearly $1 million annually. For pharmacists who work in consulting only, the salaries are good but do not start out as high as those in chain pharmacy. Consultant pharmacy has been a primary area of entrepreneurship in pharmacy since the late 1960s, and the employee who is willing to work harder can generally find an employer who is willing to pay for that dedication. However, the consultant pharmacy market consolidated during the 1990s, and entry-level pharmacists may find themselves working for large corporations that are not unlike the large chain pharmacies in many ways.

There could very well be no such thing as a typical day for a consultant pharmacist, but there are typical months. Long-term care pharmacists who provide drug distribution have daily responsibilities very similar to those of hospital pharmacists. Working with technicians, the pharmacist responds to physician orders and other requests that come in from the nursing home; communication today is usually by fax or through computerized physician order entry systems. Drugs are provided to the facility, sometimes in specialized packaging that helps nurses organize their medications according to time of intended drug administration.

Some consultant pharmacists spend most or all of their time reviewing the drug regimens of residents. They often work for larger pharmacies that only serve nursing home and long-term care facilities (closed-shop pharmacies, defined earlier in this chapter). Because these facilities may be located hundreds of miles apart, many consultant pharmacists spend a lot of time on the road, driving from one home to the next. This position can be very clinical, since all day long the pharmacist leaves notes for physicians requesting more laboratory testing, decreased medication doses, discontinuation of unnecessary or duplicative drugs, and addition of agents for previously unrecognized problems.

Other pharmacists rise into management or own consultant pharmacy operations. Their jobs are similar to managers in hospital or community pharmacy, with a very strong entrepreneurial spirit in this sector. In addition, the managers/owners are usually responsible for the never-ending process of marketing needed to maintain or expand one's business in this particular part of health care.

Many pharmacists have come to love consultant pharmacy. It combines the clinical aspects of hospital pharmacy with the patient contact and business challenges of community pharmacy. Conventions of the American Society of Consultant Pharmacists are simply exciting events, with people bubbling over to share their ideas and enthusiasm with colleagues facing similar situations. Even in the exhibits, attendees are not just looking to "fill up their bags with goodies"; instead, they genuinely seek information from exhibitors that will aid their practices. For many, consultant pharmacy is a dream come true.

Common frustrations with consultant pharmacy include the travel associated with monthly drug-regimen review and the lack of direct contact with the nurses and physicians caring for the residents. Since many residents of nursing homes are older or have incurable conditions (such as paraplegics or those with Alzheimer's disease), the work is not as dramatically rewarding as in the hospital. Nursing homes usually expect a pharmacist to be "on call" at night and on weekends, which could frustrate the pharmacist who values his or her personal time.

Copayment:
The amount of money a patient must pay when receiving certain types of health care services under insurance programs or prepaid health care plans.

With Americans living longer and the huge baby-boom generation now reaching retirement age, consultant pharmacy will be a growing field in the coming decades. For the pharmacist looking for a career that fulfills the clinical promises of pharmacy, consultant pharmacy can be the answer.

Managed care, home care, and mail-service pharmacy

Two areas of pharmacist practice have developed over the past decade or two, managed care and home care. In addition, a controversial area of practice—mail-service pharmacy—is hiring an increasing number of graduates into its pharmacies.

Managed care refers to health care provided by corporations such as health-maintenance or preferred-provider organizations (HMOs and PPOs). These corporations are really a form of insurance: They collect a prepaid premium from a consumer (or from the employer) and in return provide all needed health care services. Incentives are in place to shepherd patients to obtain the care from the organization's own employees (in the case of HMOs) or from designated physicians, hospitals, and other providers (in the case of PPOs). Also, access to certain kinds of care, especially psychiatric services or long-term care, may be limited. Other types of care, including pharmacy services, may require a **copayment** by the patient at the time of service as a way of preventing overuse of the system.

Chapter 6

Chronic conditions:
Diseases that last for more than about six months or that have long-term (usually lifelong) effects are referred to as chronic conditions. These include diabetes, hypertension (high blood pressure), and heart conditions. Also, surgery and other therapies may produce a chronic condition. For instance, a colon cancer patient may have all or some of the colon removed, with an ostomy created for the passage of waste. Or a patient whose stomach is removed because of gastric cancer may require special types of enteral nutrition rather than a normal diet of solid foods.

Managed care is a rapidly growing field because it offers a way to contain health care costs. Since pharmaceutical care is a part of these costs, many HMOs have established in-house pharmacies that enrollees can use, usually with a lower or no copayment.

PPOs contract with community pharmacies to provide prescriptions on a fee or cost-plus-fee basis. Some PPOs offer incentives to patients who are on long-term drug therapy for **chronic conditions** such as hypertension to obtain such medicines from a mail-service pharmacy. These pharmacies, often located in other states, have been very controversial among pharmacists since they offer no opportunity for face-to-face patient–pharmacist contact and they take away the kinds of prescriptions that are the bread and butter for community pharmacies. However, with the advent of toll-free telephone numbers, e-mail communications, fax machines, computerized physician order entry systems, computerized patient-specific drug information, automated drug-dispensing technology, and overnight-delivery services such as FedEx, the mail-service industry has been growing. For many elderly patients for whom travel is a major difficulty or an impossible chore, just the delivery of the medicine to the door is a critical plus—a fact that must be kept in mind by service-oriented pharmacists.

Since the PPO segment of healthcare does not directly hire pharmacists, the remainder of this section will refer only to organizations, especially HMOs, that hire pharmacists to work in in-house pharmacies, when managed care pharmacy is discussed.

The home care market is centered around the specialized needs of patients who have a short- or long-term need for products such as intravenous antibiotic solutions, intravenous nutritional solutions, or enteral (via the mouth or stomach) nutritional feedings. Home health care services require the formation of a healthcare team, with nurses who visit patients in their homes periodically, respiratory therapists who set up home oxygen equipment or provide respiratory care services at home, pharmacists and pharmacy technicians who prepare solutions and monitor the patients' care, dietitians who consult on the patients' nutritional needs, and delivery personnel who transport all these goods to the patients' homes.

Since the managed and home care markets are growing rapidly and because students are not as familiar with these settings, pharmacist positions are plentiful. HMOs, which require a substantial population base, are common in all major cities of the United States. Home care can be found everywhere, and such services are especially critical in rural areas where patients may live without transportation in remote locations. The central pharmacy operation is sometimes in a major city, with delivery personnel who travel both in the city and to the rural areas, or the pharmacy may be located in small towns. Some community independent and chain pharmacies offer home care services from within a retail location.

Mail-service pharmacies are fewer in number and more geographically dispersed. They tend to be located near population centers. Some state boards of pharmacy have banned mail-service pharmacies, so those states do not have any pharmacies of this type.

Salaries in these pharmacies are very similar to other entry-level positions. Pay scales for entry-level chain pharmacy jobs are probably higher, but independent, hospital, and consultant positions would be quite similar to the salaries found in managed care, home care, and mail-service pharmacy.

For the managed care pharmacist, a typical day would be very similar to that in community pharmacy, but with key exceptions. Since the HMO pharmacist is located in a building with prescribers and since institution-like policies and procedures are used, contact with the physician is both easy and productive. For instance, the HMO may have a **formulary** system, which is a medical staff policy that only certain drugs and drug products may be used for the HMO's patients. Thus, if a physician prescribes a nonformulary drug, the pharmacy may have been granted the authority by the medical staff to change that prescription to a safer, lower cost, or more effective drug that is on the formulary. Or, if the pharmacist wants to discuss the prescription with the prescriber, a face-to-face meeting may be only steps away.

Managers of HMO pharmacies face similar pressures as do hospital pharmacy administrators. All of these pharmacists operate within a hierarchical corporate structure that places a great deal of emphasis on costs and cost containment. Committee and department head meetings are common, and business skills are very advantageous for these administrative pharmacists.

In the home care arena, pharmacists' activities are similar to those in the intravenous product preparation area of a hospital pharmacy. If the pharmacy employs technicians, the pharmacist becomes more of a manager and clinical consultant on the care of the patients. Otherwise, the pharmacist would spend a fair amount of time in product preparation. Pharmacists in home care do travel periodically to provide pharmaceutical care to patients directly, but the distances involved limit this activity somewhat.

Staff level positions in mail-service pharmacy are largely in quality control—making sure that the automated dispensing machines have correctly filled each prescription. The pharmacist sits at a work station next to a conveyor belt, and completed prescriptions in bins queue up there. After a scanner reads a bar code on the bin, the medication order—and many times a photograph of the prescribed tablet or capsule—appears on the pharmacist's computer screen. The pharmacist makes sure that the medication and the prescription label are correct and authorizes drugs to be mailed to the patient. Using such technology, a pharmacist can dispense several hundred prescriptions in an eight-hour shift.

The opportunities for advancement in these areas are still being defined. Managed care and mail-service pharmacy seem similar to the hospital environment, since they provide job security but with somewhat limited potential for advancement. Home care is more entrepreneurial, making advancement to owning the business (or setting up a similar one) quite feasible. The pressures in each setting are just like those discussed earlier for hospital versus independent practice: The managed care pharmacist is usually part of a large department, with professional contact, schedule flexibility, and role specialization very common. The home care pharmacist is often in a smaller operation, meaning that he or she has a very diverse job. Finding someone to work on a given day may be difficult, particularly if the pharmacy is located in a rural area. But the home care pharmacy is not filled with the rules and regulations common to larger bureaucracies, such as the HMO.

For the pioneer pharmacist, managed care, home care, and mail service are currently the frontier of pharmacy practice. Depending on the direction healthcare takes, they could represent the future for an increasing number of pharmacists.

Formulary:
A list of drugs that have been selected by the medical staff of a hospital or HMO for use in that institution. Drugs are selected on the basis of efficacy, safety, cost, and quality of life. In recent years, the marketing of many "me-too" drugs by pharmaceutical industry—drugs that have no important advantage over drugs already on the market—has made cost an increasingly important factor in formulary decisions. Another important factor is the number of times per day that a medicine must be given, since in hospitals highly paid personnel must dispense and administer each dose and in HMOs patient compliance is higher with fewer doses.

Other careers for pharmacists

Three other important career paths for pharmacists are in pharmaceutical industry, government, and associations. While the skills and knowledge used in these jobs are only somewhat related to what students learn in pharmacy school, that background makes pharmacists ideal choices in many situations.

Pharmaceutical industry employs pharmacists in sales, marketing, government affairs, drug information, research, management, professional relations, and executive positions. Long-term (but maybe not starting) salaries and benefits can be higher in industry, and pharmacists who prefer a competitive, dynamic, and growing workplace like work with the industry. Many companies start pharmacists out "carrying the bag"—meaning as pharmaceutical representatives to physicians, hospitals, and pharmacies—but this is becoming less common. Promotions from sales positions are often into marketing or government affairs areas. Companies generally have a limited number of positions available in drug information, which is the part of the company that fields questions from health care professionals and the public.

For the student considering a career in pharmaceutical industry, the APhA–Academy of Student Pharmacists summer internship in industry is a must (see Table 6.1)—an absolute must! A commitment to a career in industry usually involves relocation, and re-entry into more traditional types of pharmacy practice becomes impractical quickly. Thus, these summer internships are extremely valuable in assessing industry as a career option.

A variety of positions are possible for pharmacists in government. Federal organizations such as the U.S. Public Health Service, the Food and Drug Administration, and the Drug Enforcement Administration employ pharmacists, and several pharmacists work for Senators and Representatives in the United States Congress. Related agencies such as the Congressional Office of Technology Assessment sometimes need pharmacists for specific research projects that are assigned by Congress. In state governments, the agencies responsible for Medicaid/Medicare reimbursement and the State Board of Pharmacy employ pharmacists in management and enforcement positions. No one goes to work for the government because of the salaries, or even for the job stability these days. But the opportunity to influence public policy related to pharmaceuticals and pharmacy services is all that it takes for many pharmacists to become involved as public servants.

Pharmacists are also often elected to positions of leadership by their constituents. Pharmacists have served in the U.S. Senate and House of Representatives and dozens are active in the statehouses. One pharmacist—Hubert H. Humphrey—even served as Vice President and was the Democratic nominee for President in 1968. At the local level, pharmacists are often intimately involved with politics and other positions, including mayor, school board members, and city or county commissioners. As the best educated person in any community who is directly accessible to the public, pharmacists are very well-respected people.

The COSTEP program is a valuable opportunity for the student pharmacist who wants to see more about a career in government (see Table 6.1). It provides an introduction to the U.S. Public Health Service, which is a primary path for pharmacists who would like

Table 6.3 | Summary of Key Aspects of Pharmacy Practice Areas

Practice Area	Key Satisfaction Factors[a]			
	Job Availability	**Salary**	**Advancement**	**Feeling of Accomplishment**
Independent	S	S	S	+
Chain/grocery store/ mass merchandiser	+	+	S	−
Hospital	S	S	+	+
Consulting	S	S	+	+
Managed care	S	S	S	+
Home care	S	S	+	+
Mail service	−	S	S	−
Industry	S	+	S	S
Government	−	−	S	+
Associations	S	−	+	+

[a] Shown are the author's overall opinion of the relative level of satisfaction most pharmacists have with the factors shown in each area of pharmacy practice. Key to codes: + indicates greater than average level compared with other pharmacy jobs; S indicates an average level; − indicates below average level.

a career in government work (including the Indian Health Service, which has been very progressive in its pharmacy services). The Department of Veterans Affairs has implemented some exciting changes for both pharmacists employed at VA centers and those in distant communities.[9-11]

Another potential career path is in the field of association management. As is true for government, these positions are often located in Washington, DC, or in the state capitals. In fact, most associations were started to influence the governmental oversight of a profession (see Chapters 7 and 8). Many very different kinds of positions make association work exciting: professional affairs (making policies about how pharmacists should practice or be educated), legal affairs (interfacing with the legislative, judicial, and executive branches of government to ensure the opportunity for pharmacists to provide quality pharmaceutical care), educational affairs (setting up conferences or study programs for pharmacists' continuing education), editorial work (writing or editing books, journals, software, and other pharmacy works), and executive activities (managing association offices and dealing with members who volunteer for leadership positions). Salaries in association work are not much higher than those in government, but the benefits are good, with travel to pharmacy conventions and lots of contact with colleagues a part of the "job."

While several internships are available in association management (see Table 6.1), students more often consider postgraduate, 12-month residencies in association management. These are available at ASHP, ASCP, and NCPA (see Chapter 8 for addresses and Chapter 10 for more information).

Many pharmacists find that their careers lead them into work with the industry, government, or associations. For these pharmacists, the rewards are very satisfying.

Pharmacy: A diverse profession

As described in this chapter, a degree in pharmacy opens the door to a dazzling array of career options. By studying the differences between various choices (Table 6.3), learning more about yourself (see Figure 6.1 on page 52), and going out and meeting people working in the different parts of pharmacy practice, you can select the path that is just right for you.

REFERENCES

1. Sogol EM. Career planning: gateway to future success. *US Pharm.* 1990;(Oct):98-103.
2. Lorber RL, Weltner JC. Productivity: balancing technical, people, and big picture skills. *Consult Pharm.* 1987;2:196-8.
3. National Community Pharmacists Association. Independent pharmacy today. Accessed at www.ncpanet.org/aboutncpa/ipt.php, April 5, 2008.
4. American Pharmacists Association and the National Association of Chain Drug Stores Foundation. Medication therapy management in pharmacy practice: core elements of an MTM service model, version 2.0. *J Am Pharm Assoc.* 2008;48:354-63.
5. Fera T, Bluml BM, Ellis WM, et al. The Diabetes Ten City Challenge: interim clinical and humanistic outcomes of a multisite community pharmacy diabetes care program. *J Am Pharm Assoc.* 2008;48:181-90.
6. Bunting BA, Smith BH, Sutherland SE. The Asheville Project: clinical and economic outcomes of a community-based long-term medication therapy management program for hypertension and dyslipidemia. *J Am Pharm Assoc.* 2008;48:23-31.
7. Peacock G, Kidd R, Rahman A. Patient care services in independent community pharmacies: a descriptive report. *J Am Pharm Assoc.* 2007;47:762-7.
8. Nicholas A, Divine H, Nowak-Rapp M, Roberts KB. University and college of pharmacy collaboration to control health plan prescription drug costs. *J Am Pharm Assoc.* 2007;47:86-92.
9. National Association of Chain Drug Stores Web site. Accessed at www.nacds.org/user-assets/pdfs/facts_resources/2006/Retail_Outlets2006.pdf, April 5, 2008.
10. National Association of Chain Drug Stores Web site. Accessed at www.nacds.org/wmspage.cfm?parm1=507 #membership, April 5, 2008.

Chapter 7 | Governmental and Voluntary Oversight of Pharmacy

Pharmacists are fond of saying that pharmacy is the most regulated profession in the United States, and, if it were possible to quantify this, the statement might indeed be true. Certainly no other mercantile-oriented occupation has the degree of controls on the selling of those goods as does pharmacy. But, given the inherent danger of abuse of and addiction to many of those products, society's interest in looking over pharmacy's shoulder is quite understandable and necessary.

In addition to state and federal laws, pharmacy is increasingly responsive to oversight by a number of voluntary agencies and organizations. In institutions, pharmacy must meet certain standards to qualify for federal reimbursement for health care delivered to Medicare or Medicaid patients. Colleges of pharmacy must meet criteria so that their graduates can be recognized as licensed pharmacists. Postgraduate residencies and fellowships follow standards set forth by various pharmacy associations or other accrediting agencies. And pharmacists working in specialized areas of the profession and pharmacy technicians can seek recognition for the special knowledge that they have gained.

How did this imposing structure of pharmacy regulation and oversight develop, and what does it mean today? Let's take a look.

Federal laws and regulations

A complex array of federal and state **laws** and **regulations** govern the practice of pharmacy. Some of the laws vary from state to state, and many state laws differ with federal pronouncements. A key rule to remember is that the more stringent law is the one that should be followed, regardless of its origin.

At the federal level, two agencies are of primary importance to pharmacy: the Food and Drug Administration (FDA) and the Drug Enforcement Administration (DEA). Increasingly, though, many very specific directives to pharmacy are coming through the Centers for Medicare & Medicaid Services (formerly the Health Care Financing Administration), which regulates reimbursement of health care providers under Medicare and Medicaid.

Food and Drug Administration

FDA was created through the passage of the Federal Food and Drug Act in 1906. In addition to articles in popular magazines as well as professional journals about the need for federal oversight in this area, the publication of two books were important in moving Congress to action: *The Jungle*, by Upton Sinclair, which reviewed atrocities in the meatpacking industry, and *The Great American Fraud*, by Samuel Hopkins Adams, which was

"Any movement contains the seeds of its own destruction. Gradually they may grow until the movement itself is overshadowed, until its originators find themselves in the uncomfortable position of condoning what they had condemned, and of following what they had organized to oppose. Thus, too, in pharmacy. Some organizations dedicated to avoiding legal restrictions became the initiators and, subsequently, the guardians of American pharmaceutical legislation."

—Glenn Sonnedecker, in Kremers and Urdang's *History of Pharmacy*, fourth edition, page 213

Laws:
Acts passed by a legislative body.

Regulations:
Rules promulgated by a part of the executive branch of government, usually based on a law giving the agency statutory authority for the regulation.

Misbranded:
Drug products that were not properly labeled as to contents and proper use.

Adulterated:
Products that had been changed or contaminated with impure or foreign substances.

Product labeling:
The information provided with prescription drugs, including the package insert that lists uses, precautions, adverse effects, and dosages of the drug product. The language in the product labeling must be approved by FDA.

a compilation of articles about "patent" medicines.[1] FDA initially had the authority only to pursue manufacturers of pharmaceutical products that were **misbranded** or **adulterated.**

In 1937, a terrible tragedy struck the country when a toxic preparation of Elixir Sulfanilamide caused 73 deaths.[1] This resulted in passage of the Food, Drug and Cosmetic Act of 1938, which expanded FDA's oversight to include approval of new drug products, medical devices, and cosmetics.[1]

Two important amendments have been made to the 1938 law. In 1952, Congress passed the Durham–Humphrey Amendment, which directed FDA to divide drug products into two categories, those that require a prescription issued by an authorized health professional and those that could be sold without a prescription. In 1962, Congress added more authority by passing the Kefauver–Harris drug amendments. These permitted FDA to control the research into new drugs, require that new drugs be effective for the conditions listed in **product labeling** (previously, drugs only had to be safe), remove drugs from the market more easily when necessary, and regulate advertising of prescription drugs more easily.[1]

FDA regulation of dietary supplements—which include herbal products, vitamins/minerals, and natural products such as fish oils and glucosamine/chondroitin—has been problematic. Congress in 1994 passed the Dietary Supplement Health and Education Act (DSHEA). This law permitted "structure/function claims" to be made for dietary supplements without proof of safety or efficacy by the manufacturer or distributor. This, in effect, means that FDA must prove a product to be useless or harmful to remove it from the market—the exact opposite of the system under which human drugs are approved.

FDA in 2000 issued regulations clarifying what is a permitted "structure/function claim" under DSHEA and what in its view constitutes an unacceptable "disease claim" for dietary supplements.[2] FDA included as structure/function claims effects on common conditions associated with aging, pregnancy, menopause, and adolescence. Conditions that many consumers and professionals view as "diseases"—such as morning sickness and premenstrual syndrome (PMS)—are now permissible "structure/function" claims. Thus, labels of dietary supplements might include language such as the following:
- For common symptoms of PMS
- For hot flashes

FDA also allows dietary supplements to contain "health-maintenance" claims, such as:
- Maintains a healthy circulatory system
- For muscle enhancement
- Helps you relax

Express disease claims ("prevents osteoporosis," "prevents bone fragility in postmenopausal women") remain forbidden. However, some structure/function claims (such as "prevents memory loss") will undoubtedly be confused with diseases for which those functions are hallmarks (in that case, improving cognition in Alzheimer's disease).

Following the 2003 death of a Baltimore Orioles pitcher who was taking the dietary supplement ephedra, the pendulum began swinging back to tighter regulation of this industry.[3] In 2007, FDA published final regulations that tightened the quality control over dietary supplements,[4] and these should decrease problems with what had been a perpetual source of uncertainty regarding use of these products.

After a period of activism under FDA Commissioner David Kessler, MD, in the 1990s, the federal agency encountered troubled waters in the final years of President Bill Clinton's second term and during the administration of George W. Bush, periods when FDA frequently had no Commissioner at the helm. Several highly publicized market withdrawals of medications brought scrutiny to an agency that had begun in the mid-1990s receiving a substantial portion of its funding from the pharmaceutical industry. Essentially, companies were able to pay "user fees" for expedited review of new drug applications (NDAs). This assured two things: Quick decisions about whether new drugs could be marketed (which led to a period of increased numbers of FDA drug approvals) and dependence on the industry for funding of the increased numbers of NDA reviewers employed at FDA. As some of these expedited drugs produced unanticipated adverse events and were pulled off the U.S. market, critics questioned whether FDA was moving too quickly and in general becoming too close to the powerful pharmaceutical industry.

Despite such concerns, Congress reauthorized user fees as part of the Food and Drug Administration Amendments Act of 2007, signed into law in September of that year. This legislation reauthorized user fees and encouraged research into the best use of medication in pediatric patients.[5,6]

A perpetual issue at FDA is a proposed third class of drugs that could be prescribed and dispensed by pharmacists. The term "third class" comes from the fact that drugs are currently divided into two classes: those that require a prescriber's prescription and those that can be sold over-the-counter (sometimes called informally OTCs) with no health care professional involved. Opponents of such behind-the-counter (BTC) medications include physician groups and a trade association that represents companies that sell over-the-counter medicines.

Pharmacists have been advocating for decades that BTC medications could provide a transition for prescription drugs that could be provided to patients without a physician's prescription. In recent hearings convened by FDA, pharmacy associations advocated establishment of a BTC medication category, citing successful provision of hormonal **emergency contraceptives** by pharmacists in several states.[7,8]

FDA moved emergency contraceptives from prescription to nonprescription status in 2006, but only for adult patients. Thus, these products have entered a de facto BTC category, since they must be stocked in such a way that those younger than 18 cannot obtain them without interacting with pharmacy staff. In 2007, FDA initiated a formal discussion of a BTC category of medications, but no action had occurred when this book went to print in late 2008.

Emergency contraceptives: Also known as "morning-after pills." Medications containing female hormones can be administered within 72 hours of unprotected intercourse, and pregnancy will be averted in more than 90% of women. In Washington State, California, and a few other states, pharmacists can prescribe ECs under physician-approved protocols.

Drug Enforcement Administration

DEA is responsible for the regulation of controlled substances in the United States. Controlled substances are those with abuse and addiction potential. DEA was created in 1970 by the Comprehensive Drug Abuse Prevention and Control Act and the Controlled Substances Act.

Federal law divides controlled substances into five schedules that have differing levels of requirements for handling and recordkeeping:

- *Schedule I:* These drugs have high abuse and addiction potential and have no accepted medical use in the United States. Examples are heroin, LSD, marijuana, and mescaline.
- *Schedule II:* These drugs have high abuse and addiction potential but do have medical applications. Examples include cocaine, Dilaudid (hydromorphone), Ritalin (methylphenidate), Seconal (secobarbital), and several types of amphetamines ("diet pills" or "speed").
- *Schedule III:* These drugs have abuse and addiction potential but not as much as those in Schedule II. Examples are Tylenol #3 (acetaminophen with codeine) and Fastin (phentermine).
- *Schedule IV:* These drugs have a low potential for abuse. Examples include Valium (diazepam), Halcion (triazolam), and Darvon (dextropropoxyphene).
- *Schedule V:* Drugs in this schedule have low abuse potential and have very limited amounts of drugs in each dosage form. Examples are Lomotil (diphenoxylate and atropine) and some cough syrups containing codeine. Some Schedule V products do not require a prescription (through FDA regulations), but they must be dispensed by a pharmacist because of DEA rules.

DEA today has many responsibilities for fighting the illicit drug trafficking problem, and pharmacy is only a small part of this job. DEA agents thus have two different roles, one in which they fight outright criminals who are smuggling and selling huge quantities of illegal drugs and another in which they must apprehend healthcare professionals who are diverting legal drugs into the illegal market. Different divisions of DEA work on these two aspects, but many pharmacists feel that DEA agents act inappropriately when they deal with health care professionals.

Centers for Medicare & Medicaid Services

The Centers for Medicare & Medicaid Services (CMS) is the current name for the agency that administers federal coverage of health care. It was known as the Health Care Financing Administration (HCFA) from its inception during the Great Society phase of the Johnson Administration (1965) until it was renamed during the George W. Bush Administration in 2001.

Indigent:
Unable to pay for certain basic services for oneself, including health care.

While the Medicare and Medicaid programs are very complicated, one can think of the Medicare program as paying for acute (hospital) care for the elderly and the Medicaid program as covering the **indigent**. Until 2006, Medicare paid for prescription drugs only when they were used in an acute-care institution (hospital) or in conjunction with certain medical devices such as in-dwelling catheters (tubes that go into very large veins of the body). Beginning in 2006, a Part D was added to the Medicare benefit that pays for prescription drugs for all beneficiaries. Medicaid pays for outpatient prescription drugs and other care for indigent patients in community pharmacies, nursing homes, or hospitals. Some people qualify under both Medicare and Medicaid, and they are termed "dual eligibles."

Important to note is that the Medicaid program is financed jointly by the federal and state governments, with each contributing about one half of the funds. Thus, though Medicaid is a federal program, pharmacists' interactions are usually with the agency within the state government that coordinates the program. As state budgets have been squeezed more and more recently, the Medicaid programs have been increasingly tightened. The effects of these economic constraints have been severe in many states. For example, Medicaid patients' prescriptions often must be filled off a state-approved drug list (or "formulary"), recipients may be limited to a certain number of prescriptions per month, and states have sometimes held up Medicaid payments for several months because of budgetary shortfall.

Likewise, even though Medicare Part D is a federal program, it is administered through dozens of private prescription drug providers, or PDPs. Each PDP has its own formulary, and Medicare beneficiaries can choose any PDP operating in their geographic area (usually a state). Pharmacists' interactions are generally with these intermediaries when it comes to obtaining reimbursement for prescriptions and getting approval for nonformulary medications.

As mentioned in Chapter 3, the Medicare Part D program also included a provision for medication therapy management (MTM) services. During the first three years of the program (2006–2008), PDPs were required to provide, either directly or through pharmacies, MTM services to those Medicare patients who were being treated for multiple diseases with multiple medications and who were expected to need at least $4,000 worth of medications during the year. Just how pharmacies and PDPs met this requirement is not yet clear, as efforts during these early years of the benefit focused more on the drug-distribution aspects of the new program. In the long run, CMS has stated that MTM services should become the "cornerstone" of Medicare Part D, and the associated payment aspect could enable pharmacists to further develop their pharmaceutical care and clinical pharmacy services for elderly patients. If this happens, the pharmacy technician's role in processing and preparing prescription medications will become even more important than it is today.

In addition to the daily requirements associated with processing individual prescriptions, pharmacies must comply with certain broader requirements mandated by CMS and/or state agencies. These are called "conditions of participation" because providers—including hospitals, physicians, nursing homes, and pharmacies—must agree to them in order to participate in the Medicare and Medicaid programs. Conditions for participation specify many operational, procedural, and outcome details, and you may see that your pharmacy is changing a procedure or getting a new type of hood for making intravenous fluids because of such requirements.

Serious problems with Medicare and Medicaid fraud continue to crop up for pharmacists and other types of health care providers. With spending for these programs at $300 billion annually, the possibilities for substantial amounts of graft and fraud are quite high.

In 1990, Congress passed a bill that directed CMS (then HCFA) to begin collecting rebates from pharmaceutical manufacturers based on the difference between the manufacturers' best price to any buyer of that product and the price of that drug to the government under the Medicaid program of the state. This has caused manufacturers to reassess their basic pricing structures, with detrimental results for hospitals and other institutions with nonprofit or governmental status. Beginning during World War II, manufacturers had created a separate **class of trade** for nonprofit and governmental buyers of their products, and prices for this group were sometimes only a small fraction of the price paid by community pharmacies. This gave the nonprofit/government institutions an unfair competitive advantage.

Class of trade:
Customers of a business or industry may be divided into one or more groups based on their purchasing and payment characteristics. Each of these classes of trade is dealt with differently — and may receive different prices or payment policies — because of the interplay between these characteristics and the sellers' goals and objectives relative to that part of the industry.

License:
A document issued to pharmacists and other citizens that provides special privileges based on specialized knowledge or skills. A drivers' license is one type of such document; it permits the holder to operate motorized vehicles on public roads based on a demonstration to the state of sufficient knowledge. A pharmacy license is similar; it permits the holder to engage in a specialized profession known as pharmacy following demonstration to the state of adequate knowledge. It is a privilege, not a right, and thus the state may withdraw the privilege for various reasons.

Reciprocation:
Once a pharmacist is licensed, he or she can use that license (if in good standing) to practice in other states, after the state board of pharmacy in the new state recognizes the license from the previous state.

Under current Medicaid provisions, manufacturers are encouraged to eliminate this price differential; if they do not, the Medicaid program benefits by obtaining rebates from the manufacturers for products dispensed through community pharmacies at Medicaid expense.

State laws and regulations

As has been mentioned in the above discussion of the Medicaid program, agencies of the state government are very important to pharmacists. Since the people in these agencies are much closer geographically to the pharmacy, the possibilities for frequent contacts are that much higher.

State boards of pharmacy

The division of responsibilities between the state and federal governments follows the line of reasoning known as states' rights: all responsibilities not specifically assigned to the federal government in the United States Constitution are reserved for the states. The area of drug and pharmacy regulation has been one in which the federal government has creatively enlarged its role when it felt that the public health was at risk, but the states remain an integral part of the regulatory framework.

The mechanism by which states regulate professions is through boards composed largely of members of the profession along with one or two consumer members. Federal laws generally do not deal specifically with regulation of the professions; for instance, FDA's legend drugs do not specify what types of practitioners may legally prescribe these drugs. Federal law thus depends heavily on the framework that states put in place during the last half of the nineteenth century.

State boards of pharmacy developed around 1900 after their organization had been proposed in model pharmacy laws developed by the American Pharmaceutical (now Pharmacists) Association. As Sonnedecker has described so well, pharmacy organizations and pharmacy laws have often grown together, and the organization of the state boards followed this trend.[1] However, it is important to remember that state boards of pharmacy have as their primary mission the protection of the public from the profession—not vice versa. Pharmacy associations, conversely, exist to promote the profession, which sometimes leads them along paths that are not necessarily in the best interests of the public.

State boards of pharmacy, based on authority granted to them by the various state legislatures, promulgate the specific regulations that govern the practice of pharmacy on a day-to-day basis. Boards issue **licenses** to pharmacists and pharmacies, specify by what mechanisms pharmacists can keep their licenses in force, have investigative arms that police the profession, and are the judge and jury for pharmacists who violate state pharmacy laws. For the student pharmacist, learning state pharmacy laws and preparing for the board of pharmacy examinations are major foci of activity. For the practicing pharmacist, the decisions rendered by the state board of pharmacy can drastically affect the way in which the profession must be practiced in a given state.

In 1904, a national organization of state boards of pharmacy was formed.[1] The National Association of Boards of Pharmacy (NABP) has grown to a powerful position in coordinating activities among the state boards. It now provides a national examination, called the NAPLEX®, for North American Pharmacist Licensure Examination®, for administration in all states. NABP coordinates the **reciprocation** of pharmacist licenses between states. The Association develops model pharmacy practice acts that state legislatures can consider for updating state laws to incorporate changes in pharmacy.

Other state agencies

At the state level, the other primary agency of concern to pharmacists is the one that handles the Medicaid program. Since these vary greatly, it is not possible to provide a uniform description, but talk with pharmacists in your state about what your agency is like. Also, inquire about pharmacy faculty at your school who may work with the agency in analyzing drug-use trends.

Most states have some type of controlled substances counterpart to the DEA, and pharmacists interface with those agencies as well.

Self-governance by pharmacy

Increasingly important in pharmacy is the process of **accreditation** of residency and training programs and the **certification** of individual practitioners for increased knowledge in pharmacy specialty areas. As opposed to the mandatory licensure described for pharmacists, accreditation and certification are examples of voluntary oversight by the profession. Let's look at how they work.

Accreditation of training programs

Most people are familiar with the process by which physicians enter residency programs to specialize in various medical specialty areas. But not many members of the public realize that many pharmacy graduates enter residency programs; as the entry-level PharmD movement has taken hold, an increasing number of graduates are going on for this type of specialized training.

Pharmacy residencies developed first in hospital pharmacy in the 1930s (they were called internships until 1962), and residencies in hospitals are still the most common type. The American Society of Hospital (now Health-System) Pharmacists began accrediting hospital pharmacy residencies in 1963, and it currently recognizes some 300 programs. ASHP eliminated its hospital pharmacy and clinical pharmacy residencies in 1992; all are now recognized as pharmacy practice residencies. ASHP also offers several types of specialized residencies (see Chapter 10), and in 1999 it began accrediting managed care and community pharmacy residencies with, respectively, the Academy of Managed Care Pharmacy and the American Pharmaceutical (now Pharmacists) Association.

In 2003, the Society reorganized its accreditation standards into a postgraduate year 1 (PGY1) and year 2 (PGY2). PGY1 programs can be conducted at one or more sites, and colleges of pharmacy can participate as sponsoring organizations. Residents learn about managing and improving the medication-use process, providing evidence-based, patient-centered medication therapy management with interdisciplinary teams, exercising leader-

Accreditation:
Recognition of a residency or other type of program by comparing it with standards set by the accrediting body. This standard describes the goals or ideals that each program should strive for and sets certain minimum criteria that each should maintain.

Certification:
Recognition of an individual for specialized knowledge and/or skills based on demonstration of that knowledge or those skills to the certifying body. The term certification carries the connotation that the certifying body is a nongovernmental entity, and the recognition typically carries no legally defined privileges.

ship and practice management skills, demonstrating project management skills, providing medication and practice-related education/training, and using medical informatics.[9]

PGY2 pharmacy residency programs focus on a specific area of practice, such as primary care/ambulatory, critical care, drug information, geriatrics, oncology, psychiatric, or internal medicine.[10]

ASHP also accredits technician training programs. Accredited technician training programs are based chiefly in community colleges or technical schools, but some hospitals and colleges of pharmacy also have such programs. In late 2006, ASHP recognized more than 90 accredited technician training programs, 91% of which were in community colleges or vocational/technical colleges.[11]

Certification of individuals

Certification is a term that is becoming increasingly common in pharmacy, particularly in two areas: for pharmacists who practice in highly specialized areas and for pharmacy technicians. Certification is a form of self-discipline or self-control by a profession, and the process works when employers and health care professionals are able to police themselves. For instance, any physician can legally perform brain surgery, but only those who are certified by a medical specialty board as neurosurgeons generally do so. But if a substantial number of noncertified physicians began offering services they were unqualified to perform and the public was as a result at risk of harm, the state would likely step in and set up a licensure mechanism.

In pharmacy, a Board of Pharmaceutical Specialties (BPS) was organized in 1975 to recognize what activities in pharmacy required certification and to develop processes to accomplish that certification. Since then, it has recognized five specialties[12]:
- Nuclear pharmacy
- Pharmacotherapy
- Nutrition support pharmacy practice
- Psychopharmacy
- Oncology

In addition, Infectious Diseases and Cardiology have been recognized as areas of Added Qualifications under the Pharmacotherapy Specialty. This means that Board-certified Pharmacotherapists who practice primarily in infectious diseases or cardiology can be recognized. Other areas of Added Qualifications are likely to be developed and recognized in the future.

The purpose of pharmacy certification is to demonstrate personal achievement in these specialized areas. Employers also often require applicants to have certain credentials, including certification status in one of these specialty areas.

For an area to be recognized by BPS as a specialty, one or more sponsoring organizations must submit a detailed petition outlining the specialty and related details. If approved as a specialty by BPS, the sponsoring organizations then participate in development of a certification examination that is given once or twice per year. Those attaining a certain score on the exam are designated as certified and are eligible to use certain initials after their names.

Pharmacy technicians are also becoming certified. For them, certification is a way to demonstrate accomplishment in a career that has no uniform educational or training requirements and to show employers a given level of knowledge about activities of pharmacy technicians. The Pharmacy Technician Certification Board is the certifying body for pharmacy technicians, and it had recognized more than 300,000 Certified Pharmacy Technicians by 2008,[13] more than the number of licensed pharmacists in the United States.

Employers use certification of technicians as a way of determining promotions into jobs such as those in intravenous admixture rooms or supervising other technicians.

Overregulated and loving it

As this chapter shows, pharmacy is definitely a well-regulated profession. But interestingly, pharmacists often lobby for more regulation when they want to move the profession in a certain direction. For instance, nothing made much difference in pharmacists' interest in patient counseling until national pharmacy groups caused Congress to mandate it for Medicaid recipients. For some reason, pharmacy has had more success with having the government keep the playing field level than it has with stimulating its members to raise their own professional sights. Pharmacists indeed have become the initiators and the guardians of those laws that specify sometimes very precisely what pharmacists must and must not do.

REFERENCES

1. Sonnedecker G. The rise of legislative standards. In: Kremers and Urdangs' history of pharmacy. 4th ed. Philadelphia: J. B. Lippincott Company, 1976:213-25.
2. American Dietetic Association, American Pharmaceutical Association. A healthcare professional's guide to evaluating dietary supplements. Accessed at http://www.pharmacist.com/pdf/dietary_supplements.pdf, June 2, 2003.
3. Posey LM. FDA moves on dietary supplement quality, ephedra safety. *Pharm Today.* 2003(Apr): 1, 4.
4. American Pharmacists Association. APhA Summary of Food and Drug Administration Final Rule Regarding Current Good Manufacturing, Packaging, Labeling or Holding Operations for Dietary Supplements. Accessed January 2, 2008, at http://www.pharmacist.com/AM/Template.cfm?Section=Search1&section=Other&template=/CM/ContentDisplay.cfm&ContentFileID=3615.
5. Food and Drug Administration. Law strengthens FDA. Accessed at http://www.fda.gov/oc/initiatives/advance/fdaaa.html, January 2, 2008.
6. American Pharmacists Association. Summary of the Food and Drug Administration Amendments Act of 2007. Access at http://www.pharmacist.com/AM/Template.cfm?Section=Search1&section=Breaking_Political_News&template=/CM/ContentDisplay.cfm&ContentFileID=3483, January 2, 2008.
7. Monastersky N, Landau SC. Future of emergency contraception lies in pharmacists' hands. *J Am Pharm Assoc.* 2006;46:84–8.
8. Reynolds B. Behind-the-counter drug category on the way? Time will tell. Accessed at http://www.pharmacist.com/AM/Template.cfm?Section=Search1&template=/CM/HTMLDisplay cfm&ContentID=14590, January 2, 2008.
9. American Society of Health-System Pharmacists. Accessed at http://www.ashp.org/rtp/index.cfm, January 2, 2008.
10. American Society of Health-System Pharmacists. ASHP Regulations on Accreditation of Pharmacy Residencies. Accessed at http://www.ashp.org/s_ashp/docs/files/RTP_ResidencyAccredRegulation.pdf, January 2, 2008.

11. Written communication, Janet L. Teeters, MS, of the American Society of Health-System Pharmacists, September 8, 2006.

12. Board of Pharmaceutical Specialties. Accessed at www.bpsweb.org, January 2, 2008.

13. Pharmacy Technician Certification Board. Accessed at www.ptcb.org, October 30, 2008.

Chapter 8 | Pharmacy Associations

Most major national pharmacy associations have been mentioned somewhere in Chapters 1–7 of this textbook, but a brief straightforward presentation of material is always useful. In this chapter, I will provide information about the major pharmacy practitioner organizations and their histories, current status, strengths, weaknesses, and relationships with each other.

A consortium of national pharmacy practitioner organizations, the Joint Commission of Pharmacy Practitioners, was founded in 1977, and it meets quarterly in Washington, DC. The members are listed in Table 8.1 on page 83, along with addresses and telephone numbers, and these are the primary organizations that I will discuss in this chapter.

JCPP has been an extremely effective tool for bringing to one table the leaders of American pharmacy from all sectors of the profession. People are sometimes disappointed that JCPP does not take more of an activist role, but that is not the nature of consortia. The group works through consensus building, not motions and votes. If even one member of JCPP cannot agree on a course of action about an issue, generally no action is taken, and this leaves the individual associations free to pursue their own agendas in their own ways. On the other hand, many positive joint statements, alliances, and unified actions have been facilitated because of the meetings of JCPP.

Several other non-JCPP organizations also form an important part of the framework within which pharmacists operate. These are listed in Table 8.2 on page 85 with brief descriptions of the focus of each.

With that background, here are descriptions of the pharmacy practitioner organizations that are in the JCPP.

American Pharmacists Association

Formed in 1852 as the American Pharmaceutical Association, the American Pharmacists Association (APhA) is the oldest and largest organization in pharmacy. It occupies a prominent position in the nation's capital, both politically and geographically: APhA is the organization that Congress expects to speak for pharmacy, and its historic building—with a new annex now under construction—on Constitution Avenue across from the Vietnam and Lincoln Memorials is the only private structure on that impressive boulevard.

Today's APhA is a strong organization, one that is positioned well to help pharmacists incorporate medication therapy management into their practices. APhA uses these vision, mission, and tagline statements to guide its programs and services:

"It is my firm conviction that American pharmacy will not come into its own until we have a majority of our pharmacists actively supporting their national professional organization. Someone has defined an organization as a medium for the efficient movement of groups of men towards goals to which they aspire. How can we move American pharmacists towards professional goals until we enroll them in our Association? Only when this is done will the Association, its ideals, its ethics, its concepts of professional service become ingrained in all who practice our profession."

—Donald E. Francke, in his 1953 Harvey A. K. Whitney Lecture Award Address

- *APhA's Vision for Society:* Pharmacists and patients working together to improve medica tion use and health.
- *APhA's Mission:* The American Pharmacists Association provides information, education and advocacy to help all pharmacists improve medication use and advance patient care.
- *APhA's Tag Line:* The American Pharmacists Association. Improving Medication Use. Advancing Patient Care.

APhA has more than 60,000 members (including practicing pharmacists, pharmaceutical scientists, student pharmacists, pharmacy technicians, and others interested in advancing the profession) and strong assets. As the only national organization that can claim to represent all of pharmacy, its pronouncements are respected and its activities noticed.

Members of APhA include some 30,000 members of its Academy of Student Pharmacists (APhA–ASP). It also has strong, influential membership segments of pharmacy school faculty, pharmacists who work for the federal government (e.g., in the military or the U.S. Public Health Service or for the Department of Veterans Affairs), hospital pharmacists, and community pharmacists. Membership in APhA's House of Delegates is determined by state pharmacists associations, giving a voice to pharmacists politically active at the state level. APhA seeks to represent the interests of employee pharmacists in all settings, and it has been successful in developing this concept through a new practitioner program. The idea has a lot of potential for future expansions of APhA membership, since the nation's community chain pharmacists are basically unrepresented in national pharmacy organizations.

The APhA Annual Meeting and Exposition, which includes the annual meeting of ASP, is held during the spring. Sites are rotated among the various large cities in the United States and sometimes Canada. Upwards of 2,500 student pharmacists attend the APhA annual meeting each year. In the fall, APhA–ASP's Midyear Regional Meetings are held in the group's eight regions.

Publications are an important part of APhA's services and budget. In addition to its monthly medication therapy management (MTM) magazine, *Pharmacy Today*, drug information newsletter, *APhA DrugInfoLine*, and journals, *Journal of the American Pharmacists Association* and *Journal of Pharmaceutical Sciences*, APhA publishes a number of books, including the important titles, *Handbook of Nonprescription Drugs* and *Medication Errors*.

APhA's Web site, www.pharmacist.com, offers breaking news coverage, news articles from *Pharmacy Today* and the *APhA DrugInfoLine,* legislative and regulatory updates, continuing education, and resource centers for emerging practice trends such as medication therapy management. Many parts of the site are available to everyone, while other pages are only for APhA members.

In the professional arena, APhA is quite involved in setting policy and standards of practice for pharmacy in all settings. Through its House of Delegates, many important policies express the pharmacy profession's viewpoints on controversial issues such as assisted suicide and ethics for pharmacists. These policies are communicated to other associations and policymakers in the federal and state governments by APhA's growing staff, which stands currently at 135 employees.

Table 8.1 | Members of the Joint Commission of Pharmacy Practitioners[a]

Organizations	Year Founded	No. Staff	Budget (in millions of $)	No. People (at Largest Meeting)	No. Members	Student Dues ($)	Executive (Web address)
Regular JCPP members							
APhA 2215 Constitution Ave., N.W. Washington, DC 20037	1852	135	34	7,000	60,000	35	John A. Gans[a] (www.pharmacist.com)
NCPA 205 Daingerfield Road Alexandria, VA 22314 703/683-8200	1898	200	35	4,000	23,000	25	Bruce Roberts (www.ncpanet.org)
ACA 2830 Summer Oaks Drive Bartlett, TN 38134-3811 901/383-8119	1940	6	0.6	200	1,000	15	D. C. Huffman (www.acainfo.org)
AMCP 100 North Pitt Street Alexandria, VA 22314 800/TAP-AMCP	1989	30	10	2,400	5,000	35	Judith A. Cahill (www.amcp.org)
ASHP 7272 Wisconsin Avenue Bethesda, MD 20814 301/657-3000	1942	200	41	22,000	30,000	35	Henri A. Manasse, Jr.[a] (www.ashp.org)
ASCP 1321 Duke Street Alexandria, VA 22314 703/739-1300	1968	39	9	3,800	7,000	Free	John N. Feather (www.ascp.com)
ACCP 3101 Broadway, Suite 380 Kansas City, MO 64111 816/531-2177	1979	18	4	1,300	9,000	65	Michael S. Maddux (www.accp.com)
Associate members[b]							
NABP 1300 Higgins Rd., Suite 103 Park Ridge, IL 60068 708/698-6227	1904	32	5.0	550	62[c]	N.A.	Carmen A. Catizone (www.nabp.net)
NASPA 2530 Professional Road Richmond, VA 23235 804/285-4431	~1930	1	0.065	50	52[d]	N.A.	Rebecca Snead (www.naspa.us)
AACP 1426 Prince Street Alexandria, VA 22314 703/739-2330	1900	21	10	1,450	[e]	15	Lucinda L. Maine (www.aacp.org)

[a]Has indicated intention to step down or retire from this position.

Table 8.1 | Members of the Joint Commission of Pharmacy Practitioners,[a] continued

[a] Adapted from information provided by Dr. Joseph A. Oddis, former executive vice president of the American Society of Health-System Pharmacists.

[b] Since these groups are not pharmacy practitioner organizations, they are not discussed in detail in this chapter.

[c] As was mentioned in Chapter 7, the National Association of Boards of Pharmacy (NABP) is the organization representing the state boards of pharmacy. Headquartered in suburban Chicago, NABP conducts an annual meeting for members of the state boards, prepares documents such as model pharmacy practice acts that increase consistency in pharmacy laws from state to state, and participates in committees and consortia that work on pharmacy-practice issues related to state pharmacy law (see Chapter 7).

[d] The National Alliance of State Pharmacy Associations (NASPA) is a group representing staff members who head state pharmacy associations. Currently, one statewide pharmacy association from each state is permitted to have a member in NASPA; this member is from the umbrella pharmacy organization (versus the state group of hospital, consultant, or clinical pharmacists).

[e] The American Association of Colleges of Pharmacy (AACP) is a combination individual and trade association representing the interests of the administration and faculties of 101 colleges of pharmacy and 2,500 individual members. It publishes a journal, conducts an annual meeting, and participates in many ways in dialogues within the pharmacy community about the pharmacy practice roles and how they relate to pharmacy education and research.

Medication therapy management in all settings, but especially in community independent and chain pharmacies, has been an area of particular emphasis for APhA over the past several years. Its foundation, a separate organization, has sponsored or been involved in Project ImPACT and the Asheville Project, both demonstration projects showing that pharmacists who meet one-on-one with patients with chronic diseases (e.g., diabetes, hypertension, dyslipidemias, depression, asthma) can make a tremendous difference in clinical, financial, and quality-of-life outcomes (see readings in Chapter 11). After Medicare Part D was passed by Congress, APhA convened representatives from all parts of pharmacy to develop consensus about the definition and core elements of medication therapy management, and these elements were recently revised based on the first two years of experience with this new federal benefit (see Chapter 11).

APhA also serves as a home for three other important parts of the profession: the Board of Pharmaceutical Specialties (BPS), the Pharmacy Services Support Center (PSSC), and the Pharmacy Technician Certification Board (PTCB). BPS (www.bpsweb.org), as described in Chapter 7, certifies pharmacists at the advanced practice specialty level in five specialties: nuclear pharmacy, nutrition support pharmacy, oncology pharmacy, pharmacotherapy, and psychopharmacy. PSSC (http://pssc.aphanet.org/) operates under a federal contract and endeavors to support pharmacies serving indigent patient population with lower-price drugs supplied by manufacturers under Section 340(B) of the Public Health Service Act. PTCB (www.ptcb.org), described in Chapter 7, is a separate organization that certifies pharmacy technicians.

As American society has grown more diverse, many large national associations that represent broad but splintering fields have encountered difficulties in being all things to all members. APhA is no exception. At times, in trying to meet the needs of all parts of the profession, APhA finds various subcomponents of its diverse membership in conflict with one another. More narrowly focused pharmacy organizations have sometimes pulled members away from APhA, leaving it with fewer resources to respond to problems, opportunities, and crises for the profession.

Important for pharmacists to remember is that we are all in the same boat—we will float together or we will sink together. For more than a century and a half, APhA has been our boat.

Table 8.2 | Other Pharmacy-Related Associations

Accreditation Council on Pharmacy Education
20 North Clark St., Suite 2500, Chicago, IL 60602-5109
312/664-3575 • www.acpe-accredit.org
The accrediting body for pharmacy schools and providers of pharmaceutical continuing education. Funds come from fees charged to pharmacy
schools and continuing education providers; membership on the board of directors is appointed by APhA, AACP, and other pharmacy associations.

American Association of Pharmaceutical Scientists
2107 Wilson Blvd., Suite 700, Arlington, VA 22201-3042
703/243-2800 • www.aapspharmaceutica.com
An individual membership organization representing researchers in the pharmaceutical sciences; founded as a spinoff organization from APhA during the 1980s.

American Foundation for Pharmaceutical Education
One Church St., Suite 202, Rockville, MD 20850
301/738-2160 • www.afpenet.org
Uses grants from industry and other sources to fund scholarships,
fellowships, and other grants for pharmacy students at the undergraduate and postgraduate levels.

American Institute of the History of Pharmacy
Pharmacy Building, 777 Highland Ave., Madison, WI 53705-2222
608/262-5378 • www.pharmacy.wisc.edu/aihp
An institute devoted to the study and preservation of the history of pharmacy.

Consumer Healthcare Products Association
900 19th St., N.W., Suite 700, Washington, DC 20006
202/429-9260 • www.chpa-info.org
A trade association representing the interests of companies that manufacture and distribute nonprescription drugs. Often in conflict with pharmacy associations, especially on the "third class of drugs" issue.

Healthcare Distribution Management Association
901 North Glebe Rd., Arlington, VA 22203
703/787-0000 •www.healthcaredistribution.org
A trade association representing wholesale druggists and other organizations that serve as the "middle men" in the health care product distribution chain.

International Pharmaceutical Federation
Andries Bickerweg 5, 2517 JP, The Hague, Netherlands
+31-70-3021970 • www.fip.org
An international association of pharmacists. Holds an annual session in the first week in September. Some information about FIP available from APhA and ASHP.

National Association of Chain Drug Stores
413 North Lee Street, Alexandria, VA 22313-1480
703/549-3001 • www.nacds.org

A trade association of nearly 200 chain drug stores that operate 37,000 pharmacies. Conducts an annual meeting, a pharmaceutical conference, and other meetings each year. Very involved in governmental tracking and lobbying at the national and state levels. Publishes various newsletters and informational alerts for its members.

National Council on Patient Information and Education
4915 Saint Elmo Ave., Suite 505, Bethesda, MD 20814-6082
301/656-8565 • www.talkaboutrx.org
A privately funded organization that conducts national campaigns to educate consumers about the drugs they take and that encourage pharmacists and other health care providers to provide more information to consumers. Sponsors "Talk About Prescriptions" month each October.

National Pharmaceutical Council
1894 Preston White Drive, Reston, VA 20191
703/620-6390 • www.npcnow.org
A trade association that conducts public relations activities on behalf of major research-oriented pharmaceutical firms.

Pharmaceutical Care Management Association
601 Pennsylvania Ave., NW, Suite 740, Washington, DC 20004
202/207-3610 • www.pcmanet.org
A trade association representing companies that provide pharmacy benefit managers, including mail-service pharmacies.

Pharmaceutical Research and Manufacturers of America
950 F Street, N.W., Washington, DC 20004
202/835-3400 • www.phrma.org
A trade association representing the research-oriented pharmaceutical industry. Heavily involved in lobbying at the state and federal levels.

Poison Prevention Week Council
P. O. Box 1543, Washington, DC 20013
301/504-7058 • www.poisonprevention.org
The organization that coordinates Poison Prevention Week activities during the third week of March each year.

PQA
703/690-1987 • www.PQAAlliance.org
A pharmacy quality alliance, PQA is a collaborative initiative that seeks to define quality measures for pharmacist and pharmacy services.

United States Pharmacopeial Convention
12601 Twinbrook Parkway, Rockville, MD 20852-1790
301/881-0666 • www.usp.org
The national body that sets standards for drug products in the United States. Has quasi-governmental status since its pronouncements on drug quality, assay methodology, and standards have the weight of federal law.

National Community Pharmacists Association

Founded in 1898 as the National Association of Retail Druggists, NCPA continues to build on its reputation for entrepreneurial programs that benefit community pharmacists and for championing community pharmacy on Capitol Hill. NCPA has worked with industry partners to help build the fourth largest Medicare Prescription Drug Program in the country, Community CCRx. A key part of CCRx has been an aggressive medication therapy management (MTM) program that has resulted in more than 100,000 patients benefiting from pharmacist-provided MTM programs. Pharmacists have been recognized for their work with more than $10 million in payments. NCPA's members are entrepreneurs and the association reflects those intrinsic characteristics.

NCPA is also well known and has been extremely active and effective in the governmental arena. It has been able to focus its lobbying efforts in Washington and at the state level, and the cohesiveness of its members can produce remarkably successful grassroots campaigns. And if there's one person a legislator does not want on the other side of an issue, it's the local pharmacist back home.

NCPA's members are based in the nation's 23,000 plus independent community pharmacies. As was noted in Chapter 6 on career paths, many of these pharmacies are anything but the standard corner drug store—they often have multiple locations, offer intravenous admixture services, and boast long-term care divisions that serve nursing homes. NCPA has historically been the organization of the pharmacy owners, but its memberships also includes pharmacy technicians and thousands of community staff pharmacists and pharmacy students.

NCPA conducts three meetings annually. Its Annual Convention and Trade Exposition in October includes education, exhibits, and political activity in a House of Delegates. The Multiple Locations Pharmacy Conference, held during the winter in a location with a warm climate, is focused on continuing education, networking, and exhibits. Sites of these two meetings vary each year. The NCPA National Legislation and Government Affairs Conference, held in Washington, D.C. each May, attracts members who want to know more about and make a difference in the pharmacy-related laws and regulations being debated at the federal level.

NCPA publishes *America's Pharmacist* monthly, and it contains a wealth of information of use to the practicing community pharmacist. NCPA also publishes several newsletters, including some devoted to the home health and long-term care fields. The *NCPA Digest* is an annual presentation of data and information about the professional and business aspects of community pharmacy practice.

NCPA has responded aggressively to the advent of Medicare Part D and MTM. NCPA subsidiary organizations are both serving as a national provider of Medicare Part D services (Community CCRx; http://www.communityccrx.com) and partnering with pharmacists to provide MTM services directly to patients (www.mirixa.com). NCPA, APhA, and the National Alliance of State Pharmacy Associations launched www.RxWiki.com in August 2007 to provide a Web-based drug information resource for patients, one that is written and updated by participating pharmacists.

In 1991, NCPA expanded its commitment by launching a separate organization called the National Home Infusion Association. NHIA is headquartered at NCPA and is devoted to legislative and regulatory representation, clinical continuing education, and management and marketing assistance for home infusion providers. NHIA holds an annual conference each year, and it publishes a bimonthly journal for its members, *Infusion*, as well as providing bulletins on emerging issues.

As reflected by its annual governmental conference, NCPA continues its long-standing commitment in this arena. It has been instrumental in gaining passage of several important pieces of legislation at both the federal and state levels. It was a key player in passage of federal pharmacy crime law, making robbery or burglary of a pharmacy a federal offense; the Prescription Drug Marketing Act, which combats illicit drug diversion; and the so-called Pryor legislation, requiring manufacturers to provide their best prices to the Medicaid programs and pharmacists to offer patient counseling. In addition, the association is pursuing legislation regarding prompt payment for Medicare claims, tamper-resistant prescription pads for Medicaid prescriptions, and fair reimbursement payment formula for Medicaid claims. The organization's efforts have led its political action committee (PAC) to become one of the top 50 trade association PACs in the country and to the formation of the Congressional Community Pharmacy Caucus to serve as a permanent platform for sharing ideas, news, and research on community pharmacy legislative issues on Capitol Hill.

NCPA has an aggressive student-outreach program that now features active student chapters in most of the nation's pharmacy schools. To attract more student pharmacists to community pharmacy, the Association has developed information on community pharmacy ownership, including publications such as *How to Buy a Pharmacy: A How to Guide*, a robust Management section at www.ncpanet.org, and articles published in *America's Pharmacist* about young entrepreneurs who have been successful in independent practice and tips on how to get started in purchasing one's own pharmacy.

NCPA has successfully been able to shift the solutions it provides as the times have changed community pharmacy. The organization continues to respond quickly and effectively as changes in pharmacy and health care present opportunities for its members.

American College of Apothecaries

The term *college,* when used in the name of a professional association, connotes more selective membership criteria or procedures than are used by *societies or associations*. So it is with the American College of Apothecaries (ACA).

Founded in 1940 by members of the APhA, ACA has always represented the hopes and desires of pharmacists who wanted their colleagues to focus on the professional side of practice rather than on the business aspects. Thus, ACA members must meet certain criteria, including owning or working in a pharmacy that is devoid of commercialistic trappings or advertising. ACA pharmacies would fit in the category referred to as apothecary shops: those with limited or no "front-end" merchandise and that sell primarily prescription and nonprescription drugs, medical supplies, and related materials.

Today, ACA has full-time staff members at its offices in Memphis, Tenn. It has two sister organizations, the ACA Research & Education Foundation, established in 1978, and the American College of Veterinary Pharmacists, founded in 1998. ACA's role in pharmacy politics has always been somewhat limited by its small membership and budget, but ACA members remain a very cohesive bunch.

ACA activities include the publication of several newsletters and two meetings annually, in the spring and autumn.

In many ways, ACA represents the professional aspirations of pharmacists that were dashed by the rush to commercialism and mass merchandising of the 1950s and 1960s. The same fuel that spurred the growth of outlets such as CVS, K-Mart, and Wal-Mart burned the hopes for universalization of a more professional level of pharmacy practice, one that required the half century described in Chapter 3 to re-emerge.

American Society of Health-System Pharmacists

The American Society of Health-System Pharmacists (ASHP) is the national professional society for pharmacists who practice in hospitals and health systems. Founded as the American Society of Hospital Pharmacists in 1942, the Society's 30,000 members include pharmacists who practice in inpatient, outpatient, home-care, and long-term care settings, as well as pharmacy technicians and student pharmacists.

ASHP's mission is to "advance and support the professional practice of pharmacists in hospitals and health systems and serve as their collective voice on issues related to medication use and public health." As part of that mission, ASHP strives to provide leadership and advocacy in the patient safety arena, advance the patient-care role of pharmacists, and provide education, practice guidelines, publications, and other resources for its members.

ASHP began its life in 1936 as a subsection of hospital pharmacists at APhA. Officially founded in 1942, the Society became fully autonomous in 1960 when it opened its first full-time office in Washington, D.C., and hired Joseph Oddis, ScD, as executive vice president. ASHP moved to Bethesda, Md., in 1966 and, in 1992, moved down the street to its current location on Wisconsin Avenue. In 1994, ASHP changed to its current name to reflect the changes occurring in the hospital industry as many hospitals began linking as systems and diversifying beyond inpatient care, as well as recognize that many ASHP members serve patients in outpatient clinics and home care operations associated with hospitals.

Started with an initial group of 154 charter members, the organization has grown to more than 30,000 members today. As an organization focused on serving pharmacists who practice in hospitals and health systems, the Society offers membership sections that provide tailored resources to pharmacists in specific areas of practice. The following member sections serve as a "home within a home" for members who provide input on the Society's policy-making process, educational resources, and other programs:
- Section of Inpatient Care Practitioners
- Section of Clinical Specialists and Scientists
- Section of Home, Ambulatory, and Chronic Care Practitioners

- Section of Pharmacy Practice Managers
- Section of Pharmacy Informatics and Technology

The Society also provides two membership Forums—the Student Forum and the New Practitioner's Forum—for pharmacists just starting their careers. The Forums offer resources across practice settings that can help students and new practitioners gain insights from their pharmacy peers and provide leadership opportunities.

The Society maintains affiliate relationships with state-based health-system pharmacy organizations throughout the United States. ASHP is aligned with student societies of health-system pharmacy at nearly all colleges and schools of pharmacy.

Other areas of emphasis for ASHP include accreditation of pharmacy residency and technician-training programs; publishing journals and books (including the respected reference text, the *AHFS Drug Information*); providing practitioner education; advocacy at the federal and state levels; public relations; a research and education foundation; and maintenance of a dynamic Web site.

Throughout its history, ASHP has been driven by the ideals of improving patient safety and advancing the practice of pharmacy in hospitals and health systems. Steadfast devotion to these ideals have allowed ASHP to effect practice change and provide pharmacists in hospitals and health systems with the tools they need to best care for their patients.

American Society of Consultant Pharmacists

Founded in 1969 by a group of entrepreneurs within pharmacy practice, the American Society of Consultant Pharmacists (ASCP) continues to reflect that spirit and drive. With a membership exceeding 7,000, the organization also has more than 5,700 student members. The Society has no House of Delegates; policy is developed by committees of members and approved by the Board of Directors.

ASCP members are experts in geriatric pharmacotherapy who treat medically complex and frail, elderly patients wherever they reside. As patient advocates, they are often known as "America's Senior Care Pharmacists."

ASCP is fulfilling the dream of providing advanced pharmaceutical care to improve quality of life. ASCP members practice in a multitude of diverse settings including nursing facilities (71%), assisted living facilities (49%), hospice (40%), acute care and hospital-based facilities (30%), community pharmacy (28%), mental health facilities (26%), in-home settings (20%), and adult day care (11%). Traditionally known for their federally mandated role in nursing facilities, ASCP members now are leading the way in delivering medication therapy management services both under the Medicare Part D prescription drug benefit and in private-pay situations.

ASCP has two annual conventions, both of them a good mix of clinical, business, and regulatory educational sessions, balanced with exhibits, and social networking functions. The ASCP Annual Meeting, known as "Senior Care Pharmacy," is held in mid-November and attracts about 3,000 attendees. The Midyear Conference, themed "Geriatrics," is held in May at resort locations, and attracts about 1,500 people. Both events offer pharmacy continuing education credit.

Information delivery through publications, including software and other new kinds of media, are an increasingly important service of ASCP. *The Consultant Pharmacist,* the Society's Medline-indexed, peer-reviewed journal, mixes feature articles on current developments with practice-oriented research articles and departments. Its award-winning Web site, www.ascp.com, is rich with information. ASCP offers clinical references, practice development and regulatory and policy guides, and resources on business and management.

ASCP focuses heavily on building relationships with other pharmacy, aging, and long-term care associations. ASCP holds a seat on the steering committee of PQA, a pharmacy quality alliance, with members and staff serving as cochairs of the long-term care quality metrics subcommittee.

Tertiary-care institutions:
Hospitals that provide care to patients who could not be treated adequately at the primary (community hospital) or secondary (regional referral hospitals) institutions. Tertiary-care hospitals are often affiliated with medical schools.

ASCP also works closely with officials from the Centers for Medicare & Medicaid Services. Most recently, it was ASCP that led the fight to protect the health and welfare of long-term care residents, especially those known as "dual-eligibles," under the recently enacted Medicare Modernization Act of 2005.

The future is bright for ASCP. As the aging population continues to grow and use more medications, ASCP members' unique expertise will be needed by ever larger numbers of individuals to ensure that their medications are the most appropriate, the most effective, the safest possible, and are used correctly. The entrepreneurial spirit that is the hallmark of ASCP thrives as consultant and senior care pharmacists take their unique expertise to provide medication therapy management to seniors wherever they reside.

American College of Clinical Pharmacy

Founded in 1979 by ASHP members who practiced clinical pharmacy at an advanced level, the American College of Clinical Pharmacy (ACCP) is another rapidly growing pharmacy association. Like ACA, the College's criteria for full membership are more restrictive than those of other pharmacy organizations; in these criteria, ACCP emphasizes experience in practicing or teaching patient-oriented clinical pharmacy.

With a membership approaching 10,000, ACCP has gone through several phases during its brief history. Until 1986, ACCP was closely aligned with the journal *Drug Intelligence & Clinical Pharmacy* (known today as *Annals of Pharmacotherapy*), which served as its offices and provided some staff support. Since 1986, ACCP has had paid staff based in the Kansas City, Missouri, area, and has acquired the journal *Pharmacotherapy* as its official publication. ACCP established a Washington, D.C., office in 2000, and through its Director of Government and Professional Affairs, C. Edwin Webb, the College pursues an advocacy agenda set annually by its Board of Regents.

ACCP actively recruits members who practice clinical pharmacy in a variety of settings beyond the **tertiary-care institutions** where its early members worked. This has greatly increased the College's membership rolls and provided the group with increased political clout.

Table 8.3 | Major Pharmacy Conventions

APhA–ASP .....Midyear Regional Meetings/eight locations (see www.pharmacist.com)/Fall

APhA–ASP ....APhA Annual Meeting/mid-March to early April

Upcoming sites of APhA–ASP Annual Meetings

2009 ....San Antonio

2010 ....Washington, D.C.

2011 ....Seattle

2012 ....New Orleans

NCPA ....Annual Meeting/October

NCPA ....NCPA Multiple Locations Conference/February

ACA ....Annual Conference/October or November

ASHP ....Midyear Clinical Meeting/early December

ASHP ....Summer Meeting/June

ASCP ....Senior Care Pharmacy (Annual Meeting)/November

ASCP ....Geriatrics (Midyear Conference)/May

ACCP ....Annual Meeting/October to early November

ACCP ....Spring Practice and Research Forum/April

NACDS ....Pharmacy, Managed Care, and Technology Conference/late August

NACDS ....Annual Meeting/late April

AMCP............Educational Conference/October

AMCP............Annual Meeting/April

NABP ....Annual Meeting (see www.nabp.net)/May

NASPA...........meets at the APhA and NCPA annual meetings

AACP ....Annual Meeting/July

ACCP was the driving force behind the recognition of Pharmacotherapy as a certifiable pharmacy specialty in 1988 by the Board of Pharmaceutical Specialties.

ACCP conducts two conferences per year. An annual meeting, attracting more than 1,000 people, is conducted in late October or November; the conference is heavy on continuing education about clinical practice and research and includes little political activity (the College has no House of Delegates). A midyear research forum attracts several hundred attendees in April; it also focuses on clinical practice and research.

The College has been very successful at establishing post-PharmD fellowships in advanced areas of pharmacotherapy (see Chapter 10). It is also an important part of the dialogue on such issues as the entry-level degree, the kinds of residencies and fellowships needed by pharmacy practitioners, and other issues on the interface between pharmacy education and clinical practice.

ACCP members are undoubtedly some of the best thinkers in pharmacy. They have led pharmacy to a point where society increasingly recognizes the value of the information and clinical management skills pharmacists offer patients. Their challenge today remains extending such services in such a way that all pharmacists—not just the best minds—can effectively provide them in a variety of types of pharmacy practice settings.

Academy of Managed Care Pharmacy

The Academy of Managed Care Pharmacy (AMCP) is one of pharmacy's newest and fastest-growing organizations. Founded in 1989, AMCP boasts some 5,000 members, 30 staff members, and a budget of $10 million. The organization estimates that its members provide care to more than 200 million Americans served by managed care.

The Academy conducts two meetings annually and publishes a newsletter and journal, *Journal of Managed Care Pharmacy.* Because of the rapid growth of managed care, attendance at AMCP meetings has swelled, and representatives of the pharmaceutical industry attend in large numbers to gain a better appreciation of this emerging market segment.

AMCP members strongly buy into the pharmaceutical care system. With members in health-maintenance organizations, other types of managed care groups, and pharmacy benefit management companies, AMCP members are in a prime position to help define the appropriate roles for pharmacists in the years to come.

The rapid growth of managed care bodes well for AMCP. The importance of managed care pharmacy should continue to increase as the positive influences of cost containment and quality of care are recognized and appreciated by an increasing number of health care payers.

Pharmacy's alphabet soup

In addition to these major pharmacy practitioner organizations, several dozen other groups operate within pharmacy or on its periphery. Many of these are listed at the bottom of Table 8.1 or in Table 8.2. In addition, major pharmacy conventions and the general time frames when they usually occur are shown in Table 8.3.

For the student, the message is simple: get involved. To become a successful and contributing part of the profession of pharmacy, the student pharmacist must become integrated within the profession's patchwork of organizations. Through them, the student and young pharmacist can be nurtured professionally. Someday, the new practitioner can give back to the profession through involvement as a leader in one of these groups, so that pharmacy becomes even better. This is the expectation society has of a professional, and the professional association is the most common mechanism for actualizing that goal.

Chapter 9 | Using the Pharmacy Literature— and Writing for It

One characteristic of a profession is that it has its own body of literature. Thus, a corollary to this idea is that professionals should contribute to that literature. This chapter is included so that you can begin to envision your future role as a creator of knowledge about pharmacy and to inculcate in you the idea that pharmacy professionals always share new knowledge with colleagues for the benefit of all patients.

It is never too early to begin contributing to the pharmacy literature. As a student pharmacist or even prepharmacy student, you already are experiencing a part of the culture and traditions of pharmacy. As you do so, your thoughts and ideas about pharmacy or about pharmacy education could be of interest and value to the rest of the profession. A simple letter to the editor of a state or national publication could launch a noteworthy career as a pharmacist-author.

In this chapter, I will describe the structure of the pharmacy literature, clues about ways of accessing it, and tips for contributing to it. Students who desire more information about the pharmacy or biomedical literature should check their schools' curricula for courses in drug information or talk with pharmacy faculty members who publish frequently. Also, visit the library and seek assistance with tasks such as literature searches; the librarians can be very helpful, even to experienced authors.

Structure of the biomedical literature

Much of the scientific and biomedical literature, including that of pharmacy, is divided into three categories:

- Primary literature, such as original research articles, descriptive reports, case reports, opinions, and news articles
- Secondary literature, such as review articles that summarize the primary literature on a specific topic or abstracting/indexing services that provide information about where to look in the primary literature for specific types of information
- Tertiary literature, such as books and other major summaries of broad topics, including reference books

Most of this chapter is devoted to the primary literature. Pharmacy has numerous professional journals, news magazines, practice-oriented magazines, newsletters, and other regular periodicals (Table 9.1). Many industry-sponsored publications are available as well.

Among the components of the secondary pharmacy literature, foremost is International Pharmaceutical Abstracts (IPA). Created by the American Society of Health-System Pharmacists in 1964 and acquired by Thomson Scientific in 2005, IPA electronically provides **abstracts** of pharmacy literature from around the world. It can be searched online

"Many pharmacists are good writers; to most of them, including the widely published stars, writing does not come naturally or easily. They sweat over their masterpieces, word after word, draft after crumpled draft. Although there are rare exceptions whose first drafts read with the grace and fluency of an E. B. White essay, most good writers have achieved this distinction through hard work. They have high standards and the perceptiveness to recognize when their work is only half done."

—William A. Zellmer, in "How to Write a Research Report for Publication," *Research in Pharmacy Practice: Principles and Methods*, 1981:142

Table 9.1 | Selected Pharmacy Periodical Publications

Periodical Name/Address	Editor	Publisher/Web Site
Association newsletters and journals[a]		
Journal of the American Pharmacists Association	L. Michael Posey	APhA
Pharmacy Today	L. Michael Posey	APhA
APhA DrugInfoLine	L. Michael Posey	APhA
Journal of Pharmaceutical Sciences	Ronald T. Borchardt	APhA
Student Pharmacist	Tom English	APhA–ASP
America's Pharmacist	Michael F. Conlan	NCPA
NCPA Newsletter	Michael F. Conlan	NCPA
Infusion	Jeannie Counce	NHIA
Journal of Managed Care Pharmacy	Frederic R. Curtiss	AMCP
AMCP News	Carolyn Stables	AMCP
American Journal of Health-System Pharmacy	C. Richard Talley	ASHP
ASHP Intersections	Ellen Wilcox	ASHP
The Consultant Pharmacist	H. Edward Davidson	ASCP
ASCP Update	Marlene Bloom	ASCP
Pharmacotherapy	Richard Scheife	ACCP
ACCP Report	Mary T. Roth	ACCP
American Journal of Pharmaceutical Education	Joseph T. DiPiro	AACP
AACP News	Mary B. Bassler	AACP
The Practice Memo	Ronna B. Hauser, Crystal Lennartz	NACDS
Pharmaceutical Research	Vincent H. L. Lee	AAPS
American Association of Pharmaceutical Scientists		
2107 Wilson Blvd, Suite 700		
Arlington, VA 22201-3042		
Other publications		
Annals of Pharmacotherapy	Milap C. Nahata	Harvey Whitney Books
Journal of Medical Technology	Harvey A. K. Whitney, Jr.	www.hwbooks.com
P. O. Box 42696, Cincinnati, OH 45242	513/793-3555	www.theannals.com
ComputerTalk for the Pharmacist	Will Lockwood	ComputerTalk Associates
492 Norristown Road, Suite 160, Blue Bell, PA 19422	610/825-7686	www.computertalk.com
Drug Topics	Thomas Skernivitz	Avanstar Communications
123 Tice Blvd., Woodcliff Lake, NJ 07677	440/891-2702	www. drugtopics.com
Drug Safety News (podcast/RSS)/Drug Safety Newsletter (e-mail)	Food and Drug Administration	www.fda.gov/cder/drug/
5600 Fishers Lane, Rockville, MD 20857	888-INFO-FDA	podcast/rss_podcast.xml
		www.fda.gov/emaillist.html
FDC Reports ("The Pink Sheet")/ Health News Daily	Joseph Hecker	FDC Reports, Inc.
5635 Fishers Lane, Suite 6000, Rockville, MD 20852	800/332-2181	www.fdcreports.com
Hospital Pharmacy	Dennis Cada	Wolters Kluwer Health
77 Westport Plaza, Suite 450, St. Louis, MO 63146	800/223-0554	www.factsandcomparisons.com/
		hospitalpharm/
Journal of Pharmacy Practice	Henry Cohen	Sage Publications
2671 East 64th Street, Brooklyn, NY 11234	Henry.Cohen@LIU.edu	http://jpp.sagepub.com/
Pharmacist's Letter	Jeff M. Jellin	Therapeutic Research Ctr.
3120 W. March Lane, PO Box 8190, Stockton, CA 95208	209/472-2240	www.pharmacistsletter.com
Pharmacy Times	James R. Granato	Ascend Media
103 College Road East, Princeton, NJ 08540-6612	609/524-9560	www.pharmacytimes.com
U.S. Pharmacist	Harold E. Cohen	Jobson Medical Information
One Meadowlands Plaza, 10th Floor, East Rutherford, NJ 07073	201/623-0999	www.uspharmacist.com

[a] See Chapter 8 for association addresses and Web links (Table 8.1).

Table 9.2 | Key Pharmacy References

- Remington: The Science and Practice of Pharmacy. 21st ed. University of the Sciences in Philadelphia, ed. Baltimore: Lippincott Williams & Wilkins, 2005. Updated every 5 years.
- Physicians' Desk Reference. Oradell, NJ: Medical Economics Co. Updated annually.
- American Hospital Formulary Service Drug Information. Bethesda, MD: American Society of Health-System Pharmacists. Updated annually.
- Facts and Comparisons. St. Louis, Missouri: Lippincott. Updated annually.
- Iowa Drug Information Service (microfiche). Iowa City, IA: Iowa Drug Information Service. Updated annually.
- Berardi RR, Ferreri SP, Hume AL, et al. Handbook of Nonprescription Drugs: An Interactive Approach to Self-Care. 16th ed. Washington, DC: American Pharmacists Association, 2009. Updated every 3 years.
- Drugdex/Poisondex (microfiche). Denver: Micromedex. Updated annually.
- Goodman and Gilman's The Pharmacological Basis of Therapeutics. Brunton LL, Lazo JS, Parker KL. 11th ed. New York City: McGraw-Hill, 2006. Updated every 5 years.
- Koda-Kimble MA, Young LY, Kradjan WA, Guglielmo BJ, Alldredge BK, Corelli, RL, Williams BR. Applied Therapeutics: The Clinical Use of Drugs. 9th ed. Baltimore, MD: Lippincott Williams & Wilkins, 2008. Updated every 4 years.
- DiPiro JT, Talbert RL, Yee GC, Matzke GR, Wells BG, Posey LM. Pharmacotherapy: A Pathophysiologic Approach. 7th ed. New York City: McGraw-Hill, 2008. Updated every 3 years.

---

through TOXLINE, a searchable **computerized database** available through several **vendors** (including Cambridge Scientific Abstracts, DataStar, Dialog, DIMDI, EBSCO, Optionline div. PTI, OVID, SilverPlatter, and STN) and many medical libraries.

In addition, most pharmacy journals regularly publish review articles about diseases, drugs, and other pharmacy topics. Some are devoted entirely to review and survey articles.

Two other key indexing services are very useful for pharmacists and student pharmacists. *Index Medicus* is the indexing publication of the National Library of Medicine, and it is available online as PubMed (www.pubmed.gov). *Index Medicus* includes much of the pharmacy literature and virtually all of the important medical literature; thus, it is the key source used for clinically oriented literature searches. The other publication, *Science Citation Index,* is a publication of the Institute of Scientific Information in Philadelphia. *SCI* lists previously published articles and all subsequent articles that have used the older article as a reference. Suppose, for example, that you are preparing a paper on heart transplants. You could look in *SCI* for one of the early articles from the 1960s on heart transplants, and there find all later articles that cited the original works. *SCI* thus provides a valuable check on the accuracy of computerized literature searches and provides a way to come forward in the literature.

Pharmacy's tertiary literature is also very broad. While entire libraries could be filled with these texts, a few key reference books are listed in Table 9.2.

With that background to the pharmacy literature as a whole, let's look at the process many authors go through when writing articles for publication. While examples from the primary literature will be used, the same steps and principles would apply to other kinds of professional writing, from patient newsletters to review articles for journals to chapters in books.

Abstracts:
A short (100–200 words) summary of an article. Abstracts may merely describe the scope of an article, or they may present the key points or data presented in the paper.

Computerized databases:
Used in reference to the literature, this term means computer files containing information from articles that have been published in journals, magazines, and newspapers. These databases are searchable, using either key words from the title or abstract of the article, the authors' names, or the journals' names.

Database vendors:
Companies or organizations that obtain several databases and make them available to the public or others. Examples include DIALOG and BRS; bulletin board services such as America Online, CompuServe, and Prodigy also have access to databases.

Writing for publication

When it comes right down to it, writing for publication is no different than writing in your diary. It's just that a lot more people will read it.

The biggest obstacle to writing—writer's block—is a psychological phenomenon that every writer in the world has experienced. The only real cure for it that I have found so far is a firm deadline, usually combined with pressure from an editor, publisher, coauthor, preceptor, or mentor. Since most pharmacists do not have such a person to keep them on track, we procrastinate and procrastinate and procrastinate. However, help is available—by forcing oneself to write, regardless of how painful it may seem. Write about anything, but make yourself express your thoughts through the written word. Don't worry about format or spelling or structure or organization—just write. A good editor can fix it later—the hard part is getting started.

Of course, a common form of writer's block is provided by the tortuous process of deciding what to write about. While authors of research projects have usually spelled out a great many parts of the final article at various stages of conducting the project, authors of opinion pieces or descriptive reports do not have this advantage. All I can say is this: if you can imagine that any other pharmacist in the country or even in the world might encounter the same problem or situation that you have and not know precisely how to handle it, then you have the kernel of some type of publication. In nearly 30 years of editing pharmacy journals, I have seen reports published such as the one in which the primary original thought was to cut the top off a box of intravenous fluid bottles and use the resulting cubbyholes for sorting medication orders as they came from nursing units in a hospital. I have seen scientifically questionable articles published because they were timely, and I have seen seemingly irrelevant articles published because they were scientifically valid. Simply put, most articles in the professional literature are not earth-shaking pieces of research; some of the most valuable are simply practical tips on how a pharmacist solved an everyday problem.

Also remember that several different types of articles can be published. Research articles are subjected to rigorous scientific review, but many journals and magazines have sections for descriptive reports, letters to the editor, and editorials (Table 9.3). Think about what you want to say, and then look at the journal to which you want to submit your article. Write your article like those in the section where you think the content of your article will fit.

Once a topic is identified, the next step is to read related articles that have already been published. As a pharmacy resident, I wasted two or three months growing bacteria in intravenous and parenteral nutrition solutions only to find out that microbiology researchers had published the same studies nearly 10 years earlier. One rule that editors of pharmacy journals won't usually break is that articles should not reinvent the wheel.

In preparing for the day when you want to put your hands on the keyboard, consider these tips:
- Read books about writing well (as listed in Table 9.4)
- Regularly read publications that are well written and well edited. Emulate them. They are the best models available.

Table 9.3 | Types of Articles in the Pharmacy Literature[a]

- Research paper
- Case report
- Reviews and case-series analysis

- Editorial
- Book review
- Letter to the editor

[a] For advice on how to write each type of paper, consult: Huth EJ. Writing and Publishing in Medicine. 3rd ed. Baltimore: Williams & Wilkins, 1999.

- Take courses in grammar, composition, or other skills that need improvement.
- Purchase a good style manual (Table 9.4) appropriate for your writing needs. Read it for understanding and study its preferences and principles. Write with the necessary tools at hand or available in your word-processing software—including a dictionary, thesaurus, and when appropriate, a medical dictionary and style manual.
- Always write for the specific journal and audience for which the article is intended.
- Have your writing critiqued by professors or colleagues whose skills are well developed. Heed their comments—criticism may be hard to take at first, but there is usually an element of truth in those comments that hits the hardest.
- Write every time you can. Write reports for class; prepare articles for school organizations and publications; contribute to your pharmacy college newsletter and state pharmacy journal. Analyze the feedback you receive.
- Review the instructions for authors of the publication to which you plan to submit. If you cannot find them, contact the Editor and request a copy. Read these closely before you begin writing.
- Develop a system for writing. Find a subject and make a list. Organize the list into an outline. Always write in an appropriate location or situation, or with a certain pen or color of paper, or with a certain word-processing program. Write when you are fresh, not tired or frustrated. Minimize distractions and interruptions.

Table 9.4 | Tools for Improving Writing[a]

Dictionaries
- *American Heritage Dictionary:* Includes helpful style and usage notes
- *Stedman's Medical Dictionary*, 27th ed.: Also available on disk with medical and pharmaceutical terms (including drug names) for use with many word processing programs.

Style manuals
- *Council of Biology Editors Style Manual*, 5th ed.: Very good for scientific papers.
- *American Medical Association Manual of Style*, 10th ed.: The best guide for medical and clinical manuscripts.

Writing style and grammar
- *The Elements of Style*, 3rd ed.: Also known as Strunk and White; a classic book on the philosophy of modern writing.
- *Writing and Publishing in Medicine*, 3rd ed.: An excellent discussion of how to prepare papers for biomedical journals and what happens to them after they are submitted.

[a] These books are readily available in most college bookstores, especially those on medical campuses, and online at www.amazon.com and other online book vendors.

- Write, rewrite, edit, and revise. There is one best way to express a thought. Find it.
- After a paper is perfect, have colleagues critique it. Then revise it again — cut out the fat, but leave the arteries intact. Every good writer needs an editor; use the feedback to improve accuracy and clarity of the article.

When writing an article, begin with the part of it that you find the easiest to put on paper. For instance, in a research article, the hardest part to write is often the introduction. Start with something very straightforward, such as the tables and figures or the methods. These parts involve less creativity, and they are the parts that you know best. It should be easy to put them down on paper, and seeing the article begin to coalesce will give you the drive to keep going.

After the methods, tables, and figures are done, draft the results and discussion sections. The results flow logically from the methods, and the discussion should put your results in perspective with previously published material on the same or similar subjects.

Finally, at the end, draft the conclusion and introduction sections. The conclusion should flow logically from the study objectives that you set at the beginning of the project, and you can now write the perfect introduction to the paper. Finalize your references once the introduction is in place, and get ready to provide your first draft to some friends or colleagues who can give you critical feedback.

The revision process for a manuscript is designed to accomplish two goals: to improve your paper's accuracy (conveyance of what really happened or how the research was actually conducted) and your paper's clarity (saying what happened in such a way that people not involved in the project can understand). The best technique for accomplishing these goals is to have the first draft reviewed by other people who know the situation (review for accuracy, often performed by coauthors of the paper), incorporate those comments, and then have the paper reviewed by others not familiar with the manuscript (review for clarity). If the comments from these two rounds of review are minimal, the manuscript is ready for submission for publication.

Peer review:
Analysis of submitted articles by experts who are not part of the journal's staff.

Peer review in biomedical publishing

When the editor receives your manuscript for publication, he or she has two primary questions: Is the paper of interest to the readers of this journal, and is it accurate and clear in its presentation? To answer these questions, the advice of outside reviewers who are knowledgeable in your content area is often sought.

The process of obtaining this outside review is known in biomedical publishing as the **peer-review process.** For many pharmacy journals, the process is double-blinded: neither the reviewers nor the authors know the identity of the other party. Other journals use a partially blind system in which the authors are known to the reviewers, but the reviewers' identities are masked to the authors. A few journals use a fully open process in which both parties know the identify of the other. The editors have an ethical obligation to provide the author with the contents of the reviewers' critiques, regardless of whether the editor agreed with them, but the editor does not disclose the identity of the other parties without their express permission.

The editor usually arrives at one of four decisions about submitted manuscripts:
1. Accept for publication
2. Revise before publication
3. Clarify before a decision can be reached
4. Reject

In writing to the author, the editor clearly states one of these four options. Very few papers are accepted outright with no changes requested of the author. The second option creates a kind of legal contract between the editor and the author; the editor is saying that if the author will make or agree to certain changes in the paper, then the paper will be published. Letters expressing option 3 carry no such commitment; in particular, authors receiving a letter asking for clarification often find that the editor seeks again the advice of outside reviewers before reaching a decision.

If changes to an article are made as requested, the editor will normally accept the paper and schedule it for publication.

Copyediting and steps in the production process

Following acceptance of a paper for publication, the journal's staff will **copyedit** the paper to conform with the style of that periodical. Some authors are surprised at the extent of editing, but most agree that the changes improve the clarity and accuracy of the manuscript.

The **style manual** of a publication is used by the editors to create a familiarity with the content among regular readers. In short, the editor wants the journal to be as comfortable to readers as slipping on a pair of favorite shoes. For instance, a certain term may always be used when referring to a certain disease. Common abbreviations may not be spelled out on first mention. Editors may move parts of the paper around to what they consider a clearer or more logical flow of ideas. And, of course, overt spelling or grammatical errors are corrected.

Authors of major articles in pharmacy journals will receive one or more proofs of the article before it goes to print. Some journals will provide the edited manuscript as a word-processing file, while others continue to provide a **galley proof** for approval before printing. These are often followed by a set of page proofs that show the article as it will appear in the journal. At these stages, be certain to read the article very closely, and question changes that you feel have altered the meaning of the article. Good editing is like good surgery: it removes the fat but leaves the muscles and blood vessels intact. If the editors have massacred parts of your paper, then challenge them to defend their changes. If the only answer they can provide is, "It sounds better this way," or "That's just our style," then ask them to use your version. After all, your name is on the paper!

The editors see one or more proofs of the article after the galleys and first set of page proofs, and soon the journal will be mailed to pharmacists throughout the country and around the world. You will suddenly be famous, with some people viewing you as an expert on the subject. You will certainly want to order a few reprints of the article for friends, family, and holiday gifts!

Copyediting:
Correction and preparation of a manuscript for typesetting and printing.

Style manual:
A book listing preferred ways of stating material in a field or publication.

Galley proofs:
Typeset versions of articles that are provided to editors (and usually to authors) for a final check of spelling, style, and accuracy.

Sharing your ideas with colleagues: Your ticket to fame and fortune

Even if you never pen a phrase that is printed in the pharmacy literature, the odds are still 100% that you will be called on to write something during your pharmacy career. It may be an article for the local newspaper about a new drug, a proposal for providing services to a home health agency or nursing home, a memorandum for employees of a pharmacy, or simple instructions on how to administer a prescription. Whatever the time and place, the principles spelled out in this chapter will apply, and the quality of your written presentation will affect the response of the readers. Writing is simply a skill that all pharmacists must hone in today's practice environment.

Chapter 10 | Postgraduate Educational Opportunities

While the end of pharmacy school may seem a lifetime away, now is the time to begin planning your postgraduate education. Even for the decreasing number of you who will graduate and enter practice immediately, your education cannot end then. Pharmacy school provides an excellent basis for entering practice, but there is more to learn after you graduate—much, much more.

The purpose of this chapter is to stimulate you to begin exploring the various postgraduate opportunities that are available. Among the formal educational options open to the new pharmacy graduate are residencies, fellowships, traineeships, and graduate school. Let's look at what each of these entails.

Residencies

Student pharmacists are increasingly choosing to go into **residency** programs after graduation. This path may soon be just as common for a pharmacist to pursue a residency as it has been for physicians.

Residencies are valuable experiences because they offer a systematic educational focus in a real-world setting using a Socratic method of teaching. Each residency program is headed by a preceptor who takes personal responsibility for assuring that each resident has a quality learning experience. Through rotations in various clinical or other areas, pharmacy residents have the opportunity to learn about differet types of patients and how various parts of the pharmacy or facility work by talking directly with patients, physicians, nurses, and pharmacy managers or supervisors. While it is possible to gain these skills and knowledge in other ways, the residency facilitates their acquisition in a short amount of time.[1,2]

Pharmacy residency programs are now available in the areas shown in Table 10.1. Sources of current information about residency programs are the ASHP (www.ashp.org, under the Accreditation heading) and APhA Web sites (www.pharmacist.com, under the Student Pharmacist heading). A comprehensive list of available residencies and fellowships is maintained on the ACCP Web site (www.accp.com/resandfel/directorynon.php).

Residencies have been common in hospital and health-system pharmacy since the 1960s, and they are now spreading to community pharmacies. First begun in the mid-1980s, community pharmacy residencies have grown in prominence and number since the late 1990s. Several dozen community pharmacy residency programs are now accredited, and they offer a growing number of slots for innovative student pharmacists who want to expand medication therapy management into the nation's chain and independent community pharmacies.[3-7] In addition to the ASHP and APhA Web sites mentioned above, a good source of information about community pharmacy residencies is www.communires.com,

"The true value of a residency is that it provides you with an unparalleled opportunity to gain competence, confidence, and a competitive edge. There is no other choice that you could make for that first year out of school that would give you the same comprehensive results in so short a time.... The career-long value of the residency experience is irreplaceable. It more than offsets the short-term financial sacrifice that is required."

—David Vogel and Anne Blake
Why pursue a residency?
Am J Hosp Pharm. 1991; 48:1878.

Table 10.1 | Types of Pharmacy Residency Programs

Postgraduate year 1 residencies

- Community pharmacy
- Pharmacy

- Managed care pharmacy

Postgraduate year 2 residencies

- Ambulatory care pharmacy
- Critical care pharmacy
- Emergency medicine pharmacy
- Infectious disease pharmacy
- Internal medicine pharmacy
- Medication-use safety
- Nutrition support pharmacy
- Pediatric pharmacy
- Health-system pharmacy administration
- Solid organ transplant pharmacy
- Drug information

- Cardiology pharmacy
- Drug information
- Geriatric pharmacy
- Informatics
- Managed care pharmacy systems
- Nuclear pharmacy
- Oncology pharmacy
- Pharmacotherapy
- Psychiatric pharmacy

---

a Web site managed by the Midwestern University College of Pharmacy–Glendale under a grant from the Institute for the Advancement of Community Practice.[6]

Residency:
A postgraduate program of organized training that meets the requirements of a residency-accreditation body.

In 2003, ASHP reorganized its accreditation standards into a postgraduate year 1 (PGY1) and year 2 (PGY2). PGY1 programs can be conducted at one or more sites, and colleges of pharmacy can participate as sponsoring organizations. Residents learn about managing and improving the medication-use process, providing evidence-based, patient-centered medication therapy management with interdisciplinary teams, exercising leadership and practice management skills, demonstrating project management skills, providing medication and practice-related education/training, and using medical informatics.

PGY2 pharmacy residency programs focus on a specific area of practice, such as primary care/ambulatory, critical care, drug information, geriatrics, oncology, psychiatric, internal medicine, and other areas listed in Table 10.1.

ASHP uses a resident-matching program in which both programs and applicants submit lists of their preferences; programs are then matched with their selected applicants who rank them the highest. Because of this national program, the deadlines for making application are not flexible, and interviews must be completed so that a program will be able to rank each person adequately before the deadline for rankings to be submitted.

Stipends for residencies are generally about one half of what a starting pharmacist would earn. Benefits of employment are usually provided.

Other kinds of residencies are also available (Table 10.2); these were mentioned in Chapter 6 in the discussion of alternative career paths in industry, government, and associations.

Table 10.2 | Nonpractice Residencies/Internships Available to Pharmacists

Association management

APhA, ASHP, ASCP, NCPA, and NASPA Executive Residencies

Yearlong residences available to student pharmacists after graduation. Contact the organizations at the addresses shown in Table 8.1 for more information.

Editing and writing

George P. Provost Editorial Internship

Deadline: February 1 of each year

Contact: C. Richard Talley, ASHP,

7272 Wisconsin Avenue, Bethesda, MD 20814

Fellowships and traineeships

The important distinction between a residency and a **fellowship** is that the residency is practice-oriented while the fellowship has a research focus. Also, where there might be several residents in a given pharmacy training under one preceptor, there is usually only one fellow, thereby further increasing the **Socratic style of teaching**. In recent years, **traineeships** have grown in number and popularity, as practicing pharmacists have sought ways to enhance their knowledge and skills without interrupting their practices for an extended (usually one year) residency or fellowship.

Many different areas—most of them clinical—are now available for pharmacists interested in completing a fellowship (Table 10.3). The major sponsor of fellowships is the ACCP Research Institute. It uses grants from the pharmaceutical industry to support the fellowship programs. Note that fellowships are not conducted at the sponsoring companies; hospitals and institutions apply for funding and then select an individual for the fellowship.

As with residencies, stipends for fellowships are about one half of a starting pharmacist's salary. Employment benefits are usually provided. Fellowships, which may last for one or two years, are intensive research-oriented experiences and are therefore excellent ways to prepare for a career in academia or pharmaceutical industry. The fellow generally spends the entire time on a small number of research projects, including formulating the methods, conducting the research, and writing a manuscript for publication.

Traineeships are generally conducted for a few days (often from Sunday through Friday) at leading institutions or facilities specializing in the disease or area of interest. A limited number of pharmacists are accepted for each session, and they learn the latest concepts in clinical areas such as those listed in Table 10.3.

Using this intensive experience as a springboard, the practitioners then take their new skills and knowledge back to their practice setting, where they implement what they have learned in the traineeships. In some cases, pharmacists continue their training through interactions with local groups with interests in that disease or condition.

Graduate studies

For the student who wishes to pursue a research-oriented career in academia or pharmaceutical industry, graduate school is often the best path to take. Graduate studies are academically based experiences that focus on the student's research abilities, including literature review and analysis, statistical expertise, language skills, and in-depth knowledge of the field of study.

Fellowship:
A postgraduate program, usually research-oriented, often in a narrow field of study that relies on a Socratic teaching method.

Socratic teaching method:
The transfer of knowledge that relies on a person teaching one or a few students in a highly individualized manner. Named after Socrates of ancient Greece.

Traineeship:
Short-term programs, usually of one week in duration, that provide intensive information and demonstrations about one disease or a small group of similar conditions.

Table 10.3 | Available Fellowships and Sponsoring Organizations Type of Fellowship or Traineeship (funding sponsor)[a]

ASHP Research and Education Foundation
- Anticoagulation traineeship (DuPont Pharma)
- Asthma care traineeship (Merck)
- Stem cell transplantation traineeship
- Diabetes patient care traineeship (GlaxoSmithKline)
- Oncology patient care traineeship (Chiron Therapeutics and SuperGen)
- Pain management traineeship (Endo Pharmaceuticals)

American College of Clinical Pharmacy Research Institute
- Cardiovascular (Merck)
- Critical care (Bayer)
- Infectious disease therapeutics (Aventis and Ortho-McNeil)
- Oncology (Aventis)
- Pharmacoecomics and Outcomes (Merck)
- Psychopharmacy (Wyeth-Ayerst)
- Transplantation (Roche)

American Society of Consultant Pharmacists Research and Education Foundation
- Alzheimer's/dementia traineeship (Pfizer and Eisai)
- Disease pharmacotherapy traineeship in heart failure, osteoporosis, and osteoarthritis (Merck Human Health Division)
- HIV/AIDS pharmacotherapy traineeship (GlaxoSmithKline)
- GeroPsych/behavioral disorders traineeship (Lilly)
- Pain management traineeship (Johnson & Johnson Long-Term Care Group, Janssen Pharmaceutica, Ortho-McNeil Pharmaceutical)
- Parkinson's disease traineeship
- Thrombosis prevention and management traineeship (Aventis)

[a] The ASHP Research and Education Foundation, ACCP Research Institute, and ASCP Research and Education Foundation fund these fellowships and traineeships with support from the companies shown. Fellowships are conducted at teaching or health care institutions, not at the sponsoring company. The organizations may be contacted at the addresses shown in Table 8.1 on page 83.

The lack of students entering graduate studies—especially American-born student pharmacists—has been a concern of some in the profession. The concern relates to the fact that most pharmacy school faculty are products of such graduate work, and without pharmacists who have completed masters or doctor of philosophy degrees to mix with the nonpharmacists in those positions, the coursework offered may become less relevant to practice. Various techniques for increasing the interest of student pharmacists in graduate work have been proposed and tested.[8]

Many strong graduate programs are available in pharmacy and related disciplines. A PDF document listing graduate programs at U.S. colleges of pharmacy is available under the "Current Pharmacy Student" option on the AACP Web site (www.aacp.org). If you wish to write to these schools, your instructor or dean can provide you with addresses, or you can find most schools by searching on the Web.

In addition to the pharmacy graduate courses listed, many pharmacists have chosen to enter business, law, or medical schools. Depending on your overall career objectives, you may wish to consult with a career-counseling office at your school or university for more information about such options.

To apply to most graduate schools, you will need to take the Graduate Records Examination or other national tests and provide the school with transcripts and references. The graduate school to which you plan to apply can provide information about these items.

Pharmacy education: A lifelong experience

As was noted at the beginning of this book, change is a constant part of today's pharmacy world. Not only does pharmacy school *not* teach its students everything they need to know for pharmacy practice, but the amount of information known by the human race is now doubling every few years. No one—in any field—can leave school and assume that they know everything they will need to be a good practitioner for a lifetime. There are always new drugs, new diseases, new ideas, and new laws. The learning really never stops, and the potential opportunities offered by residencies, fellowships, traineeships, and graduate school should be seriously considered by every pharmacy graduate as a means of being well prepared to deal with the pharmacy world of today and tomorrow.

REFERENCES

1. Vogel D, Blake A. Why pursue a residency [student & resident forum]? *Am J Hosp Pharm.* 1991; 48:1878.

2. Miller WA. Postgraduate residency education and training: a call for action [president's section]. *Am J Pharm Educ.* 1989; 53:310-1.

3. Posey LM. Rachel Henderson: ensuring pharmacy's role in MTM services. *Pharm Today.* 2006 (Sept);12(9):20–4.

4. Egervary A. Pharmacy professor and Rite Aid collaborate on community MTM. *Pharm Today.* 2007 (Sept);14(9):36–9.

5. Pruchnicki MC, Rodis JL, Beatty SJ, et al. Practice-based research network as a research training model for community/ambulatory pharmacy residents. *J Am Pharm Assoc.* 2008;48:191–202.

6. Unterwagner WL, Zeolla MM, Burns AL. Training Experiences of Current and Former Community Pharmacy Residents, 1986–2000. *J Am Pharm Assoc.* 2003;43:201–6.

7. Rupp MT. Program planning for a community pharmacy residency support service using the nominal group technique. *J Am Pharm Assoc.* 2002;42:646–51.

8. Draugalis J, Bootman JL, McGhan WF, Larson LN. Attitudes of pharmacy students toward graduate education and research activities: suggestions for recruitment activities. *Am J Pharm Educ.* 1989; 53:111-20.

Chapter 11 | Current Issues in Pharmacy

This final chapter of *Pharmacy: An Introduction to the Profession* provides selected readings from recent pharmacy literature. Its purpose is to give the future pharmacist an appreciation for contemporary discussions of areas of controversy and detailed information on topics presented in other chapters of this textbook.

A list of updated readings is available through the Publications page of APhA's Web site, www.pharmacist.com. Please check it to access articles published after this book was printed.

Medication Therapy Management

Gans JA. Fulfilling pharmacy's destiny: a project for the ages. Pharm Today. 2008(May):14. (textbook page 109)
In this editorial, APhA's Executive Vice President comments on plans to transform community pharmacies into health care centers.

American Pharmacists Association and the National Association of Chain Drug Stores Foundation. Medication therapy management in pharmacy practice: Core elements of an MTM service model (version 2.0). J Am Pharm Assoc. 2008;48:341–53. (textbook pages 110–122)
This document updates the five basic services—the "core elements"—pharmacists should uniformly provide when delivering MTM services to patients: medication therapy review, personal medication record, medication-related action plan, intervention and referral, and documentation and follow-up.

Schommer JC, Planas LG, Johnson KA, Doucette WR. Pharmacist-provided medication therapy management (part 1): provider perspectives in 2007. J Am Pharm Assoc. 2008;48:354–63. (textbook pages 123–132)
The diffusion of MTM services into pharmacy practice is documented in this report on the second year of coverage under the Medicare Part D prescription drug benefit.

Schommer JC, Planas LG, Johnson KA, Doucette WR. Pharmacist-provided medication therapy management (part 2): payer perspectives in 2007. J Am Pharm Assoc. 2008;48:478–86. (textbook pages 133–141)
In this complementary article, payers add their perspective on the value of MTM services and plans for expanded coverage in the future.

Fera T, Bluml BM, Ellis WM, et al. The Diabetes Ten City Challenge: interim clinical and humanistic outcomes of a multisite community pharmacy diabetes care program. J Am Pharm Assoc. 2008;48:181–90. (textbook pages 142–151)
The American Pharmacists Association Foundation has been instrumental in demonstrating the impact of pharmacists' MTM services to employees and their dependents.

This report shows that the professional practice model can be scaled up from local demonstration projects and replicated in a wide variety of employer and geographic settings.

Somma McGivney M, Meyer SM, Duncan–Hewitt W, et al. Medication therapy management: its relationship to patient counseling, disease management, and pharmaceutical care. J Am Pharm Assoc. 2007;47:620–8. (textbook pages 152–160)
Pharmacy has had a succession of buzzwords to describe its approach to clinical practice. This article compares and contrasts the concepts of patient counseling, disease management, pharmaceutical care, and MTM.

Posey LM. Stebbins integrates MTM Core Elements into office-based practice. Pharm Today. 008(Mar):56–62. (textbook pages 161–167)
Working in a 120-physician group practice in Sacramento, Calif., Marilyn Stebbins, PharmD, exemplifies the new frontier of pharmacists providing MTM to patients day in and day out.

Challenges in the Pharmacy Workplace

Knapp KK, Cultice JM. New pharmacist supply projections: lower separation rates and increased graduates boost supply estimates. J Am Pharm Assoc. 2007;47:463–70. (textbook pages 168–175)
While the supply of pharmacists has been increased by the recent trends documented in this article, demand continues to be healthy, and salaries are higher than ever.

Walton SM, Knapp KK, Miller L, Schumock GT. Examination of state-level changes in the pharmacist labor market using Census data. J Am Pharm Assoc. 2007;47:348–57. (textbook pages 176–185)
When there's a pharmacist shortage, some states are more affected than others, as this article demonstrates.

Brown CM, Cantu R, Corbell Z, Roberts K. Attitudes and interests of pharmacists regarding independent pharmacy ownership. J Am Pharm Assoc. 2007;47:174–80. (textbook pages 186–192)
Once a profession dominated by owners of independent pharmacies, pharmacy is now more of a profession of employees of large corporations and health systems. This article quantifies that shift in pharmacists' priorities and preferences.

Egervary A. Preparing health care for baby boomers' golden years. Pharm Today. 2008(May):36. (textbook page 193)
As mentioned in Chapter 1, the baby boomers are reaching retirement age, and the health care system is inadequately prepared for the coming onslaught of seniors.

Assuring Quality in Health Care

Sheffer J. Paving the way for high-quality health care. Pharm Today. 2008(Jan):49–50. (textbook pages 194–195)
This article discusses mechanisms that might someday reimburse pharmacies and pharmacists based on outcomes rather than specific services rendered. "Pay for performance," a trend in health care financing known by the acronym P4P, could one day change the face of pharmacy.

editorial

Fulfilling pharmacy's destiny: A project for the ages

Even in a world where change is a daily occurrence, inertia remains strong. Pharmacists are wont to focus on the "way we have always done it," some physicians hold on to a patriarchal model of health care, and patients may come into the pharmacy with a set of expectations that center around how little time and money they need to spend there.

Given these realities, APhA, the National Association of Chain Drug Stores (NACDS), and the National Community Pharmacists Association (NCPA) began talking some time ago about what it would take for community chain and independent pharmacies to become and to be recognized as health care centers rather than mercantile outlets. The effort, Project Destiny (see article, page 46) has a simple but ambitious mission: develop a replicable, scalable, measurable, and economically viable future model for community pharmacy.

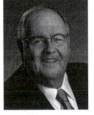

John A. Gans, PharmD, APhA Executive Vice President and CEO

Why pursue such a mission? In short, because our patients need us to and because we as pharmacists can do so and are uniquely accessible for doing so. The scope of adverse medication events among ambulatory Americans is simply unacceptable. Every day, preventable medication-related adverse events, toxicities, hospitalizations, and deaths affect thousands of our patients, even as others suffer from diseases and conditions that could have been prevented by appropriate treatment. Patients lack adequate understanding of how to take their medications properly and why adhering to and persisting with therapy is so important. As pharmacists, we all know of patients whose lives we have changed through the simple act of counseling about a prescription or OTC medication. Imagine how much more we could accomplish if we could provide a full set of medication therapy management (MTM) services to all patients with chronic diseases and complicated drug regimens.

The strategic plan we have developed through Project Destiny emphasizes the need for viability of MTM programs. This model must be replicable; it can't be something that only works in a few pharmacies with unique practices or circumstances. The way of caring for patients must be scalable, in that pharmacy education—including our schools and colleges of pharmacy, as well as our continuing education providers—must be prepared to ensure that pharmacists in all community pharmacies have the required knowledge and skills. Outcomes we can effect through MTM services must be measurable so that payers will cover them, our colleagues in other health professions will accept them, and, in the long run, our patients will demand them. Finally, the economic viability of this model is a given, as the health care system in our country is built around strong independent health care providers, group practices, and regional and national companies that must make ends meet to survive.

Project Destiny is supported financially by several pharmaceutical companies that recognize the key role that pharmacists can play in the clinical and financial success of their products. I would like to personally thank our partners in this effort: sanofi-aventis, GlaxoSmithKline, Boehringer Ingelheim Pharmaceuticals, Pfizer U.S. Pharmaceuticals, and Wyeth.

Since pharmacy's earliest days as purveyor of medicinal pastes, roots, and herbs, our profession has been centered economically around the provision of product. Only in recent times have we realized that we have always—and freely—shared our knowledge of medications and the information about the importance of pharmacotherapy in the prevention and treatment of their ailments. We now know that many patients and payers recognize the value of that service and are willing to reward it financially. Through Project Destiny, APhA, NACDS, and NCPA seek to establish the corner pharmacy as a health care center and community pharmacists as key partners in the management of the complicated and powerful drug regimens that are now the mainstay of disease therapy for people everywhere. These are exciting times, and the Project Destiny partners look forward to working with you in developing a new pharmacy for the future.

www.pharmacytoday.org

SPECIAL FEATURE

Medication therapy management in pharmacy practice: Core elements of an MTM service model (version 2.0)

American Pharmacists Association and the National Association of Chain Drug Stores Foundation

Abstract

Objective: To further develop the service model for medication therapy management (MTM) delivery by pharmacists in settings where patients or their caregivers can be actively involved in managing their medications.

Data sources: Peer-reviewed literature, structured discussions with pharmacy leaders from diverse patient care settings, input from pharmacists and pharmacy associations, recommendations on patient-centered documents (personal medication record and medication-related action plan) from experts in the field of health literacy, and incorporation of extensive feedback received during an extended public comment period open to all MTM stakeholders and interested parties.

Summary: Built on an MTM consensus definition adopted by 11 national pharmacy organizations in July 2004, Medication Therapy Management in Community Pharmacy Practice: Core Elements of an MTM Service (Version 1.0) described core elements of an MTM service model that can be provided by pharmacists across the spectrum of community pharmacy. Version 2.0 of that model, presented in this article, maintains the original five core elements of an MTM service: medication therapy review (MTR), a personal medication record (PMR), a medication-related action plan (MAP), intervention and referral, and documentation and follow-up. The MTR can be comprehensive or targeted, depending on the needs of the patient. In Version 2.0, the PMR and MAP have been redesigned with the assistance of a health literacy expert to be more "patient friendly," effective, and efficient for patients to use in medication self-management.

Conclusion: The developing service model presented in this article for use by pharmacists involved in providing MTM services in diverse patient care settings consists of five core elements. The service model provides a consistent and recognizable framework for MTM service delivery by pharmacists that enhances efficient delivery of the service and improves patient outcomes.

Keywords: Medication therapy management, Medicare, pharmaceutical care, medication self-management, coordination of care.

J Am Pharm Assoc. 2008;48:341–353.

doi: 10.1331/JAPhA.2008.08514

Developed through a joint initiative of the American Pharmacists Association and the National Association of Chain Drug Stores Foundation.

Correspondence: Anne Burns, BPharm, American Pharmacists Association, 1100 15th St., NW, Suite 400, Washington, DC 20005. Fax: 202-628-0443. E-mail: aburns@aphanet.org

Disclosure: The organizations declare no conflicts of interest regarding products or services discussed in this manuscript. The authors declare no conflicts of interest or financial interests in any product or service mentioned in this article, including grants, employment, gifts, stock holdings, or honoraria.

Acknowledgments: Individuals and organizations participating in the review of this document are listed in Appendices 1 and 2.

Eleven national pharmacy organizations achieved consensus on a definition of medication therapy management (MTM) in July 2004 (Appendix 3). Building on the consensus definition, the American Pharmacists Association (APhA) and the National Association of Chain Drug Stores (NACDS) Foundation developed a model framework for implementing effective MTM services in a community pharmacy setting by publishing Medication Therapy Management in Community Pharmacy Practice: Core Elements of an MTM Service (version 1.0). The original Version 1.0 document described the foundational or core elements of MTM services that could be provided by pharmacists across the spectrum of community pharmacy.[1]

Medication Therapy Management in Pharmacy Practice: Core Elements of an MTM Service Model (version 2.0) is an evolutionary document that focuses on the provision of MTM services in settings where patients[a] or their caregivers can be actively involved in managing their medications. This service model was developed with the input of an advisory panel of pharmacy leaders representing diverse pharmacy practice settings (listed in Appendix 1). While adoption of this model is voluntary, it is important to note that this model is crafted to maximize both effectiveness and efficiency of MTM service delivery across pharmacy practice settings in an effort to improve continuity of care and patient outcomes.[b]

At a Glance

Synopsis: Working with an expert advisory panel, and with input from national pharmacy organizations and other stakeholders, the American Pharmacists Association and the National Association of Chain Drug Stores Foundation have refined version 1.0 of the core elements of a medication therapy management (MTM) service model. The resulting version 2.0 contains the five core elements from the version 1.0 model: medication therapy review (MTR), a personal medication record (PMR), a medication-related action plan (MAP), intervention and referral, and documentation and follow-up. The new version can be implemented in more diverse patient care settings and places a greater emphasis on patient transitions of care, health care provider collaboration, and documentation requirements.

Analysis: As reflected in environmental scans of providers and payers being published in this and the next issue of JAPhA, MTM is taking hold in cities and towns across the country. The adoption of these core elements by pharmacists when providing MTM will advance comprehension by prescribers and patients of what they can expect during and following MTM visits. The result will be widespread availability of a consistent MTM service that increases opportunities for pharmacists and improves care for patients.

Medication Therapy Management in Pharmacy Practice: Core Elements of an MTM Service Model (Version 2.0) is designed to improve collaboration among pharmacists, physicians, and other health care professionals; enhance communication between patients and their health care team; and optimize medication use for improved patient outcomes. The MTM services described in this model empower patients to take an active role in managing their medications. The services are dependent on pharmacists working collaboratively with physicians and other health care professionals to optimize medication use in accordance with evidence-based guidelines.[2,3]

MTM services, as described in this model, are distinct from medication dispensing and focus on a patient-centered, rather than an individual product–centered, process of care.[4,c]

MTM services encompass the assessment and evaluation of the patient's complete medication therapy regimen, rather than focusing on an individual medication product. This model framework describes core elements of MTM service delivery in pharmacy practice and does not represent a specific minimum or maximum level of all services that could be delivered by pharmacists.[5]

Medication-related problems are a significant public health issue within the health care system. Incidence estimates suggest that more than 1.5 million preventable medication-related adverse events occur each year in the United States, accounting for an excess of $177 billion in terms of medication-related morbidity and mortality.[6,7] The Institute of Medicine advocates that health care should be safe, effective, patient centered, timely, efficient, and effective to meet patients' needs and that patients should be active participants in the health care process to prevent medication-related problems.[3,7]

MTM services, as described in this service model, may help address the urgent public health need for the prevention of medication-related morbidity and mortality.[3] MTM services may contribute to medication error prevention, result in improved reliability of health care delivery, and enable patients to take an active role in medication and health care self-management.[7] The MTM services outlined in this model are aligned with the expectations of the Centers for Medicare & Medicaid Services, as stated in the Medicare Prescription Drug, Improvement, and Modernization Act of 2003, that MTM services will enhance patient understanding of appropriate drug use, increase adherence to medication therapy, and improve detection of adverse drug events.[8]

MTM programs are demonstrating positive clinical, economic, and humanistic outcomes across diverse patient populations in various patient care settings.[9–15] MTM services are currently being delivered in both the public and private sectors. In the public sector, some state Medicaid and Medicare Part D plans have focused on a comprehensive medication therapy review as the foundation of their MTM programs. Pharmacists participating in these programs often provide patients with an initial comprehensive assessment and ongoing follow-up assessments to identify and resolve medication-related problems.[11,16–20]

In the private sector, MTM programs are beginning to emerge nationwide, offering MTM services to traditional insured groups, managed care populations, self-insured employers, and self-paying individual patients.[9,10,12]

Any patient who uses prescription and nonprescription medications, herbal products, or other dietary supplements could potentially benefit from the MTM core elements outlined in this model. As part of the effort to effectively address the urgent public health issue of medication-related morbidity and mortality, MTM services should be considered for any patient with actual or potential medication-related problems, regardless of the number of medications they use, their specific disease states, or their health plan coverage. Although MTM program structure and the needs of individual patients may vary, the use of a consistent and recognizable framework for core MTM services, as described in this model, will enhance their efficient delivery and effective quality measurement. As new opportunities arise, pharmacists in all practice settings must share a common vision for patient-centered MTM services that improve medication therapy outcomes and provide value within our nation's health care system.

Framework for pharmacist-provided MTM services

This framework for MTM service delivery in pharmacy practice is designed to facilitate collaboration among the pharmacist, patient, physician, and other health care professionals to promote safe and effective medication use and achieve optimal patient outcomes. MTM services in all patient care settings should include structures supporting the establishment and maintenance of the patient–pharmacist relationship.

Providing MTM services in various patient care settings

Patients with a potential need for MTM services can be identified by the pharmacist, physician, or other health care professionals; the health plan; or patients themselves when medication-related problems are suspected. Appendix 4 provides considerations for identification of patients who may benefit from MTM services. Patients may be especially vulnerable to medication-related problems during transitions of care, such as when their health care setting changes, when they change physicians, or when their payer status changes.[d]

These transitions of care often result in medication therapy changes that may be due to changes in the patient's needs or resources, the patient's health status or condition, or formulary requirements. It is important that systems be established so that pharmacist-provided MTM services can focus on reconciling the patient's medications and ensuring the provision of appropriate medication management during transitions of care.

For ambulatory patients, MTM services typically are offered by appointment but may be provided on a walk-in basis. MTM services should be delivered in a private or semiprivate area, as required by the Health Insurance Portability and Accountability Act, by a pharmacist whose time can be devoted to the patient during this service.[21] In other patient care settings (e.g., acute care, long-term care, home care, managed care), the environment in which MTM services are delivered may differ because of variability in structure and facilities design. Even so, to the extent that MTM core elements are implemented, a consistent approach to their delivery should be maintained.

The delivery of MTM services by the pharmacist

Within the MTM core elements service model, the patient receives an annual comprehensive medication therapy review and additional medication therapy reviews according to the patient's needs. The patient may require ongoing monitoring by the pharmacist to address new or recurring medication-related problems.

The total number of reviews required to successfully manage a patient's therapy will vary from patient to patient and will be ultimately determined by the complexity of the individual patient's medication-related problems. The extent of health plan benefits or other limitations imposed by the patient's payer may affect coverage for MTM services; however, this would not preclude additional services provided by the pharmacist for which the patient pays on a fee-for-service basis.

To perform the most comprehensive assessment of a patient, personal interaction with direct contact between a health care professional and a patient is optimal. A face-to-face interaction optimizes the pharmacist's ability to observe signs of and visual cues to the patient's health problems (e.g., adverse reactions to medications, lethargy, alopecia, extrapyramidal symptoms, jaundice, disorientation) and can enhance the patient–pharmacist relationship.[22] The pharmacist's observations may result in early detection of medication-related problems and thus have the potential to reduce inappropriate medication use, emergency department visits, and hospitalizations. It is recognized, however, that alternative methods of patient contact and interaction, such as telephonic, may be necessary for those patients for whom a face-to-face interaction is not possible or not desired (e.g., homebound patients) or in pharmacy practice settings in which the pharmacist serves in a consultative role on the health care team. Irrespective of whether the MTM service is provided by the pharmacist to the patient face to face or by alternative means, the service is intended to support the establishment and maintenance of the patient–pharmacist relationship.

Core elements of an MTM service model in pharmacy practice

The MTM service model in pharmacy practice includes the following five core elements:

- Medication therapy review (MTR)
- Personal medication record (PMR)
- Medication-related action plan (MAP)

- Intervention and/or referral
- Documentation and follow-up

These five core elements form a framework for the delivery of MTM services in pharmacy practice. Every core element is integral to the provision of MTM; however, the sequence and delivery of the core elements may be modified to meet an individual patient's needs.

Medication therapy review

The medication therapy review (MTR) is a systematic process of collecting patient-specific information, assessing medication therapies to identify medication-related problems, developing a prioritized list of medication-related problems, and creating a plan to resolve them.

An MTR is conducted between the patient and the pharmacist. Pharmacist-provided MTR and consultation in various settings has resulted in reductions in physician visits, emergency department visits, hospital days, and overall health care costs.[9,10,12,14,20,23–25] In addition, pharmacists have been shown to obtain accurate and efficient medication-related information from patients.[10,26,27] The MTR is designed to improve patients' knowledge of their medications, address problems or concerns that patients may have, and empower patients to self-manage their medications and their health condition(s).

The MTR can be comprehensive or targeted to an actual or potential medication-related problem. Regardless of whether the MTR is comprehensive or targeted, patients may be identified as requiring this service in a variety of ways. Commonly, patients may be referred to a pharmacist by their health plan, another pharmacist, physician, or other health care professionals. Patients may also request an MTR independent of any referral. Additional opportunities for providing an MTR include when a patient is experiencing a transition of care, when actual or potential medication-related problems are identified, or if the patient is suspected to be at higher risk for medication-related problems.

In a comprehensive MTR, ideally the patient presents all current medications to the pharmacist, including all prescription and nonprescription medications, herbal products, and other dietary supplements. The pharmacist then assesses the patient's medications for the presence of any medication-related problems, including adherence, and works with the patient, the physician, or other health care professionals to determine appropriate options for resolving identified problems. In addition, the pharmacist supplies the patient with education and information to improve the patient's self-management of his or her medications.

Targeted MTRs are used to address an actual or potential medication-related problem. Ideally, targeted MTRs are performed for patients who have received a comprehensive MTR. Whether for a new problem or subsequent monitoring, the pharmacist assesses the specific therapy problem in the context of the patient's complete medical and medication history. Follow-

ing assessment, the pharmacist intervenes and provides education and information to the patient, the physician or other health care professionals, or both, as appropriate. The MTR is tailored to the individual needs of the patient at each encounter.

Depending on its scope, the MTR may include the following:

- Interviewing the patient to gather data, including demographic information, general health and activity status, medical history, medication history, immunization history, and patients' thoughts or feelings about their conditions and medication use[28]
- Assessing, on the basis of all relevant clinical information available to the pharmacist, the patient's physical and overall health status, including current and previous diseases or conditions
- Assessing the patient's values, preferences, quality of life, and goals of therapy
- Assessing cultural issues, education level, language barriers, literacy level, and other characteristics of the patient's communication abilities that could affect outcomes
- Evaluating the patient to detect symptoms that could be attributed to adverse events caused by any of his or her current medications
- Interpreting, monitoring, and assessing the patient's laboratory results
- Assessing, identifying, and prioritizing medication-related problems related to
  —The clinical appropriateness of each medication being taken by the patient, including benefit versus risk
  —The appropriateness of the dose and dosing regimen of each medication, including consideration of indications, contraindications, potential adverse effects, and potential problems with concomitant medications
  —Therapeutic duplication or other unnecessary medications
  —Adherence to the therapy
  —Untreated diseases or conditions
  —Medication cost considerations
  —Health care/medication access considerations
- Developing a plan for resolving each medication-related problem identified
- Providing education and training on the appropriate use of medications and monitoring devices and the importance of medication adherence and understanding treatment goals
- Coaching patients to be empowered to manage their medications
- Monitoring and evaluating the patient's response to therapy, including safety and effectiveness
- Communicating appropriate information to the physician or other health care professionals, including consultation on the selection of medications, suggestions to address identified medication problems, updates on the patient's progress, and recommended follow-up care[29]

In this service model, a patient would receive an annual comprehensive MTR and additional targeted MTRs to address new or ongoing medication-related problem(s). Significant events such as important changes in the patient's medication therapy, changes in the patient's needs or resources, changes in the patient's health status or condition, a hospital admission or discharge, an emergency department visit, or an admission or discharge from a long-term care or assisted-living facility could necessitate additional comprehensive MTRs.

Personal medication record

The personal medication record (PMR) is a comprehensive record of the patient's medications (prescription and nonprescription medications, herbal products, and other dietary supplements).

Within the MTM core elements service model, the patient receives a comprehensive record of his or her medications (prescription and nonprescription medications, herbal products, and other dietary supplements) that has been completed either by the patient with the assistance of the pharmacist or by the pharmacist, or the patient's existing PMR is updated. Ideally, the patient's PMR would be generated electronically, but it also may be produced manually. Whether the pharmacist provides the PMR manually or electronically, the information should be written at a literacy level that is appropriate for and easily understood by the patient. In institutional settings, the PMR may be created at discharge from the medication administration record or patient chart for use by the patient in the outpatient setting. The PMR contains information to assist the patient in his or her overall medication therapy self-management. A sample PMR is shown in Figure 1.

The PMR, which is intended for use by the patient, may include the following information[30]:

- Patient name
- Patient birth date
- Patient telephone number
- Emergency contact information (name, relationship, and telephone number)
- Primary care physician (name and telephone number)
- Pharmacy/pharmacist (name and telephone number)
- Allergies (e.g., What allergies do I have? What happened when I had the allergy or reaction?)
- Other medication-related problems (e.g., What medication caused the problem? What was the problem I had?)
- Potential questions for patients to ask about their medications (e.g., When you are prescribed a new drug, ask your doctor or pharmacist...)
- Date last updated
- Date last reviewed by the pharmacist, physician, or other health care professional
- Patient's signature
- Health care provider's signature
- For each medication, inclusion of the following:
  —Medication (e.g., drug name and dose)
  —Indication (e.g., Take for...)
  —Instructions for use (e.g., When do I take it?)
  —Start date
  —Stop date
  —Ordering prescriber/contact information (e.g., doctor)
  —Special instructions

The PMR is intended for patients to use in medication self-management. The maintenance of the PMR is a collaborative effort among the patient, pharmacist, physician, and other health care professionals. Patients should be encouraged to maintain and update this perpetual document. Patients should be educated to carry the PMR with them at all times and share it at all health care visits and at all admissions to or discharges from institutional settings to help ensure that all health care professionals are aware of their current medication regimen.

Each time the patient receives a new medication; has a current medication discontinued; has an instruction change; begins using a new prescription or nonprescription medication, herbal product, or other dietary supplement; or has any other changes to the medication regimen, the patient should update the PMR to help ensure a current and accurate record. Ideally, the pharmacist, physician, and other health care professionals can actively assist the patient with the PMR revision process.

Pharmacists may use the PMR to communicate and collaborate with physicians and other health care professionals to achieve optimal patient outcomes. Widespread use of the PMR will support uniformity of information provided to all health care professionals and enhance the continuity of care provided to patients while facilitating flexibility to account for pharmacy- or institution-specific variations.

Medication-related action plan

The medication-related action plan (MAP) is a patient-centric document containing a list of actions for the patient to use in tracking progress for self-management.

A care plan is the health professional's course of action for helping a patient achieve specific health goals.[31] The care plan is an important component of the documentation core element outlined in this service model. In addition to the care plan, which is developed by the pharmacist and used in the collaborative care of the patient, the patient receives an individualized MAP for use in medication self-management. Completion of the MAP is a collaborative effort between the patient and the pharmacist. The patient MAP includes only items that the patient can act on that are within the pharmacist's scope of practice or that have been agreed to by relevant members of the health care team. The MAP should not include outstanding action items that still require physician or other health care professional review or approval. The patient can use the MAP as a simple guide to track his or her progress. The Institute of Medicine has advocated the need for a patient-centered model of health care.[7] The patient MAP, coupled with education, is an essential element for incorporating the patient-centered approach into the MTM service model. The MAP reinforces a sense of patient empowerment and

SPECIAL FEATURE MTM CORE ELEMENTS, VERSION 2.0

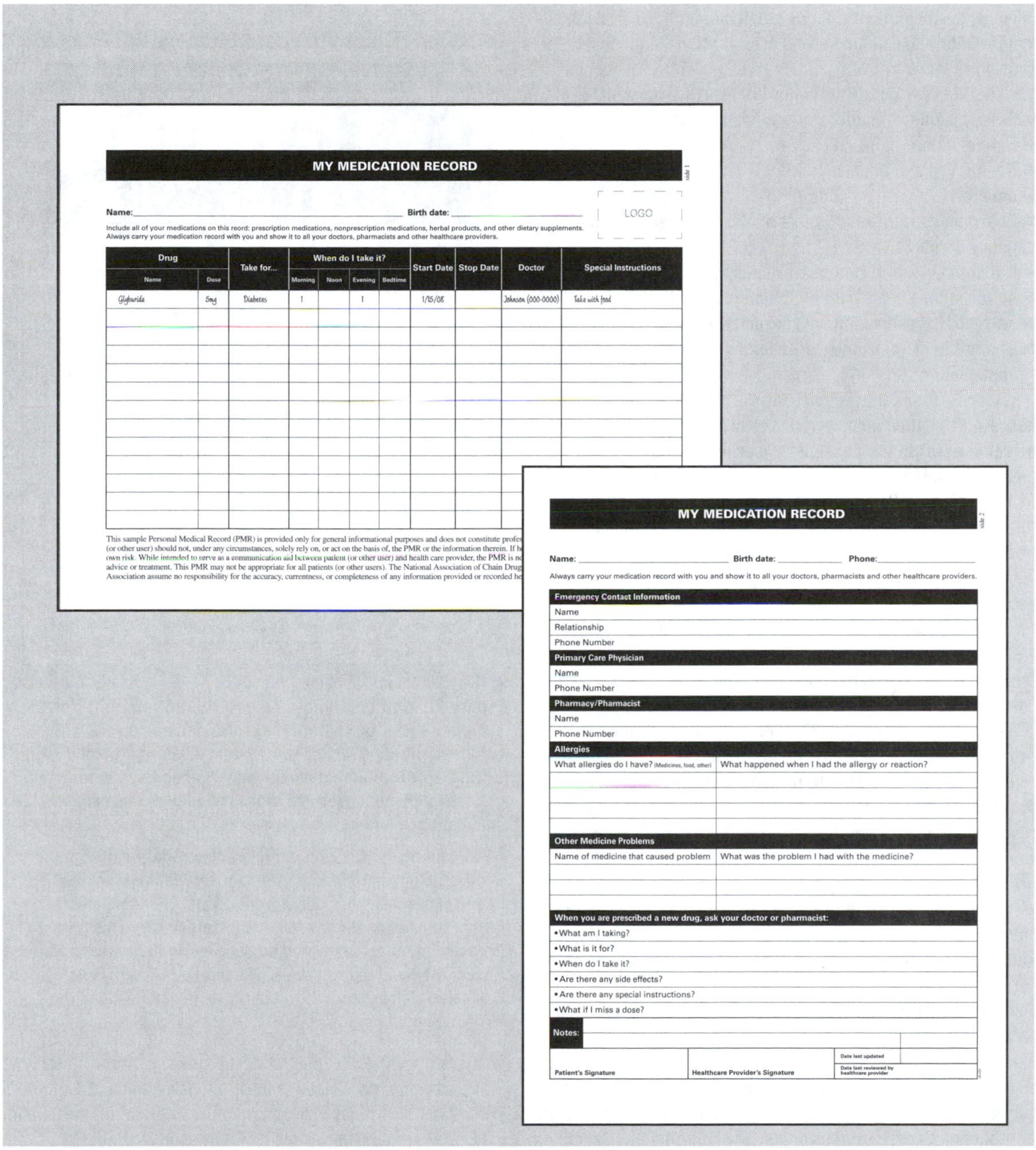

Figure 1. Sample personal medication record. Patients, professionals, payers, and health information technology system vendors are encouraged to develop a format that meets individual needs, collecting elements such as those in this sample personal medication record.

APhA and the NACDS Foundation encourage the use of this document in a manner and form that serves the individual needs of practitioners. All reproductions, including modified forms, should include the following statement: "This form is based on forms developed by the American Pharmacists Association and the National Association of Chain Drug Stores Foundation. Reproduced with permission of APhA and the NACDS Foundation."

encourages the patient's active participation in his or her medication-adherence behavior and overall MTM. A sample MAP is shown in Figure 2.

The MAP, which is intended for use by the patient, may include the following information:

- Patient name
- Primary care physician (doctor's name and telephone number)
- Pharmacy/pharmacist (pharmacy/pharmacist name and telephone number)
- Date of MAP creation (date prepared)
- Action steps for the patient: "What I need to do..."
- Notes for the patient: "What I did and when I did it..."
- Appointment information for follow-up with pharmacist, if applicable

Specific items that require intervention and that have been approved by other members of the health care team and any new items within the pharmacist's scope of practice should be included on a MAP distributed to the patient on a follow-up visit. In institutional settings, the MAP could be established at the time the patient is discharged for use by the patient in medication self-management.

Intervention and/or referral

The pharmacist provides consultative services and intervenes to address medication-related problems; when necessary, the pharmacist refers the patient to a physician or other health care professional.

During the course of an MTM encounter, medication-related problems may be identified that require the pharmacist to intervene on the patient's behalf. Interventions may include collaborating with physicians or other health care professionals to resolve existing or potential medication-related problems or working with the patient directly. The communication of appropriate information to the physician or other health care professional, including consultation on the selection of medications, suggestions to address medication problems, and recommended follow-up care, is integral to the intervention component of the MTM service model.[29]

The positive impact of pharmacist interventions on outcomes related to medication-related problems has been demonstrated in numerous studies.[32-37] Appropriate resolution of medication-related problems involves collaboration and communication between the patient, the pharmacist, and the patient's physician or other health care professionals.

Some patients' medical conditions or medication therapy may be highly specialized or complex, and their needs may extend beyond the core elements of MTM service delivery. In such cases, pharmacists may provide additional services according to their expertise or refer the patient to a physician, another pharmacist, or other health care professional.

Examples of circumstances that may require referral include the following:

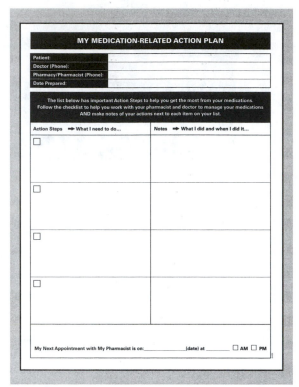

Figure 2. Sample medication-related action plan (for the patient). Patients, health care professionals, payers, and health information technology system vendors are encouraged to develop a format that meets individual and customer needs, collecting elements such as those included in this sample medication-related action plan.

APhA and the NACDS Foundation encourage the use of this document in a manner and form that serves the individual needs of practitioners. All reproductions, including modified forms, should include the following statement: "This form is based on forms developed by the American Pharmacists Association and the National Association of Chain Drug Stores Foundation. Reproduced with permission of APhA and the NACDS Foundation."

- A patient may exhibit potential problems discovered during the MTR that may necessitate referral for evaluation and diagnosis.
- A patient may require disease management education to help him or her manage chronic diseases such as diabetes.
- A patient may require monitoring for high-risk medications (e.g., warfarin, phenytoin, methotrexate).

The intent of intervention and/or referral is to optimize medication use, enhance continuity of care, and encourage patients to avail themselves of health care services to prevent future adverse outcomes.

Documentation and follow-up

MTM services are documented in a consistent manner, and a follow-up MTM visit is scheduled based on the patient's medication-related needs or the patient is transitioned from one care setting to another.

Documentation is an essential element of the MTM service model. The pharmacist documents services and intervention(s) performed in a manner appropriate for evaluating patient progress and sufficient for billing purposes. Proper documentation of MTM services may serve several purposes, including, but not limited to, the following:

- Facilitating communication between the pharmacist and the patient's other health care professionals regarding recommendations intended to resolve or monitor actual or potential medication-related problems
- Improving patient care and outcomes
- Enhancing the continuity of patient care among providers and care settings
- Ensuring compliance with laws and regulations for the maintenance of patient records
- Protecting against professional liability
- Capturing services provided for justification of billing or reimbursement (e.g., payer audits)
- Demonstrating the value of pharmacist-provided MTM services
- Demonstrating clinical, economic, and humanistic outcomes

MTM documentation includes creating and maintaining an ongoing patient-specific record that contains, in chronological order, a record of all provided care in an established standard health care professional format (e.g., the SOAP [subjective observations, objective observations, assessment, and plan] note[38]).

Ideally, documentation will be completed electronically or, alternatively, on paper. The inclusion of resources such as a PMR, a MAP, and other practice-specific forms will assist the pharmacist in maintaining consistent professional documentation. The use of consistent documentation will help facilitate collaboration among members of the health care team while accommodating practitioner, facility, organizational, or regional variations.

Documentation elements for the patient record may include, but are not limited, to the items listed in Table 1.[22,29,38–40]

External communication of MTM documentation

Following documentation of the MTM encounter, appropriate external communication should be provided or sent to key audiences, including patients, physicians, and payers. Providing the patient with applicable documentation that he or she can easily understand is vital to facilitating active involvement in the care process. Documentation provided to the patient at the MTM encounter may include the PMR, MAP, and additional education materials. Documentation to physicians and other health care professionals may include a cover letter, the patient's PMR, the SOAP note, and the care plan. Communicating with payers and providing appropriate billing information may also be necessary and could include the name of the pharmacist or pharmacy and appropriate identifier, services provided, time spent on patient care, and appropriate billing codes.

Table 1. Examples of documentation elements for patient record

Patient demographics/basic information: Address, telephone number, e-mail address, gender, age, ethnicity, educational status, patient's special needs, health plan benefit/insurance coverage
Subjective observations: Pertinent patient-reported information: previous medical history, family history, social history, chief complaints, allergies, previous adverse drug reactions
Objective observations: Known allergies, diseases, conditions, laboratory results, vital signs, diagnostic signs, physical exam results, review of systems
Assessment: Problem list, assessment of medication-related problems
Plan: A care plan is the health care professional's course of action for helping a patient achieve specific health goals
Education: Goal setting and instruction provided to the patient with verification of understanding
Collaboration: Communication with other health care professionals: recommendations, referrals, and correspondence with other professionals (cover letter, SOAP note)
PMR: A record of all medications, including prescription and nonprescription medications, herbal products, and other dietary supplements
MAP: Patient-centric document containing a list of actions to use in tracking progress for self-management
Follow-up: Transition plan or scheduling of next follow-up visit
Billing: Amount of time spent on patient care, level of complexity, amount charged

Abbreviations used: MAP, medication-related action plan; PMR, personal medication record; SOAP, subjective observations, objective observations, assessment, and plan.

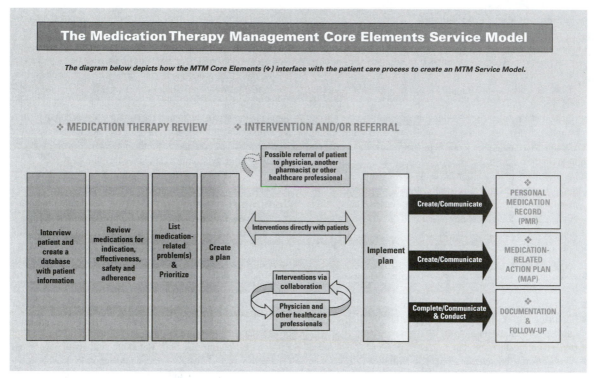

Figure 3. Flow chart of a medication therapy management service model

Abbreviation used: MTM, medication therapy management.

Follow-up

When a patient's care setting changes (e.g., hospital admission, hospital to home, hospital to long-term care facility, home to long-term care facility), the pharmacist transitions the patient to another pharmacist in the patient's new care setting to facilitate continued MTM services. In these situations, the initial pharmacist providing MTM services participates cooperatively with the patient's new pharmacist provider to facilitate the coordinated transition of the patient, including the transfer of relevant medication and other health-related information.

If the patient will be remaining in the same care setting, the pharmacist should arrange for consistent follow-up MTM services in accordance with the patient's unique medication-related needs. All follow-up evaluations and interactions with the patient and his or her other health care professional(s) should be included in MTM documentation.

Conclusion

The MTM core elements, as presented in this document, are intended to be applicable to patients in all care settings where the patients or their caregivers can be actively involved with managing their medication therapy, taking full advantage of the pharmacist's role as the "medication therapy expert." Figure 3 presents a flow chart of the core elements of an MTM service

model contained in this document. As the core elements service model continues to evolve to meet diverse patient needs, pharmacists are encouraged to make the most of the framework provided to improve patient outcomes and medication use.

---

[a]In this document, the term *patient* refers to the patient, caregiver, or other persons involved in the care of the patient.

[b]Notice: The materials in this service model are provided for general informational purposes only and do not constitute business or legal advice. The NACDS Foundation and APhA assume no responsibility for the accuracy or timeliness of any information provided herein. The reader should not under any circumstances solely rely on, or act on the basis of, the materials in this service model. These materials and information are not a substitute for obtaining business or legal advice in the appropriate jurisdiction or state.

The materials in this service model do not represent a standard of care or standard business practices. This service model may not be appropriate for all pharmacists or pharmacies. Service programs should be designed based on unique needs and circumstances, and model examples should be modified as appropriate.

Nothing contained in this service model shall be construed as an express or implicit invitation to engage in any illegal or anticompetitive activity. Nothing contained in this service model shall, or should be, construed as an endorsement of any particular method of treatment or pharmacy practice in general.

[c]MTM services are built on the philosophy and process of pharmaceutical care that was first implemented in pharmacy practice in the early 1990s. As pharmacy education, training, and practice continue to evolve to a primarily clinical "patient-centered" focus, pharmacists are gaining recognition from other health care professionals and the public

as "medication therapy experts." Recognizing the pharmacist's role as the medication therapy expert, the pharmacy profession has developed a consensus definition for MTM and is increasingly using this term to describe the services provided by pharmacists to patients.

dExamples of transitions of care may include but are not limited to changes in health care setting (e.g., hospital admission, hospital to home, hospital to long-term care facility, home to long-term care facility), changes in health care professionals and/or level of care (e.g., treatment by a specialist), or changes in payer status (e.g., change or loss of health plan benefits/insurance).

Appendix 1. Medication therapy management model advisory panel

Medication Therapy Management in Pharmacy Practice: Core Elements of an MTM Service Model (Version 2.0) was developed with the input of an advisory panel of pharmacy leaders representing diverse pharmacy practice settings. The pharmacy practice setting areas represented by members of the advisory panel included ambulatory care, community, government technical support services, hospital, long-term care, managed care health systems, managed care organization plan administration, and outpatient clinics. Advisory panel members provided expert advice. The content of this document does not necessarily represent all of their opinions or those of their affiliated organizations.

Marialice S. Bennett, BPharm, FAPhA
Ohio State University

Rebecca W. Chater, BPharm, MPH, FAPhA
Kerr Drug, Inc.

Kimberly Sasser Croley, PharmD, CGP, FASCP
Knox County Hospital

Rachael Deck, PharmD
Walgreen Co.

Jeffrey C. Delafuente, MS, FCCP, FASCP
Virginia Commonwealth University School of Pharmacy

Susan L. Downard, BPharm
Kaiser Permanente of the Mid-Atlantic States, Inc.

Margherita Giuliano, BPharm
Connecticut Pharmacists Association

Zandra Glenn, PharmD
HRSA Pharmacy Services Support Center

Melinda C. Joyce, PharmD, FAPhA, FACHE
The Medical Center

Sandra Leal, PharmD, CDE
El Rio Community Health Center

Macary Weck Marciniak, PharmD, BCPS
Albany College of Pharmacy

Randy P. McDonough, PharmD, MS, CGP, BCPS
Towncrest and Medical Plaza Pharmacies

Melissa Somma McGivney, PharmD, CDE
University of Pittsburgh School of Pharmacy

Rick Mohall, PharmD
Rite Aid Corporation

Anthony Provenzano, PharmD, CDE
SUPERVALU Pharmacies, Inc.

Michael Sherry, BPharm
CVS Caremark

Steven T. Simenson, BPharm, FAPhA
Goodrich Pharmacies

Donna S. Wall, BPharm, PharmD, BCPS, FASHP
Clarian Healthcare Partners, Indiana University Hospital

Winston Wong, PharmD
CareFirst BCBS

Staff
Ben Bluml, BPharm
American Pharmacists Association Foundation

Anne Burns, BPharm
American Pharmacists Association

Ronna Hauser, PharmD
National Association of Chain Drug Stores

Crystal Lennartz, PharmD, MBA
National Association of Chain Drug Stores

James Owen, PharmD
American Pharmacists Association

Afton Yurkon, PharmD
National Association of Chain Drug Stores

Abbreviations used: BCBS, BlueCross BlueShield; HRSA, Health Resources and Services Administration.

Appendix 2. Organizations contributing to medication therapy management model

APhA and the NACDS Foundation respectfully acknowledge the contributions of all individuals and organizations that participated in the development of Medication Therapy Management in Pharmacy Practice: Core Elements of an MTM Service Model (Version 2.0). This service model is supported by the following seven organizations:

- American Association of Colleges of Pharmacy
- American College of Apothecaries
- American College of Clinical Pharmacy
- American Society of Consultant Pharmacists
- American Society of Health-System Pharmacists
- National Alliance of State Pharmacy Associations
- National Community Pharmacists Association

Appendix 3. Definition of medication therapy management[a]

Medication therapy management (MTM) is a distinct service or group of services that optimize therapeutic outcomes for individual patients. MTM services are independent of, but can occur in conjunction with, the provision of a medication product. MTM encompasses a broad range of professional activities and responsibilities within the licensed pharmacist's or other qualified health care provider's scope of practice. These services include but are not limited to the following, according to the individual needs of the patient:

- Performing or obtaining necessary assessments of the patient's health status
- Formulating a medication treatment plan
- Selecting, initiating, modifying, or administering medication therapy
- Monitoring and evaluating the patient's response to therapy, including safety and effectiveness
- Performing a comprehensive medication review to identify, resolve, and prevent medication-related problems, including adverse drug events
- Documenting the care delivered and communicating essential information to the patient's other primary care providers
- Providing verbal education and training designed to enhance patient understanding and appropriate use of his/her medications
- Providing information, support services, and resources designed to enhance patient adherence with his/her therapeutic regimens
- Coordinating and integrating MTM services within the broader health care management services being provided to the patient

A program that provides coverage for MTM services shall include the following:

- Patient-specific and individualized services or sets of services provided directly by a pharmacist to the patient.[b] These services are distinct from formulary development and use, generalized patient education and information activities, and other population-focused quality-assurance measures for medication use
- Face-to-face interaction between the patient[b] and the pharmacist as the preferred method of delivery. When patient-specific barriers to face-to-face communication exist, patients shall have equal access to appropriate alternative delivery methods. MTM programs shall include structures supporting the establishment and maintenance of the patient[b]–pharmacist relationship
- Opportunities for pharmacists and other qualified health care providers to identify patients who should receive MTM services
- Payment for MTM services consistent with contemporary provider payment rates that are based on the time, clinical intensity, and resources required to provide services (e.g., Medicare Part A and/or Part B for CPT and RBRVS)
- Processes to improve continuity of care, outcomes, and outcome measures

Approved July 27, 2004, by the Academy of Managed Care Pharmacy, the American Association of Colleges of Pharmacy, the American College of Apothecaries, the American College of Clinical Pharmacy, the American Society of Consultant Pharmacists, the American Pharmacists Association, the American Society of Health-System Pharmacists, the National Association of Boards of Pharmacy,[c] the National Association of Chain Drug Stores, the National Community Pharmacists Association, and the National Council of State Pharmacy Association Executives (now the National Alliance of State Pharmacy Associations).

Abbreviations used: CPT, Current Procedural Terminology; MTM, medication therapy management; RBRVS, resource-based relative value scale.

[a]Bluml BM. Definition of medication therapy management: development of professionwide consensus. J Am Pharm Assoc. 2005;45:566–72.

[b]In some situations, MTM services may be provided to the caregiver or other persons involved in the care of the patient.

[c]Organization policy does not allow the National Association of Boards of Pharmacy to take a position on payment issues.

Appendix 4. Considerations for identification of patients who may benefit from MTM services

Any patients using prescription and nonprescription medications, herbal products, and other dietary supplements could potentially benefit from the medication therapy management (MTM) services described in the core elements outlined in this service model, especially if medication-related problems or issues are discovered or suspected. Patients may be evaluated for MTM services regardless of the number of medications they use, their specific disease state(s), or their health plan coverage.

Opportunities for the identification of patients targeted for MTM services may result from many sources, including, but not limited to, pharmacist identification, physician referral, patient self-referral, and health plan or other payer referral. Pharmacists may wish to notify physicians or other health care professionals in their community or physicians within their facility, if applicable, of their MTM services, so that physicians may refer patients for MTM services.

To provide assistance in prioritizing who may benefit most from MTM services, pharmacists, health plans, physicians, other health care professionals, and health systems may consider using one or more of the following factors to target patients who are likely to benefit most from MTM services:

- Patient has experienced a transition of care, and his or her regimen has changed
- Patient is receiving care from more than one prescriber
- Patient is taking five or more chronic medications (including prescription and nonprescription medications, herbal products, and other dietary supplements)
- Patient has at least one chronic disease or chronic health condition (e.g., heart failure, diabetes, hypertension, hyperlipidemia, asthma, osteoporosis, depression, osteoarthritis, chronic obstructive pulmonary disease)
- Patient has laboratory values outside the normal range that could be caused by or may be improved with medication therapy
- Patient has demonstrated nonadherence (including underuse and overuse) to a medication regimen
- Patient has limited health literacy or cultural differences and therefore requires special communication strategies to optimize care
- Patient wants or needs to reduce out-of-pocket medication costs
- Patient has experienced a loss of or significant change in health plan benefit or insurance coverage
- Patient has recently experienced an adverse event (medication- or non–medication-related) while receiving care
- Patient is taking high-risk medication(s), including narrow therapeutic index drugs (e.g., warfarin, phenytoin, methotrexate)
- Patient self-identifies and presents with perceived need for MTM services

Abbreviation used: MTM, medication therapy management.

References

1. American Pharmacists Association, National Association of Chain Drug Stores Foundation. Medication therapy management in community pharmacy practice: core elements of an MTM service (version 1.0). J Am Pharm Assoc. 2005;45:573–9.
2. Wagner EH. Chronic disease management: what will it take to improve care for chronic illness? Eff Clin Pract. 1998;1(1):2–4.
3. Institute of Medicine. Crossing the quality chasm: a new health system for the 21st century. Washington, D.C.: Institute of Medicine; 2001.
4. Cipolle RJ, Strand LM, Morley PC. Pharmaceutical care practice: the clinician's guide. New York: McGraw Hill; 2004.
5. McGivney MS, Meyer SM, Duncan-Hewitt W, et al. Medication therapy management: its relationship to patient counseling, disease management, and pharmaceutical care. J Am Pharm Assoc. 2007;47:620–8.
6. Ernst FR, Grizzle AJ. Drug-related morbidity and mortality: updating the cost-of-illness model. J Am Pharm Assoc. 2001;41:192–9.
7. Institute of Medicine. Report brief: preventing medication errors. Accessed at www.iom.edu/Object.File/Master/35/943/medication%20errors%20new.pdf, September 1, 2007.
8. Centers for Medicare & Medicaid Services. Medicare Prescription Drug Benefit final rule: 42 CFR parts 400, 403, 411, 417, and 423 Medicare Program. Federal Register. 2005;70(18):January 28. Accessed at http://a257.g.akamaitech.net/7/257/2422/01jan20051800/edocket.access.gpo.gov/2005/pdf/05-1321.pdf, September 1, 2007.
9. Garrett D, Bluml B. Patient self-management program for diabetes: first-year clinical, humanistic, and economic outcomes. J Am Pharm Assoc. 2005;45:130–7.
10. Cranor CW, Bunting BA, Christensen DB. The Asheville Project: long-term clinical and economic outcomes of a community pharmacy diabetes care program. J Am Pharm Assoc. 2003;43:173–90.
11. Chrischilles EA, Carter BL, Lund BC, et al. Evaluation of the Iowa Medicaid pharmaceutical case management program. J Am Pharm Assoc. 2004;44:337–49.
12. Bunting BA, Cranor CW. The Asheville Project: long-term clinical, humanistic, and economic outcomes of a community-based medication therapy management program for asthma. J Am Pharm Assoc. 2003;43:133–47.
13. Jameson J, VanNoord G, Vanderwould K. The impact of a pharmacotherapy consultation on the cost and outcome of medical therapy. J Fam Pract. 1995;41:469–72.
14. Lipton HL, Bero LA, Bird JA, et al. The impact of clinical pharmacists' consultations on physicians' geriatric drug prescribing. Med Care. 1992;30:646–58.
15. Schumock GT, Butler MG, Meek PD, et al. Evidence of the economic benefit of clinical pharmacy services: 1996–2000. Pharmacotherapy. 2003;23:113–32.
16. Minnesota Department of Human Services. MHCP enrolled providers. Accessed at www.dhs.state.mn.us/main/idcplg?IdcService=GET_DYNAMIC_CONVERSION&RevisionSelectionMethod=LatestReleased&dDocName=id_000090, February 5, 2007.
17. Traynor K. Wyoming program brings pharmacist consultations home. Am J Health Syst Pharm. 2004;61:760.
18. North Carolina Department of Health and Human Services. North Carolina Medicaid: medication therapy management program (MTMP). Accessed at www.dhhs.state.nc.us/dma/Forms/mtmpinstructions.pdf, September 1, 2007.

19. Touchette DR, Burns AL, Bough MA, et al. Survey of medication therapy management programs under Medicare Part D. J Am Pharm Assoc. 2006;46:683–91.

20. Galt KA. Cost avoidance, acceptance, and outcomes associated with a pharmacotherapy consult clinic in a Veterans Affairs medical center. Pharmacotherapy. 1998;18:1103–11.

21. Rovers J, Currie J, Hagel H, et al. Re-engineering the pharmacy layout. In: A practical guide to pharmaceutical care. 2nd ed. Washington, D.C.: American Pharmacists Association; 2003:261–6.

22. Rovers J, Currie J, Hagel H, et al. Patient data collection. In: A practical guide to pharmaceutical care. 2nd ed. Washington, D.C.: American Pharmacists Association; 2003:26–51.

23. Borgsdorf LR, Miano JS, Knapp KK. Pharmacist-managed medication review in a managed care system. Am J Hosp Pharm. 1994;51:772–7.

24. Bond CA, Raehl CL, Franke T. Clinical pharmacy services, pharmacy staffing, and the total cost of care in the United States hospitals. Pharmacotherapy. 2000;20:609–21.

25. Christensen D, Trygstad T, Sullivan R, et al. A pharmacy management intervention for optimizing drug therapy for nursing home patients. Am J Geriatr Pharmacother. 2004;2:248–56.

26. Gurwich EL. Comparison of medication histories acquired by pharmacists and physicians. Am J Hosp Pharm. 1983;40:1541–2.

27. Nester TM, Hale LS. Effectiveness of a pharmacist-acquired medication history in promoting patient safety. Am J Health Syst Pharm. 2002;59:2221–5.

28. Rovers J, Currie J, Hagel H, et al. The case for pharmaceutical care. In: A practical guide to pharmaceutical care. 2nd ed. Washington, D.C.: American Pharmacists Association; 2003:3–4.

29. Berger BA. Interacting with physicians. In: Communication skills for pharmacists. 2nd ed. Washington, D.C.: American Pharmacists Association; 2005:131–9.

30. American Society of Health-System Pharmacists. Executive summary of the American Society of Health--System Pharmacists (ASHP) and ASHP Research and Education Foundation Continuity of Care in Medication Use Summit. Am J Health Syst Pharm. In press.

31. Rovers J, Currie J, Hagel H, et al. Patient care plan development. In: A practical guide to pharmaceutical care. 2nd ed. Washington, D.C.: American Pharmacists Association; 2003:69.

32. Rupp MT. Value of the community pharmacists' interventions to correct prescribing errors. Ann Pharmacother. 1992;26:1580–4.

33. McMullin ST, Hennenfent JA, Ritchie D, et al. A prospective randomized trial to assess the cost impact of pharmacist-initiated interventions. Arch Intern Med. 1999;159:2306–9.

34. Knapp KK, Katzman H, Hambright JS, et al. Community pharmacist intervention in a capitated pharmacy benefit contract. Am J Health Syst Pharm. 1998;55:1141–5.

35. Dobie RL, Rascati KL. Documenting the value of pharmacist interventions. Am Pharm. 1994;NS34(5):50–4.

36. Hepler CD, Strand LM. Opportunities and responsibilities in pharmaceutical care. Am J Hosp Pharm. 1990;47:533–43.

37. Bootman JL, Harrison DL, Cox E. The healthcare cost of drug-related morbidity and mortality in nursing facilities. Arch Intern Med. 1997;157:2089–96.

38. Zierler-Brown S, Brown TR, Chen D, et al. Clinical documentation for patient care: models, concepts, and liability considerations for pharmacists. Am J Health Syst Pharm. 2007;64:1851–8.

39. Currie JD, Doucette WR, Kuhle J, et al. Identification of essential elements in documentation of pharmacist-provided care. J Am Pharm Assoc. 2003;43:41–9.

40. Culhane N, Brooks A, Cohen V, et al. Medication therapy management services: application of the core elements in ambulatory settings. Accessed at www.accp.com/position/pos_AmCare.pdf, September 1, 2007.

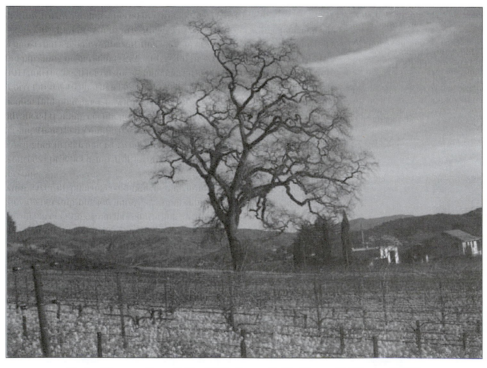

Mustard Season • Napa, Calif. • 2008 • George E. MacKinnon III, BPharm, FASHP

RESEARCH

Pharmacist-provided medication therapy management (part 1): Provider perspectives in 2007

Jon C. Schommer, Lourdes G. Planas, Kathleen A. Johnson, and William R. Doucette

Abstract

Objectives: To collect and describe information from providers of medication therapy management (MTM) services regarding (1) implementation strategies used for providing MTM services to patients/clients; (2) specific measures, if any, used to quantify the costs and benefits of MTM; (3) how the value of MTM services was tracked during 2007; and (4) barriers to offering MTM services to patients/clients.

Design: Descriptive, nonexperimental, cross-sectional study.

Setting: United States during 2007.

Participants: Of the 6,873 providers who presumably received an e-mail invitation to participate in the survey, 687 (10%) responded and were included for analysis.

Interventions: Self-administered online survey.

Main outcome measures: Implementation and monitoring of MTM.

Results: 65% of survey respondents were involved in providing MTM services as defined in the consensus definition used. Of these, 47% reported that they were contracted with programs to provide MTM services. Of respondents, 35% indicated that these contracts provided a positive return on investment (ROI), 31% reported that they did not provide a positive ROI, and 34% reported that they did not know. Providers varied widely on how they implemented MTM service offerings and typically did not use specific measures to quantify the costs and benefits of MTM. In addition, they did not use systematic methods for assessing value from providing MTM services to their patients.

Conclusion: This descriptive environmental scan can serve as a baseline measure and be used for future comparisons.

Keywords: Medication therapy management, cost analysis, pharmacy services, surveys, return on investment.

J Am Pharm Assoc. 2008;48:354–363.
doi: 10.1331/JAPhA.2008.08012

Received January 28, 2008. Accepted for publication March 7, 2008.

Jon C. Schommer, PhD, is Professor, College of Pharmacy, University of Minnesota, Minneapolis. **Lourdes G. Planas, PhD,** is Assistant Professor, College of Pharmacy, University of Oklahoma Health Sciences Center, Oklahoma City. **Kathleen A. Johnson, PhD,** is Associate Professor, School of Pharmacy, University of Southern California, Los Angeles. **William R. Doucette, PhD,** is Professor, College of Pharmacy, and Director, Center for Improving Medication Use in the Community, College of Pharmacy, University of Iowa, Iowa City.

Correspondence: Jon C. Schommer, PhD, Professor, College of Pharmacy, University of Minnesota, 308 Harvard Street, SE, Minneapolis, MN 55455. Fax: 612-625-9931. E-mail: schom010@umn.edu

Disclosure: The authors declare no conflicts of interest or financial interests in any product or service mentioned in this article, including grants, employment, gifts, stock holdings, or honoraria.

Acknowledgments: To American Pharmacists Association (APhA) staff with whom we collaborated for this project: Anne Burns, Maria Gorrick, James Owen, Deborah Ruddy, and Margaret Tomecki.

Funding: By APhA through an unrestricted grant from Wyeth. Data were collected and made available for analysis by APhA.

The expansion of the U.S. Medicare program through the Medicare Prescription Drug, Improvement, and Modernization Act of 2003 (MMA) began an important new chapter in national health policy.[1] MMA provided not only an outpatient prescription drug benefit but also new medication therapy management (MTM) programs for eligible beneficiaries. MTM services were conceived so that therapeutic outcomes would be optimized through improved medication use and through reduced risk of adverse events.[1] During approximately the same period of time, state-based Medicaid programs and self-

At a Glance

Synopsis: A total of 687 individuals who were likely to be involved directly with pharmacist-provided medication therapy management (MTM) services or to be responsible for individuals who provided MTM services completed a self-administered online survey assessing implementation and monitoring of MTM during 2007. Based on a consensus definition provided to these potential MTM service providers, 65% indicated that they provided, 27% indicated that they did not provide, and 8% indicated that they did not know whether they provided MTM. Of the 65% of respondents reporting that they provided MTM services, 47% indicated that they were contracted with programs to provide MTM services. Methods for implementing, quantifying the costs and benefits of, and assessing the value of providing MTM services varied considerably among respondents. Barriers to providing MTM included lack of pharmacist time, insufficient staffing, devoting large amounts of time to dispensing activities, and difficulties in billing for MTM.

Analysis: Diffusing an emerging service such as MTM involves, for example, identifying and recruiting new patient groups, adopting new methods of service provision, using new patient care processes, and adopting new documentation and billing systems. Widespread uptake may be curtailed if current business models are sufficiently profitable and a transition to offering MTM services is viewed as risky. Individual providers are urged to let employers and organizations know that investing in MTM services has merit and that active approaches to implementation and monitoring would be in their best interest. Professional enthusiasm and advocacy for services such as pharmacist-provided MTM can help persuade organizational decision makers to take more active approaches to implementing and evaluating such services. In addition, actively lobbying for MTM could increase the likelihood that practitioners are included in decision making and help ensure that MTM is successfully integrated into practice.

insured employer groups used similar approaches and focused on improving medication therapy outcomes.

These goals of MTM and similar programs are consistent with, and central to, modern pharmacy practice concepts.[2] In light of the strong link between MTM services and modern pharmacy practice, and the specific naming of pharmacists as providers of MTM services for Medicare beneficiaries,[1] the pharmacy profession adopted the terminology and assumed leadership for planning and implementing MTM services for all patients. For example, pharmacy organizations provided leadership for developing business and payment models,[3] consensus definitions,[4] core element frameworks,[5,6] and procedural terminology codes for billing third-party payers,[7–10] therefore enabling the profession to offer a consistent approach for providing MTM services to patients qualifying for and wishing to receive them.

A consensus definition for MTM was achieved among 11 national pharmacy organizations in July 2004,[4] and core elements for providing MTM services were established in 2005 to "maximize both effectiveness and efficiency of MTM service delivery across pharmacy settings in an effort to improve continuity of care and patient outcomes."[5,6] The published definition has served as a foundation for the pharmacy profession and was our focus of inquiry. Thus, for our study, MTM was defined as "a distinct group of services that optimize therapeutic outcomes for individual patients. MTM services are independent of, but can occur in conjunction with, the provision of a medication product. MTM encompasses a broad range of professional activities and responsibilities within the licensed pharmacist's or other qualified health care provider's scope of practice. MTM services encompass those services being provided either via face-to-face contact or telephonically by a pharmacist or other qualified health care professional, but do not include mailings to a patient."[2–6] For clarification, we note that some MTM services provided by companies contracted by the Centers for Medicare & Medicaid Services under Medicare Part D are not considered MTM by this definition and, thus, are not investigated in this study (most notably, e-mail/Internet-based information or educational information mailed to patients and/or practitioners).

Recent reports in the literature describe how MTM services have been implemented in the United States.[11–14] To date, the literature contains information about the initial planning and implementing of MTM services. However, we are not aware of any published reports regarding the value of MTM services to providers and payers of these services. Such information would be useful for future planning and for implementation decisions regarding the use of pharmacist-provided MTM services.

Objectives

To add to what is known about the initial implementation phases of these services and related programs, the purpose of this study was to conduct an environmental scan of pharmacist-provided MTM services during 2007 in which the opinions of payers for these services and providers of these services would be collected and summarized regarding how service implementation is being monitored and value is being assessed. We sought to answer from both payer and provider perspectives these specific questions:

■ What implementation strategies were used for providing MTM services to patients/clients?

■ What specific measures, if any, were used to quantify the costs and benefits of MTM?

■ How was the value of MTM services tracked during 2007?

■ What were the barriers to offering MTM services to patients/clients?

We used the professionwide consensus definition of MTM[4–6] for our study so that the findings could be applied to a diverse array of patient populations and would not be limited to patients who are eligible for MTM services under the Medicare Part D program. Furthermore, we chose to focus specifically on pharmacist-provided MTM for several reasons. First, pharmacists were the health professional group specifically named as MTM providers in MMA.[1] Second, by using this focus, we sought to add to reports in the pharmacy literature on pharmacist-provided MTM.[1–14] Finally, this focus would allow the sponsor of the project (American Pharmacists Association [APhA]) to use the findings in making decisions about how to serve its members and the pharmacy profession. The purpose of the remainder of this article is to report findings from the provider perspective. An article in the July/August issue of *JAPhA* will describe payer perspectives for the study questions; it is available at www.japha.org in advance of print publication.

Methods

Study sample: Providers

The provider sample was selected in a nonrandom purposive manner. The goal was to select the sample members based on those who either were likely to have had direct involvement with pharmacist-provided MTM services as part of their practice or had responsibility for individuals who provided such services. Individuals were identified from APhA databases and included both APhA members and nonmembers involved in (1) pharmacy residency programs, (2) executive pharmacy management, (3) clinical coordinator positions, (4) MTM certificate training programs, (5) MTM advisory panels, (6) MTM best-practices programs, or (7) general practice settings. After removing any individuals from this list who had requested not to receive e-mails from APhA or who had an undeliverable e-mail address, a total of 6,873 individuals were included in the provider sample. Institutional review for treatment of human subjects was conducted internally by APhA. The Association also conducted data collection and served as final repository for the data.

Data collection

Data were collected via a self-administered online survey. FormSite services were used for creating and administering the survey (www.formsite.com). FormSite is a self-service tool that

enables the creation of HTML forms using a Web browser. Survey forms for this study were created using an Internet connection and stored on secure FormSite servers located in Chicago. Form results were stored on these servers and were available for review by research personnel in secure format 24 hours per day. Respondent names were not identified in the data files. The invitation to participate in the survey was sent to sample members via e-mail with an open participation period from November 14, 2007, through December 3, 2007.

Questions for the survey were developed by a geographically diverse expert advisory panel convened by APhA staff via a series of conference calls during fall 2007. The resulting survey form included questions regarding (1) provision of MTM services, (2) patient participation in MTM services, (3) investment into MTM services, (4) value of MTM services, (5) payment for MTM services, (6) future considerations for providing MTM services, and (7) respondent background information. A copy of the survey form is available upon request from the corresponding author.

Data analysis

Data files from the FormSite data repository were converted to SPSS version 16.0 for analysis (www.spss.com). Descriptive statistics were used for summarizing responses, and open-ended responses were selected to provide further insight for answering the research questions. To learn more about several responses, we conducted subanalyses in which we investigated differences in response patterns among categories of work position and practice setting. Because we conducted these multiple comparisons in a post hoc fashion, and in light of relatively large standard deviations for the variables tested, we set the level of statistical significance at $P < 0.01$.

Results

Of the 6,873 providers who presumably received an e-mail invitation to participate in the survey, 687 (10%) responded and were included in the analysis. The respondents had diverse pharmacy-related training backgrounds and were distributed throughout the United States. A summary of job titles and organization classifications for respondents is presented in Table 1.

For the question, "Do you or your organization provide MTM services as defined in the consensus definition?" 65% reported "yes," 27% "no," and 8% "don't know." The distributions of job titles and organization classifications for respondents who reported "yes" to this question were similar to those summarized in Table 1. Of respondents who reported that they provided MTM services, 47% reported that they contracted with programs for providing MTM services, while 28% reported that they did not and 26% that they did not know.

Implementation strategies for MTM services

For respondents who indicated that they were implementing MTM services, 50% reported that they actively identified

Table 1. Job titles and organization classifications for MTM survey respondents (n = 687)[a]

Job title	% Reporting
Staff pharmacist	30
Pharmacy manager	17
Pharmacy owner	13
Clinical pharmacist	13
Director of pharmacy	6
Clinical services coordinator	5
Consultant pharmacist	4
Corporate executive manager	3
Regional manager	1
Federal pharmacist	1
Pharmacy benefits manager	1
Other[b]	6
Organization classification	
Independent community	21
National chain	18
Regional chain	7
Health system: inpatient	7
Supermarket: regional	7
Acute care inpatient	6
Ambulatory care clinic	6
Supermarket: national	6
Long-term care	4
Federal pharmacy	2
Health system: outpatient	2
Managed care	2
Mass merchandiser	2
Pharmacy benefit management	1
Supermarket independent	1
Small chain, up to 10 locations	1
Community health center	1
Contracted external MTM provider	<1
Hospice/home care	<1
Insurance company	<1
Mail service	<1
Other[c]	5

Abbreviation used: MTM, medication therapy management.
[a]Online survey respondents.
[b]Included job titles such as clinical specialist, consultant, faculty member, and resident.
[c]Included organization classifications such as compounding/infusion specialty, consulting, outreach programs, physician office, specialty clinic, and university.

patients as potential candidates for MTM services, 41% reported that they did not, and 9% reported they did not know. Those who did not identify patients themselves relied on health plans, Part D plans, employer groups, referrals from other professionals, patient self-referral, or chance.

Respondents who reportedly identified patients as potential candidates for MTM services typically used multiple strategies within their organizations, including, but not limited to, number of medications taken, specific medications, number of diseases, specific diseases, specific health plan, specific level of drug spend, emergency department or hospital discharges, suspected adverse drug reaction, history of nonadherence, or suspected medication-related problem. When asked to whom they actively marketed MTM services, more than one-half of respondents indicated "no one" or that "they did not know if they

did or not" (31% and 20%, respectively). The remaining 49% reported marketing to multiple groups, including, but not limited to, commercial insurance, Medicare supplement plans, Medicare Advantage plans, Medicare stand-alone prescription drug plans, managed care, preferred provider organizations, health indemnity plans, self-insured groups, home care/hospice, long-term care, federal government, and state Medicaid programs. Written comments revealed several themes regarding this topic, as follows: (1) providers used widely varying strategies ranging from marketing to any person who might benefit from their services to marketing only to their own employees who had diabetes, (2) providers planned to expand their marketing efforts in 2008, and (3) marketing activities often were coordinated only at the corporate office level with none occurring at the individual pharmacy level.

For providers who reported billing for MTM services, multiple billing methods typically were used at each site. The most commonly used methods were Internet (proprietary Web portal) and the pharmacy's own computer system. However, paper (claim form/invoice) and fax methods also were used. When asked about what billing format(s) their organizations used for MTM claims submission (e.g., 1500 form, X12 837 electronic, National Council for Prescription Drug Programs), 57% reported they did not know.

Based on 83 usable responses, the most commonly reported methods on which to base payment for MTM services are summarized in Table 2. The most common response was time only (24%), followed by time/type of MTM service/level of complexity (23%). Time was mentioned alone or in combination with other methods by 74% of respondents. Type of MTM service was mentioned alone or in combination with other methods by 61% of respondents. Level of complexity was mentioned alone or in combination with other methods by 34% of respondents.

When those who used a fee-for-service basis for billing were asked about their average rate, almost all respondents reported that they did not know. For the 19 respondents who provided an answer, the fees ranged from $1 to $3 per minute ($60–$180/hour).

Measures used to quantify costs and benefits of MTM

In terms of learning about measures used for quantifying costs, 69% of respondents reported that they incurred costs for offering MTM services in their organization, while 18% reported that they incurred no costs and 13% that they did not know. Of those reporting that they incurred costs, most were related to staff training or addition of staff. To a lesser extent, costs for remodeling facilities, installing technology, or purchasing equipment/supplies were reported. Only 4 of 289 respondents who answered a question requesting specific average dollar amount invested for each individual location where MTM services were provided were able to report an amount. All others (285 of 289) reported "don't know." Based on written comments, reasons for not knowing this information were associated with (1) viewing

RESEARCH MTM PROVIDER PERSPECTIVES

Table 2. Methods upon which to base fees for MTM services (n = 83)[a]

Methods used in setting fees[b]				% Reporting
Time	Type of MTM service	Level of complexity of service provided	Other/ don't know	
■				24
■	■	■		23
■	■			19
		■		17
■		■		7
			■	5
		■		2
	■	■		1
■	■	■	■	1

Abbreviation used: MTM, medication therapy management.
[a]83 respondents, as a result of item nonresponse. Percentages do not sum to 100% due to rounding.
[b]Respondents could report multiple methods. The table summarizes combinations of methods as reported by respondents.

MTM as something already being done as part of routine practice using existing staff, (2) not having the resources for quantifying costs, (3) knowing only some cost information for their organization, and (4) reporting that the primary costs for MTM services were for personnel.

Regarding measures used for quantifying benefits, respondents were asked to report any quality indicators that were improved from provision of MTM services and to respond to a series of questions about (1) revenue generated from MTM, (2) increased prescription volume, (3) increased prescription sales, (4) increased patient traffic, and (5) any other measures of value used. The results revealed that 70% of the respondents did not know of any quality indicators that were improved from MTM services. Of the remaining 30% who did report indicators, two-thirds (20% of all respondents) indicated quality indicators of a general nature, such as patient satisfaction, quality, professional satisfaction, adherence, and improved interactions with others. One-third of those reporting indicators (10% of all respondents) indicated specific quality indicators such as glycosylated hemoglobin, blood pressure, lipid profile, weight control, absenteeism, length of stay in health facilities, cost of medications, smoking cessation, overall health care costs, number of medications, dosing adjustment, and adverse drug reactions

When asked to report the monthly dollar revenue generated by MTM, 97% of respondents indicated that they did not know. Of the eight respondents who provided an answer, the amounts ranged from –$1,500 to $1,500 per month per location. Regarding percentage increase in prescription volume, only 2% of the responders (n = 7) provided an answer other than "don't know." Of the seven who answered, five reported none/unimportant, with one person reporting 0% to 2% and the other reporting

2% to 3%. Only four respondents chose to answer the question regarding percentage increase in prescription sales. Of these, three reported no increase and one reported a decrease in prescription sales. A similar response was given for a question about the percent increase in patient traffic: two of the four responders reported no increase, and the other two reported "<5%" and "increased."

Providers were also asked to report any other measures used to quantify benefits. Two-thirds (67%) of respondents provided specific answers that included cost savings, cost avoidance, number of drug-related problems identified, number of interventions provided, decreased inappropriate therapy, patient satisfaction scores, decreased hospitalizations, pain management, diabetes management, profit increase of 4%, wait times in pharmacy, prescription drug cost per member per month, data library generation, and nurse, physician, and/or patient education.

One-third (33%) of the respondents to this question did not provide specific answers but, instead, commented that (1) providers may consider MTM to be part of the care they have given to all of their patients and do not quantify benefits, (2) they do not have the resources or expertise for quantifying benefits from MTM services, or (3) the services are too new for them to detect any quantifiable impact at this point in time. These comments were evenly distributed (11% for each answer).

Assessing value of MTM services during 2007

To help learn how the value of MTM services was assessed during 2007, respondents were asked to rate, using a Likert-type scale (1, very unimportant, to 5, very important) six criteria in reference to their importance in providing value to their organization as a result of MTM services. Those who reported that they were providing MTM services were asked about actual value, and those who reported that they were not, or did not know whether they were, providing MTM services were asked about the potential value to their organization. Results for this question are presented in Table 3 and show that the most important criteria were (1) increased professional satisfaction (overall mean 3.7), (2) increased quality of care (3.7), and (3) increased patient satisfaction (3.7). Other criteria were rated as being less important (revenue generated from MTM services, increased patient traffic, increased prescription volume, and increased prescription sales). Table 3 also reveals that the pattern of responses was significantly different for those who reported providing MTM services compared with those who did not. Those providing MTM services typically reported lower scores (actual value scores) than other responders (potential value scores) (Table 3).

To learn more about how the value of MTM services was assessed during 2007, we conducted a subanalysis in which we investigated differences in response patterns among categories of work position (management or staff) and practice setting (large chain of >10 units, independent/small chain, or inpatient

Table 3. Importance of selected criteria in providing value to pharmacy organizations that did or did not provide MTM services in 2007

Criteria	Provided MTM[a]	Mean ± SD (range 1–5)	Distribution of responses (%)				
			1: Very unimportant	2: Somewhat unimportant	3: Neither	4: Somewhat important	5: Very important
Increased professional satisfaction							
n = 353	Yes	3.5 ± 1.6	24	8	4	23	41
n = 183	No	4.2 ± 1.1	6	4	8	30	53
n = 536	Overall	3.7 ± 1.5	18	7	6	25	45
		t test P < 0.001	χ² P < 0.001				
Increased quality of care							
n = 353	Yes	3.5 ± 1.6	21	9	7	25	37
n = 183	No	4.1 ± 1.1	6	5	7	39	44
n = 536	Overall	3.7 ± 1.5	16	8	7	30	39
		t test P < 0.001	χ² P < 0.001				
Increased patient satisfaction							
n = 353	Yes	3.5 ± 1.7	26	6	5	22	41
n = 183	No	4.1 ± 1.1	7	4	11	35	44
n = 536	Overall	3.7 ± 1.5	20	5	7	26	42
		t test P < 0.001	χ² P < 0.001				
Revenue generated from MTM services							
n = 353	Yes	2.9 ± 1.3	21	17	26	21	14
n = 183	No	3.7 ± 1.2	8	7	21	39	25
n = 536	Overall	3.2 ± 1.3	17	14	25	27	18
		t test P < 0.001	χ² P < 0.001				
Increased patient traffic							
n = 353	Yes	2.8 ± 1.3	24	16	31	18	11
n = 183	No	3.4 ± 1.2	10	9	32	29	20
n = 536	Overall	3.0 ± 1.3	19	14	31	22	14
		t test P < 0.001	χ² P < 0.001				
Increased prescription volume							
n = 353	Yes	2.8 ± 1.2	21	18	37	15	10
n = 183	No	3.3 ± 1.1	10	10	36	30	15
n = 536	Overall	2.9 ± 1.2	17	15	36	20	12
		t test P < 0.001	χ² P < 0.001				
Increased prescription sales							
n = 353	Yes	2.8 ± 1.2	21	17	36	16	10
n = 183	No	3.3 ± 1.2	11	10	35	28	15
n = 536	Overall	2.9 ± 1.2	18	15	36	20	12
		t test P < 0.001	χ² P < 0.001				

Abbreviation used: MTM, medication therapy management.
[a]Yes: Reported that his or her organization provided MTM services as defined in the consensus definition listed in the survey. No: Reported that his or her organization had not provided MTM services or did not know if it had.
Total number does not equal 687 as a result of item nonresponse.

settings) while controlling for provision of MTM services (yes or no). Of the 536 respondents shown in Table 3, we were able to categorize 457 of them into these post hoc categories for analysis. The results showed that work position did not significantly affect the pattern of responses for any of the variables in Table 3. However, practice setting significantly affected three of the six variables, namely, increased patient traffic, increased prescription volume, and increased prescription sales. For each of these three variables, respondents categorized as working in large chain settings reported these as more important in providing value to their organization than those working in independent/small chain settings, who, in turn, rated the variables as more important than respondents working in inpatient settings (P <

0.01 for each comparison).

Asking those who were offering MTM services how important several factors were in their organization's decision to begin providing MTM services was another way we gained insight into how providers assessed the value of MTM services to their organization. Table 4 summarizes the results for this question and shows that the most important factors were (1) patient needs, (2) responsibility as a health provider, (3) recognized a need to improve health care quality, (4) contribution to health care team, and (5) professional satisfaction. Of lesser importance were reducing health care system costs, primary business mission, reducing health insurer costs, provider needs, need for other revenue sources, competitive pressure, and decreased

RESEARCH MTM PROVIDER PERSPECTIVES

Table 4. Importance of selected factors in pharmacy organizations' decisions to begin providing MTM services (n = 381)

Factor	Mean ± SD (range 1–4)	Distribution of responses (%)			
		1: Not important at all	2: Not too important	3: Somewhat important	4: Very important
Patient needs	3.8 ± 0.5	1	1	18	80
Responsibility as health provider	3.7 ± 0.6	2	2	19	77
Recognized a need to improve health care quality	3.7 ± 0.6	1	3	21	76
Contribution to health care team	3.6 ± 0.6	1	4	27	68
Professional satisfaction	3.6 ± 0.6	2	4	27	67
Reducing health care system costs	3.3 ± 0.8	3	11	37	49
Primary business mission	3.1 ± 0.9	7	17	39	37
Reducing health insurer costs	2.9 ± 1.0	11	20	37	32
Provider needs	2.8 ± 0.9	9	23	45	23
Need for other revenue sources	2.7 ± 1.1	20	17	36	27
Competitive pressure	2.4 ± 1.0	22	32	31	15
Decreased prescription volume	2.0 ± 1.0	35	36	18	10

Abbreviation used: MTM, medication therapy management.
Results are based on responses from respondents who reported that they were providing MTM services to their patients. Percentages may not sum to 100% due to rounding.

prescription volume.

To learn more about how important these factors were in an organization's decision to begin providing MTM services, we conducted a subanalysis in which we investigated differences in response patterns among categories of work position (management or staff) and practice setting (large chain of >10 units, independent/small chain, or inpatient settings). Of the 381 respondents in Table 4, we were able to categorize 313 of them into these post hoc categories for analysis. The results showed that practice setting exerted a significant main effect on 4 of the 12 variables and that the interaction term (work position × practice setting) exerted a significant effect on one of the variables ($P < 0.01$). Regarding the significant main effects of practice setting, the results showed that large chain settings rated the variable "patient needs" as less important than the other two practice setting categories. For the variable, "need for other revenue sources," both large chain and independent/small chain settings rated this variable as more important compared with respondents categorized as working for "inpatient settings." Respondents in large chain settings rated "competitive pressure" as more important compared with the other two practice settings. Finally, "decreased prescription volume" was rated as most important by large chain settings, followed by independent/small chain and inpatient settings.

The interaction term (work position × practice setting) significantly affected the variable "recognized a need to improve health care quality" ($P < 0.01$). The interaction occurred because those in staff positions rated this as more important than those in management positions for the independent pharmacy practice setting (mean 4.8 and 4.7, respectively). For the other two practice settings, the relationship was reversed; those in management positions rated the variable as more important (4.8 for large chains and 4.9 or inpatient settings) compared with those in staff positions (4.4 for large chains and 4.8 for inpatient settings).

Finally, we investigated value in terms of return on investment (ROI). Of those who reported that they were contracted with programs for MTM services provision, 35% reported that the contracts provided a positive ROI, 31% reported that they did not provide a positive return, and 34% reported that they did not know.

Barriers to providing MTM services

Another goal of our study was to gain insight about factors that may have prevented providers from offering MTM services to their patients. To do this, we asked respondents who reported that they were not providing MTM to report how important (1, very unimportant, to 5, very important) 15 factors were in preventing them from offering MTM. Table 5 provides a summary of the results and shows that the most important factors were (1) pharmacists have inadequate time, (2) staffing levels insufficient, (3) dispensing activities too heavy, and (4) billing for MTM is difficult. Respondents also were asked to write in any comments they had about this section in the survey, and 41 respondents did so. Most comments revealed that respondents would like to be more actively engaged in patient care services such as MTM but that they viewed their current work environment as not being conducive to providing MTM. Of note, respondents who were offering MTM services were not asked these questions.

To learn more about these barriers to offering MTM services (for those not offering them), we conducted a subanalysis in which we investigated differences in response patterns among categories of work position (management or staff) and practice setting (large chain of >10 units, independent/small chain, or inpatient settings). Of the 186 respondents in Table 5, we were able to use 171 of them for the subanalysis. The results showed that work position did not significantly affect the pattern of responses for any of the variables in Table 5 and that practice setting affected only 2 of the 15 variables. For the variables "inadequate training/experience to provide MTM" and

Chapter 11

Table 5. Importance of factors in preventing providers from offering MTM services to their patients (n = 186)

Factor	Mean ± SD (range 1–5)	1: Very unimportant	2: Somewhat unimportant	3: Neither	4: Somewhat important	5: Very important
		Distribution of responses (%)				
Pharmacists have inadequate time	4.1 ± 1.1	4	9	11	29	47
Staffing levels insufficient	4.0 ± 1.2	5	8	11	30	46
Dispensing activities too heavy	3.7 ± 1.2	7	8	17	29	40
Billing for MTM is difficult	3.7 ± 1.1	7	8	26	33	26
Inadequate training/experience to provide MTM	3.5 ± 1.2	8	13	21	39	20
Documentation for MTM is difficult	3.5 ± 1.1	8	9	25	41	17
Inadequate space available for providing MTM	3.4 ± 1.3	12	12	20	29	26
Management does not support provision of MTM	3.2 ± 1.3	12	16	33	20	19
Technology barriers	3.1 ± 1.2	12	16	35	23	13
Too few MTM patients to justify cost of provision	3.1 ± 1.1	10	18	37	25	10
Too difficult to determine patient eligibility	3.0 ± 1.1	9	20	38	26	8
Unable to collect patient information needed to provide MTM	3.0 ± 1.2	14	20	27	28	11
Patients aren't interested or decline to participate	2.9 ± 1.1	12	18	45	17	8
Local physician resistance expressed	2.8 ± 1.1	15	20	44	15	8
Eligible patients for MTM don't really need it	2.5 ± 1.0	23	20	45	9	3

Abbreviation used: MTM, medication therapy management.
Results are based on responses from respondents who reported that they were not offering MTM services to their patients. The question was not applicable to those who were offering MTM.
Percentages may not sum to 100% due to rounding.

"inadequate space available for providing MTM," respondents categorized as working in large chain settings reported these as more significant in preventing them from providing MTM compared with respondents in the other two practice setting categories ($P < 0.01$).

Discussion

The results showed that 65% of the respondents to this survey were involved in MTM provision as defined in the consensus definition. Based on the nonrandom sampling method we used, we suspect that this proportion is higher than that which would be found for the overall population of providers in the United States. Of the respondents who were involved in providing MTM services, 47% reported that they were contracted with programs for providing MTM services. Such contracts reportedly provided a positive ROI for 35% of these respondents, while 31% reported that they did not provide a positive ROI and 34% that they did not know.

Findings related to implementation strategies for MTM services revealed wide variation in what was reported. Some responses revealed a "passive" approach to implementation, in which the services may have been provided to patients as part of normal care but that little or nothing was done to promote, develop, or monitor MTM service offerings. Other responses revealed an approach we describe as one of "pursuit and exploration." In this implementation strategy, multiple strategies and ideas were used concurrently. Finally, some responses revealed

an "unsure" approach to implementation in which the respondent deferred to others for decisions or reported that they did not have access to information to respond to our questions.

Providers typically did not use specific measures to quantify the costs and benefits of MTM. As of 2007, providers did not use systematic methods for assessing value from providing MTM services to their patients. Rather, they associated value with provision of such services as being part of their professional role in the health care system and society.

The most common barriers to offering MTM services (for respondents not currently offering them) were lack of time, insufficient staffing, heavy medication dispensing responsibilities, and difficulty in billing for MTM. Most of these barriers relate to staffing and workflow within the pharmacy practice. These are operational issues that need attention whenever new services are brought into practice.

With no apparent business case being reported for MTM services, providers' reluctance or unwillingness to allocate resources to provide them is understandable. Financial performance of new pharmacy services needs to be tracked for the services to be evaluated, monitored, and sustained. In our view, MTM services are relatively new and adoption of business models for provision of such services may be slow.[15,16] Unlike the adoption of a close substitute, such as a new type of seed for planting in agriculture, MTM services differ substantially from traditional pharmacist work activities. Using the seed example from agriculture, a new hybrid seed can be adopted quickly

RESEARCH MTM PROVIDER PERSPECTIVES

because the same land plots, planting equipment, growing procedures, harvesting equipment, and transportation methods can be used for either type of seed. Thus, adoption of a new type of seed can be rapid and tracking its value is straightforward because the same metrics can be used from one type of seed to the next.

In contrast, the diffusion of an emergent service offering such as MTM services involves new patient groups to be identified and recruited, new methods of service provision to be adopted, new patient care procedures to be used, new documentation and billing systems to be developed, and new ways for distributing the service to be established compared with traditional pharmacist work activities such as medication product dispensing and associated consultation. In addition, metrics for monitoring ROI are different and difficult to compare between MTM services and medication dispensing services. Such disparity may be making it difficult for providers to assess the opportunity costs of maintaining the status quo for the short term versus transitioning into MTM services provision. The transition may be especially slow if current business models are sufficiently profitable and a transition to offering MTM services is viewed as uncertain and risky.

Our finding that the primary reasons for providing MTM services were "meeting patient needs" and "fulfilling one's responsibility as a health provider" supports the notion that the transition into MTM services provision is not primarily for financial gain but, rather, for professional fulfillment and satisfaction as a patient care provider. These findings may be reflecting pharmacists' current motivation for providing MTM as one of meeting patient needs because models for measuring or justifying success in business terms are not widely available.

Concurrent developments may help speed the diffusion of MTM services as a standard of patient care and the advancement of a more systematic and sophisticated understanding of metrics for assessing ROI for such services. These developments include the efforts already completed within the pharmacy profession regarding business and payment models for MTM,[3] consensus definitions,[4] core element frameworks,[5,6] current procedural terminology codes for billing third-party payers,[7–10] and documentation systems (www.pharmacist.com/AM/Template.cfm?Section=Documentation_and_Billing). In our opinion, these resources serve as a solid foundation for provision of MTM services that are effective, efficient, consistent, applicable across pharmacy practice settings, widely accepted, and conducive for continuity of patient care within the health care system. We suggest that building on these initial efforts through continued development, broad dissemination, and objective evaluation would establish an even stronger foundation for modern pharmacy practice.

Other emerging efforts may help speed the diffusion of MTM services and create incentives for providers to develop more systematic and sophisticated metrics for evaluating these services. For example, PQA, a pharmacy quality alliance (www.

pqaalliance.org), is working to "improve health care quality and patient safety through a collaborative process in which key stakeholders agree on a strategy for measuring performance at the pharmacy and pharmacist levels; collecting data in the least burdensome way; and reporting meaningful information to consumers, pharmacists, employers, health insurance plans, and other health care decision makers to help make informed choices, improve outcomes and stimulate the *development of new payment models*" (emphasis ours).

Another example of a concurrent effort is the National Committee for Quality Assurance (NCQA; http://web.ncqa.org), which develops "quality standards and performance measures for a broad range of health care entities. These measures and standards are the tools that organizations and individuals can use to identify opportunities for improvement. The annual reporting of performance against such measures has become a focal point for the media, consumers, and health plans, which use these results to set their improvement agendas for the following year."

External metrics and standards generated by organizations such as PQA or NCQA can serve as the basis for a business case for services such as MTM so that allocation of planned and defined resources can be approved and applied by organizations. In addition, financial performance evaluation for new services such as MTM could mirror performance standards generated by national consensus groups such as PQA and NCQA. Through the generation of consensus standards and metrics, services such as MTM could be evaluated, monitored, and sustained from an ROI perspective.

We suggest that professional pharmacy associations can play active roles for research, demonstration projects, training, professional resources, and advocacy as evidentiary and analytical standards are established for MTM services and programs. In addition, our findings show that individual practitioners provided MTM services for professional fulfillment and satisfaction as patient care providers rather than for financial gain. We propose that individual providers should actively try to persuade their employers/organizations that investment in MTM services has merit and that active approaches to implementation and monitoring would be in the organization's self-interest. Furthermore, information gained from monitoring MTM financial and health outcomes would be useful for organizations when negotiating contracts with payer programs. Individual practitioners also could express an interest in becoming more involved in demonstrating successful business models to promote MTM service delivery. In the health care domain, tensions commonly develop between direct patient practice models and financial considerations or limitations. Individual practitioners may feel that they do not have decision-making authority within their practice. However, we suggest that professional enthusiasm and advocacy for emergent services such as pharmacist-provided MTM can help inform and persuade organizational decision makers to take more active approaches to implementing and evaluating such services. In addition, such activities could increase the likelihood that individual practitioners would be included in decision making and could help ensure successful integration of MTM into practice.

Limitations

The findings of this study should be interpreted in light of the study's limitations. First, we applied a pharmacy profession consensus definition for MTM. Other definitions or perspectives for MTM services could lead to different findings. Second, we used a purposive sampling technique in which we sought to survey individuals who either were likely to have had direct involvement with providing MTM services or had responsibility for individuals who provided MTM services. This approach allowed for "informed opinions" from "engaged key opinion leaders" in our data collection, but the findings cannot be generalized to the overall provider population in the United States. Third, respondents appeared to be able to answer questions that were site specific but less able to answer questions that asked about the characteristics of overall corporations or organizations. Conducting surveys at the corporate level to answer some of the questions posed in our study may be necessary. Finally, the use of an online survey provided both time and cost advantages. However, this survey method suffers from poor response rates. We were willing to accept this limitation because our goal was to gain insights and informed opinions from engaged key opinion leaders. However, the findings cannot be extrapolated to the broader MTM provider population.

Conclusion

The results of this study showed that providers varied widely on how they implemented MTM service offerings and typically did not use specific measures to quantify the costs and benefits of MTM. In addition, they did not use systematic methods for assessing value from providing MTM services to their patients. Rather, they associated value with provision of such services as being part of their professional role in the health care system and society.

References

1. Smith SR, Clancy CM. Medication therapy management programs: forming a new cornerstone for quality and safety in Medicare. Am J Med Qual. 2006;21:276–9.
2. McGivney MS, Meyer SM, Duncan-Hewitt W, et al. Medication therapy management: its relationship to patient counseling, disease management, and pharmaceutical care. J Am Pharm Assoc. 2007;47:620–8.
3. The Lewin Group. Medication therapy management services: a critical review. J Am Pharm Assoc. 2005;45:580–7.
4. Bluml BM. Definition of medication therapy management: development of professionwide consensus. J Am Pharm Assoc. 2005;45:566–72.
5. American Pharmacists Association, National Association of Chain Drug Stores Foundation. Medication therapy management in community pharmacy practice: core elements of an MTM service (version 1.0). J Am Pharm Assoc. 2005;45:573–9.
6. American Pharmacists Association, National Association of Chain Drug Stores Foundation. Medication therapy management in pharmacy practice: core elements of a MTM service model (version 2.0). J Am Pharm Assoc. In press.
7. Thompson CA. National billing codes announced for pharmacists' clinical services. Am J Health Syst Pharm. 2005;62:1640–2.
8. Thompson CA. Pharmacists' CPT codes become permanent. Am J Health Syst Pharm. 2007;64:2410–2.
9. Zingone MM, Malcolm KE, McCormick SW, Bledsoe KR. Analysis of pharmacist charges for medication therapy management services in an outpatient setting. Am J Health Syst Pharm. 2007;64:1827–31.
10. Isetts BJ, Buffington DE, Pharmacist Services Technical Advisory Coalition. CPT code-change proposal: national data on pharmacists' medication therapy management services. Am J Health Syst Pharm. 2007;64:1642–6.
11. Touchette DR, Burns AL, Bough MA, Blackburn JC. Survey of medication therapy management programs under Medicare Part D. J Am Pharm Assoc. 2006;46:683–91.
12. Touchette DR, Burns AL, Bough MA, Blackburn JC. Effective Health Care Research Reports: survey of Medicare Part D plans' medication therapy management programs. Accessed at http://effectivehealthcare.ahrq.gov/repFiles/Medication_Therapy_Management_Programs.pdf, February 1, 2008.
13. Doucette WR, Witry MJ, Alkhateeb F, et al. Attitudes of Medicare beneficiaries toward pharmacist-provided medication therapy management activities as part of the Medicare Part D benefit. J Am Pharm Assoc. 2007;47:758–62.
14. Moczygemba LR, Barner JC, Roberson K. Texas pharmacists' opinions about and plans for provision of medication therapy management services. J Am Pharm Assoc. 2008;48:38–45.
15. Rogers EM. New product adoption and diffusion. J Consum Res. 1976;2:290–301.
16. Rogers EM. Diffusion of innovations. 5th ed. New York: Free Press; 2003.

RESEARCH

Pharmacist-provided medication therapy management (part 2): Payer perspectives in 2007

Jon C. Schommer, Lourdes G. Planas, Kathleen A. Johnson, and William R. Doucette

Abstract

Objectives: To collect and describe payer perspectives regarding (1) implementation strategies used for providing medication therapy management (MTM) services to patients/clients; (2) specific measures, if any, used to quantify the costs and benefits of MTM; (3) how the value of MTM services was tracked during 2007; and (4) barriers to offering MTM services to patients/clients.

Design: Descriptive, nonexperimental, cross-sectional study.

Setting: United States during 2007.

Participants: Of the 1,898 payers who presumably received an e-mail invitation to participate in the survey, 132 (7%) responded. In addition to the online survey, 20 individuals who reported that they developed or used MTM for their organization participated in a telephone interview consisting of open-ended questions.

Interventions: Self-administered online survey and telephone interview.

Main outcome measures: Implementation and monitoring of MTM.

Results: The results showed that 20% (n = 26) of the e-mail survey respondents offered MTM services to their members as described in the consensus definition of MTM. Payers for MTM services varied widely on how they implemented and monitored their organization's MTM programs. For 2008, MTM payer organizations plan to expand their use of face-to-face pharmacist–patient interaction.

Conclusion: During 2008, plans may have greater opportunity to measure outcomes in a longitudinal fashion and make adjustments to MTM provision strategies. Some evidence for this was suggested in respondent comments to our survey, but future validation is needed before reaching a firm conclusion.

Keywords: Medication therapy management, cost analysis, pharmacy services, surveys, return on investment.

J Am Pharm Assoc. 2008;48:478–486.
doi: 10.1331/JAPhA.2008.08023

Received February 9, 2008. Accepted for publication March 10, 2008.

Jon C. Schommer, PhD, is Professor, College of Pharmacy, University of Minnesota, Minneapolis. Lourdes G. Planas, PhD, is Assistant Professor, College of Pharmacy, University of Oklahoma Health Sciences Center, Oklahoma City. Kathleen A. Johnson, PhD, is Associate Professor, School of Pharmacy, University of Southern California, Los Angeles. William R. Doucette, PhD, is Professor, College of Pharmacy, and Director, Center for Improving Medication Use in the Community, College of Pharmacy, University of Iowa, Iowa City.

Correspondence: Jon C. Schommer, PhD, Professor, College of Pharmacy, University of Minnesota, 308 Harvard Street, SE, Minneapolis, MN 55455. Fax: 612-625-9931. E-mail: schom010@umn.edu

Disclosure: The authors declare no conflicts of interest or financial interests in any product or service mentioned in this article, including grants, employment, gifts, stock holdings, or honoraria.

Acknowledgments: To American Pharmacists Association (APhA) staff with whom we collaborated for this project: Anne Burns, Maria Gorrick, James Owen, Deborah Ruddy, and Margaret Tomecki.

Funding: By APhA through an unrestricted grant from Wyeth. Data were collected and made available for analysis by APhA.

Medication therapy management (MTM) has been defined as "a distinct service or group of services that optimize therapeutic outcomes for individual patients.

At a Glance

Synopsis: A total of 132 individuals who, during 2007, were likely to be involved directly with providing payment for medication therapy management (MTM) services or to have responsibility for individuals who provided payment completed a self-administered online survey; another 20 individuals who reported developing or using MTM for their organization participated in a telephone interview consisting of open-ended questions. Using the pharmacy profession's MTM consensus definition as guidance, 20% (n = 26) of participants indicated they were offering such services to their members. The results confirmed that the MTM services and programs offered by payer organizations varied widely. Payers associated value of MTM programs with cost avoidance/minimization, increased member satisfaction, improved member medication adherence, and quality indicators. In general, these findings indicate that MTM services offered by payer organizations during 2007 are still in the development stages and that organizations are willing to expand their service offerings as they develop more familiarity with these services and programs.

Analysis: The cost of providing MTM services under Medicare Part D guidelines during 2007 stemmed from health plans' administrative costs, which produced economic pressure to provide minimally acceptable levels of MTM to contain costs. To increase options and intensity for MTM services, the Centers for Medicare & Medicaid Services could consider basing reimbursement for MTM on continuous quality improvement, instead of making these services an administrative cost of the program. Evidence indicates that pharmacist-provided MTM results in better outcomes and return on investment compared with other methods that use impersonal approaches and could emerge as a preferred strategy for payers. Standard-setting organizations such as PQA (a pharmacy quality alliance) and the National Committee for Quality Assurance are actively working to cultivate quality metrics for gauging MTM services and outcomes. Core MTM services (i.e., comprehensive, evidence-based, generalist practices) and prioritized MTM services (i.e., targeted, evidence-based, specialist practices) are expected to emerge as viable models for payers as experience with providing MTM grows. Building consensus models for provision, payment, and pay-for-performance evaluation of pharmacist-provided MTM is one suggestion for moving away from cost avoidance/minimization models to quality improvement models.

MTM services are independent of, but can occur in conjunction with, the provision of a medication product. MTM encompasses a broad range of professional activities and responsibilities within the licensed pharmacist's, or other qualified health provider's, scope of practice."[1–5] Standards for billing and reimbursement purposes have been developed for these services[6–9] that are applicable for all pharmacy practice environments and all patient types.[10–16] However, providers and payers who use these standards still determine their own fee structures, rates, and payment guidelines for a diverse array of MTM service types.

For example, during early implementation of MTM services covered by the Medicare Part D program,[4] broad definitions were used for MTM that allowed impersonal approaches such as mailings to help suppress costs because the cost of providing MTM service benefits typically arose from a plan's administrative costs.[17,18] Evidence showing that information pamphlets or telephonic interventions are useful for meeting goals of MTM programs is lacking.[19–22] Nonetheless, these methods served as the foundation for most Medicare Part D MTM programs during 2006. A national survey of MTM programs showed that such interventions were offered to an estimated three-quarters of all MTM beneficiaries during 2006 and that 90% of the health plans elected to provide some or all of their MTM services in house.[17,18] In contrast, however, all but one of the programs involved pharmacists in some aspect of MTM services and 19% of MTM programs reported contracting with pharmacies to provide some or all of their MTM services via face-to-face methods.[17,18] The health plans that contracted with pharmacies tended to be relatively large and accounted for approximately 7.5 million lives.

In light of these early findings, questions arise about the evidence supporting the effectiveness of various interventions and about how the value of MTM is assessed and monitored by providers and payers of these services. Without an acceptable return on investment (ROI) for MTM programs, such programs would not be sustainable over the long term.

Objectives

To help understand how providers and payers might be monitoring and assessing the value of pharmacist-provided MTM, an environmental scan was conducted during 2007.[23] For this project, we used the professionwide consensus definition of MTM[1–3] so that the findings could be applied to a diverse array of patient populations and would not be limited to patients who are eligible for MTM services under the Medicare Part D program. Furthermore, we chose to focus specifically on pharmacist-provided MTM for several reasons. First, pharmacists were the health professional group specifically named as MTM providers in the Medicare Prescription Drug, Improvement, and Modernization Act of 2003.[4] Second, by using this focus, we sought to add to reports in the pharmacy literature on pharmacist-provided MTM.[1–18,23–27] Finally, this focus would allow the sponsor of the project (American Pharmacists Association [APhA]) to use the findings in making decisions about how to serve its members and the pharmacy profession.

For the overall project, the opinions of payers for these services and providers of these services were collected and summarized regarding how service implementation was being monitored and value was being assessed during 2007. The specific questions we sought to answer from both payer and provider perspectives were as follows.

■ What implementation strategies were used for providing MTM services to patients/clients?
■ What specific measures, if any, were used to quantify the costs and benefits of MTM?
■ How was the value of MTM services tracked during 2007?
■ What were the barriers to providing MTM services to patients/clients?

This article is the second of a two-part series. In part one, provider perspectives of pharmacist-provided MTM services were described.[23] The results from the provider survey showed that 65% of the respondents were involved with providing MTM services as defined in the consensus definition presented in the survey. Of these, 47% reported that they contracted with programs for providing MTM services. Such contracts reportedly provided a positive ROI for 35% of respondents, while 31% reported that they did not provide a positive ROI and 34% said they did not know.

As of 2007, most providers did not use systematic methods for assessing value from providing MTM services to their patients. Rather, they perceived the value from provision of such services as part of their professional role in the health care system and society. For part two of our project, payer perspectives of MTM were studied and are the focus of the remainder of this article.

Methods
Study sample: Payers
The payer sample was selected in a nonrandom purposive manner. The goal was to select sample members who either were likely to have had direct involvement with providing payment for MTM services or had responsibility for individuals who provided payment. Candidates for the self-administered online survey were identified from public Web sites, APhA staff members' knowledge, and a purchased list of 1,804 e-mail contacts for insured groups covering between 5,000 and 150,000 lives nationally. Sample members worked for group insurers, benefits coalition groups, state Medicaid programs, Medicare Advantage Prescription Drug plans, private prescription drug plans, prescription/pharmacy benefit management organizations, claims administrators, the Centers for Medicare & Medicaid Services (CMS), or MTM contract vendors. After removing any individuals from this list who had requested not to receive e-mails from APhA or who had an undeliverable e-mail address, a total of 1,898 individuals were included in the payer sample.

Another sample for participation in telephone interviews

was identified from the complete list described above. Individuals known to be involved with MTM by APhA staff or researchers and assumed to be likely to participate in this project were identified for initial contact. These individuals worked for group insurers, business coalition groups, self-insured payers, state Medicaid programs, Part D plans, pharmacy benefit managers, and MTM vendors. Of 32 individuals contacted, 21 were recruited for participation and their contact information was forwarded to a contract survey company for scheduling and conducting telephone interviews. In addition to these individuals, four others indicated in their online survey that they would be willing to participate in a follow-up interview. Thus, contact information for 25 individuals was forwarded to the contract survey company.

Data collection
Data were collected via a self-administered online survey and telephone interviews. For creating and administering the online survey, FormSite.com was used (www.formsite.com).[23] The invitation to participate in the survey was sent to sample members via e-mail with an open participation period from November 14, 2007, through December 14, 2007.

In addition to the online survey, which served as the primary data collection method, 20 of the 25 individuals contacted for a telephone interview were reached and interviews completed. The telephone interviews consisted of open-ended questions that were similar to the online survey but allowed for more in-depth answers in respondents' own words. Responses to the telephone interviews helped in interpreting findings, provided validation for responses to the online survey, and gave insights for addressing our research questions. Phone interviews were coordinated and conducted by Strategic Business Research, Inc., between November 21, 2007, and December 21, 2007. To maintain respondent confidentiality, we did not attempt to link data from telephone interviews to online survey data for any individuals who participated in both.

Questions for the survey and interviews were developed by a geographically diverse expert advisory panel convened by APhA staff via a series of conference calls during fall 2007. The resulting survey form and telephone interviews included questions about (1) offering of MTM programs, (2) member participation in MTM programs, (3) investment into MTM programs, (4) value of MTM programs, (5) payment for MTM services, (6) future considerations for providing MTM services, and (7) respondent background information. A copy of the survey form is available upon request from the corresponding author.

For the purposes of this project, we included the following description of MTM in the surveys and interviews.

"In a consensus definition, the pharmacy profession has defined medication therapy management (MTM) to be a distinct group of services that optimize therapeutic outcomes for individual patients. MTM services are independent of, but can occur in conjunction with, the provision of a medication product.

MTM encompasses a broad range of professional activities and responsibilities within the licensed pharmacist's or other qualified health provider's scope of practice.

"Please note: It is acknowledged that some health plans/organizations use different terms than medication therapy management (MTM) to describe the same services as those in the definition above. Other terms readily used include drug therapy management, medication use management, among others, and for the purposes of this survey are considered synonymous with MTM.

"In this survey, MTM services encompass those services being provided either via face-to-face contact or telephonically by a pharmacist or other qualified health professional, but do not include mailings to members."[23]

As a result of using this definition, some CMS-defined and -approved MTM services offered to Medicare Part D beneficiaries were not considered in our study.

Data analysis

Data files from the Formsite data repository that contained payer responses were converted to SPSS version 16.0 for analysis (www.spss.com). Descriptive statistics were used to summarize responses, and open-ended responses were selected to help address our research questions. Interview transcripts were converted to PDFs for review. Analysis was exploratory in nature and focused on gaining insights rather than on description or prediction.

Results

Of the 1,898 payers who presumably received an e-mail invitation to participate in the survey, 132 (7%) responded and were included in the analysis. The online survey respondents represented diverse plan types and were distributed throughout the United States. A summary of job titles and organization classifications for the 132 online respondents is presented in Table 1. The number of people covered by each organization varied considerably (median 48,000, range 0–14 million).

For the question, "As described in the consensus definition of MTM, does your organization currently offer medication therapy management (MTM) services to members?" 20% reported "yes," 7% "no," and 5% "don't know," while 68% did not provide an answer. The relatively high proportion of survey participants who did not answer the question had already discontinued answering the online survey a few questions earlier. Those questions asked about medical plan and pharmacy plan characteristics of respondents' organizations and presumably did not apply to those who discontinued the survey. Thus, we surmised that the question asking about offering MTM services also did not apply to their situation and/or organization.

For answering our research questions, we used responses from the 26 respondents (20% of the 132 responders to the online survey) whose organizations reportedly offered pharmacist-provided MTM services to members. In addition, we

Table 1. Job titles and organization classifications for MTM survey respondents (n = 132)[a]

Category	% Reporting
Job title	
Pharmacy director	22
Corporate executive	13
Clinical services director	10
Pharmacy benefits manager/executive	9
State Medicaid director/administrator	8
Other[b]	38
Organization classification	
HMO/managed care organization	22
State Medicaid program	15
Prescription benefit management company	13
Self-insured employer	12
Other single-entity company[c]	27
Multifaceted organization (combination of at least two of the categories above)	11

Abbreviations used: HMO, health maintenance organization; MTM, medication therapy management.
[a]Online survey respondents.
[b]Included titles such as clinical pharmacist, compliance/regulatory, quality management, provider network manager, marketing manager, MTM specialist, pharmacist, project consultant.
[c]Included classifications such as academia, behavior change company, consulting organization, distribution and software development, MTM contract vendor company, program evaluation research company, quality improvement organization.

used responses from the 20 individuals who agreed to participate in a telephone interview. (A total of 25 individuals were contacted for telephone interviews.) The distributions of these respondents' job titles and organization classifications were similar to those summarized in Table 1. Of note, although these respondents offered pharmacist-provided MTM services and were asked questions related to those services, their responses likely reflected all types of MTM services offered by their organization.

Implementation strategies for MTM services

Results from both the online survey and phone interviews confirmed that payer organizations were providing multiple types of MTM services and programs to their clients. All respondents reported that their MTM services included patient education. Nearly all respondents also reported that patient medication adherence, monitoring of medication-related problems, physician consultations, medication therapy review, and patient monitoring were components of their MTM services. Approximately one-half of respondents reported that their MTM services were developed to target patients with chronic illnesses such as hypertension, diabetes, chronic obstructive pulmonary disease, depression, asthma, and dyslipidemia.

The percentage of total covered members in respondents' organizations who were eligible for MTM services varied considerably (range 1%–100%). Of those responding to this question in the online survey, 47% reported that 100% of their members were eligible for MTM services, 30% reported 1% to 5% were eligible, and 23% reported 7% to 60% were eligible.

When asked how members are determined to be eligible for MTM services, 60% of the online respondents were unique in their answers; examples of responses included "all members are eligible" and "varies, depending on program administered." Factors that were used for determining eligibility included number of medications, specific medication use (e.g., warfarin), number of diseases, specific diseases (e.g., asthma), type of health plan, specific level of drug spend, history of hospitalization, documented adverse drug reaction, and history of nonadherence. Both specific disease types and specific drug types were used to determine eligibility for MTM by 40% of respondents.

Variation among online respondents also was found regarding the percentage of total MTM eligible members who received MTM services by phone (median 10.5%, range 0%–100%; 24% reported 0%, 19% reported 100%), the percentage who received MTM services in person (median 3%, range 0%–100%; 45% reported 0%, 14% reported 100%), and the percentage of members who were eligible for MTM services who participate in them (median 25%, range 0%–100%; 5% reported 0%, 10% reported 100%).

Payer organizations also varied in terms of who identified members for eligibility for MTM services (e.g., health plan, physician, pharmacist, other), how members are enrolled (e.g., opt-in, opt-out, both), and who recruits members to participate in MTM services (e.g., health plan, physician, pharmacist, self-referral). Regarding the most common answers to these questions, 60% of online respondents reported that health plans identified members for eligibility, 64% used opt-out enrollment, and 60% reported that health plans were used for recruitment of members to participate in MTM.

Table 2 summarizes provider types that were used for MTM service delivery by the 21 respondents who answered this online survey question. Contracted pharmacists were used by the majority of plans for MTM service provision. According to responses to the telephone interviews, providers for MTM service provision were selected based on expertise and availability of the providers. Respondents considered licensed pharmacists to have the greatest expertise regarding drug therapy, formularies, and drug interactions, and most payers did not apply specific training standards for determining level of expertise. Regarding availability, pharmacists were considered more accessible than physicians, in-house providers were considered more accessible than others, and providers selected for MTM provision needed to demonstrate that they were able to devote time to the MTM program.

Table 3 summarizes claims processing for MTM services. Internet (Web portal) claims processing was the most commonly used method, followed by processing done through another party such as a pharmacy benefit management organization or an MTM contractor. The X12 837 standard was used most often for electronic claims submission.

In both the online survey and the telephone interviews, approximately one-half of respondents reported using *Current*

Table 2. Types of providers used for MTM service delivery (n = 21)[a]

Provider type	% Reporting
Contracted pharmacists + contracted MTM provider organization	24
Contracted pharmacists	19
Contracted pharmacists + pharmacist in-house	10
Pharmacist in-house	10
Contracted pharmacists + pharmacist in-house + nurses in-house	5
Contracted pharmacists + pharmacist in-house + contracted nurses	5
Contracted pharmacists + disease management vendor	5
Pharmacist in-house + disease management vendor	5
Nurses in-house	5
Prescription benefit management organization	5
Don't know	7

Abbreviation used: MTM, medication therapy management.
[a]Online survey respondents who reported that they developed or used MTM for their organization. Number does not equal 26, as a result of item nonresponse.

Procedural Terminology (CPT) codes for claims processing and were ready to use the following "permanent" codes when they became effective on January 1, 2008: 99605 (initial 15 minutes of MTM services, including assessment and intervention, if appropriate, for a new patient), 99606 (initial 15 minutes of MTM services, including assessment and intervention, if appropriate, for an established patient), and 99607 (each additional 15 minutes; used in addition to 99605 or 99606). However, some respondents reported that their MTM providers use reason–action–result

Table 3. Claims processing for MTM service delivery (n = 21)[a]

How claims are accepted	% Reporting
Internet (Web portal)	29
Don't accept claims directly (done through PBM or MTM contractor)	24
Paper	14
Don't know	13
Internet (Web portal) + fax	5
Internet (Web portal) + paper	5
Paper + fax	5
Internal agreement with human resources department	5
Billing standards used for electronic claims submission	
X12 837 electronic	29
No specific standard	24
Don't know	17
NCPDP	10
X12 837 electronic + NCPDP	5
X12 837 electronic + proprietary billing system	5
Proprietary billing system	5
MTM vendor fields	5

Abbreviations used: MTM, medication therapy management; NCPDP, National Council for Prescription Drug Programs; PBM, pharmacy benefits management.
[a]Online survey respondents who reported that they developed or used MTM for their organization. Number does not equal 26, as a result of item nonresponse.

codes that then map to MTM CPT codes within their organization. In the future, these respondents expected to convert to *CPT* codes.

Measures used to quantify costs and benefits of MTM

Nineteen respondents to the online survey reported that it cost their organization between $0 and $300 per member per month to provide MTM services (median $1.92). Of these respondents, 21% reported $0, 37% reported a value between $0.01 and $5.00, 21% reported a value between $5.01 and $40.00, and 21% reported a value greater than $40 per member per month.

For quantifying benefits from provision of MTM services, more than 70% of respondents to both the online survey and phone interviews reported that they measured the following outcomes: (1) drug interactions identified/resolved, (2) improved medication adherence, (3) medication over/underuse, (4) therapeutic duplications resolved, and (5) overall medication costs. Table 4 summarizes the pattern of responses for both the online survey and telephone interview.

Organizations that routinely analyzed medication-related problems used methods such as reports from pharmacy benefit management companies, electronic alerts (e.g., drug use review programs), and claims data analysis. We also learned from one Medicaid program that it used a systems analysis of aggregated data from both medical and pharmacy claims. This program monitored emergency department visits, hospitalization, and frequency of laboratory tests; it focused on disease and had a stated goal of decreasing total health care costs by 6% to 8% through the use of MTM in its program.

Tracking value of MTM services during 2007

Ten of the 26 respondents to the online survey who provided MTM services also reported that their organization attributed a financial return value for their programs. Of these, seven reported that the ratio of return to costs ranged from 2:1 to 12:1 (median 3:1). Those who did not report a ratio of return commented that this analysis was too complex for an evaluation, that participation in MTM programs was too small for conducting the evaluation, or that they were not ready to publicly report their findings.

In both the online survey and telephone interviews, respondents were asked to describe how they would define and assess value. The question was not answered consistently; some respondents used a pre/postanalysis of claims, clinical outcomes, and/or patient satisfaction for defining and assessing value. Others reported using cost avoidance or minimization models. One respondent outlined an "estimated cost avoidance" model in which the pharmacist selects a cost avoidance amount with each claim submission. The claim is then subject to an external quality assurance process before the cost avoidance amount is used for reimbursement purposes. Some respondent comments revealed that they did not assess value for MTM pro-

grams during 2007 because their services and programs were quite minimal and relied on mailings or phone interventions.

Some respondents' comments revealed that their organizations planned to make adjustments during 2008 based on their experiences to date. Most of the adjustments would increase the involvement of pharmacists and face-to-face interventions in MTM programs. For example, one respondent plans to contract with a local vendor for face-to-face interventions that would "provide better outcomes in 2008." Another respondent commented that benefit design changes will be targeted to best practices and will use medical evidence to target interventions. Another comment revealed that the government entitlements the respondent's organization services do not require sophisticated MTM programs at this time. However, the organization plans to implement programs using pharmacists and then provide information to the entitlements. One respondent's comment showed that the organization's MTM programs were aiming to empower the community pharmacist so that during the encounter, the pharmacist can resolve "green flags" (cost-saving opportunities) and interact with "red flags" (i.e., drug–drug interactions, drug–disease interactions, other adverse events).

Barriers to providing MTM services

Respondents to the phone interview reported that the primary barrier they experienced for providing MTM services was lack of a perception of need by patients. Some comments to this question suggested that patients may mistake MTM calls for sales calls. Also, patients might become confused when their pharmacist and physician provide conflicting recommendations. Still others might not understand the importance of MTM for their care.

The next most frequently reported barrier was lack of acceptance by physicians. Some comments revealed that physicians might be skeptical of pharmacists making therapeutic recommendations that could conflict with the physician's recommendation. Six of 14 respondents who added comments for this question felt that physicians' skepticism regarding the tangible value of MTM services was a barrier.

In the online survey, four of the respondents who reportedly did not offer MTM services during 2007 provided written comments about the information they would find helpful for making a decision about providing MTM services in the future. All four reported that more information about the cost of providing these services would be helpful for decision making and would overcome some barriers to providing or covering MTM services for clients.

Discussion

In general, respondents reported that MTM services offered by their organizations were still in the development stages and that health plans varied widely in their implementation strategies. For example, our findings showed that the percentage of the total covered members in respondents' organizations that were eligible for MTM services ranged from 1% to 100%. Furthermore, the percentage of members who were eligible for MTM services who actually participated in them ranged from 0% to 100% across respondents' plans. Such variation may decrease over time as plans learn from each other or, perhaps, CMS sets tighter standards for MTM services and programs.

Respondents consistently reported that drug interactions, medication adherence, medication use, therapeutic duplications, and costs were monitored for MTM programs (Table 4). Also, respondents consistently reported that the primary barriers to providing MTM services were lack of perception of need by patients and lack of acceptance by physicians. However, methods for measuring MTM outcomes differed across organizations. The results showed various assessment strategies such as pre/postanalysis of claims, clinical outcomes monitoring, patient satisfaction surveys, and/or cost avoidance or minimization monitoring. The results also showed that plans differed widely in terms of their use of contracted pharmacists for MTM programs, claims processing approaches, and use of CPT codes for claims processing (Tables 2 and 3).

Our interpretation of these findings is that Medicare Part D guidelines likely were used as a standard to follow for many MTM programs and that cost avoidance remained a primary goal for implementation of MTM services during 2007. However, our findings showed that all MTM programs described in our study provided basic services related to patient education and that nearly all provided MTM services related to patient medication adherence, monitoring of medication-related problems, physician consultations, medication therapy review, and patient monitoring. Furthermore, approximately one-half of the respondents developed MTM services targeted to specific treatment areas such as hypertension, diabetes, chronic obstructive pulmonary disease, asthma, and dyslipidemia.

Respondents' comments suggested that an increase in face-to-face pharmacist–patient interactions may occur in the future. Contract year 2007 for Medicare Part D likely had a greater number of beneficiaries who qualified earlier for MTM, considering that health plans had historical data from 2006 with which to identify beneficiaries for MTM services. Also, beneficiaries who continued to meet the eligibility criteria for program year 2007 could have been offered MTM services on the first of the year to avoid gaps in MTM services. Such experience over time might be a contributing factor for plans to increase the use of face-to-face pharmacist–patient interaction. During 2008, plans will have an even greater opportunity to measure outcomes in a longitudinal fashion and make adjustments to MTM provision strategies. While some evidence for this was suggested in respondent comments to our survey, future validation is needed before reaching a firm conclusion. Findings from the provider survey[23] also revealed that providers were in the early stages of offering MTM services and that they were, for the most part, willing to expand their service offerings as they develop more familiarity with these services and programs.

Table 4. Types of outcomes measured by payers for measuring benefits from MTM

Measure	% Online survey respondents answering yes (n = 22)[a]	% Telephone interview respondents answering yes (n = 14)[b]
Drug interactions identified/resolved	91	79
Improved medication adherence	91	79
Medication over/underuse	82	79
Therapeutic duplications resolved	73	79
Overall medication costs	73	71
Member satisfaction	45	71
Nontreated conditions identified and appropriately treated	45	64
Number of medication-related problems resolved	64	57
Treatment changes to bring therapy in line with guidelines	64	57
Overall health care costs	68	50
Quality measure scores (e.g., HEDIS)	45	43
Number of high-risk medications	45	29
Costs associated with adverse drug events	14	29

Abbreviations used: HEDIS, Healthcare Effectiveness Data and Information Set; MTM, medication therapy management.
[a]Online survey respondents who reported that they developed or used MTM for their organization. Number does not equal 26, as a result of item nonresponse.
[b]Telephone interview respondents who reported that they developed or used MTM for their organization. Number does not equal 20, as a result of item nonresponse.

We suggest that pharmacist intervention could emerge as a preferred MTM strategy for payers. Based on our findings, this may be a result of evidence/experience showing that pharmacist-provided MTM results in better outcomes and ROI than other strategies that use impersonal approaches.[19–22] In time, CMS expects MTM to drive improvements in quality of care and health outcomes. CMS; the National Quality Forum (NQF); the Agency for Healthcare Research and Quality (AHRQ); PQA, a pharmacy quality alliance; the National Committee for Quality Assurance (NCQA), and other standard-setting organizations are actively working on cultivating the quality measures that will be used to gauge MTM services and outcomes. However, the effect of quality improvement organizations' efforts may only be seen after years of monitoring and reporting.[27] We propose that our findings (particularly respondent comments and reported use of contracted pharmacists for MTM) are evidence that payers may make adjustments to their MTM programs during 2008 to help improve the likelihood of achieving measurable outcomes from MTM provision.

With more experience over time, we believe that core MTM services (i.e., comprehensive, evidence-based, generalist practices) and prioritized MTM services (i.e., targeted, evidence-based, specialist practices) may both emerge as viable models for payers.[2,3] In our project, we found evidence that both of these approaches are being used and developed by payers.

We propose that future development of MTM services would be enhanced through developing and applying (1) quality standards and pay-for-performance goals that emerge from evidence-based practice, (2) best practices, (3) data-identified opportunities for improving medication use in defined populations, (4) targeted medication therapy reviews for patients, (5) accessible electronic medical records, (6) referral networks, and (7) continuity-of-care processes. With experience and development of well-defined processes over time, we believe that both comprehensive and targeted MTM approaches would provide value and ROI for payers.

As of 2008, the cost of providing MTM service programs under Medicare Part D guidelines still stems from health plans' administrative costs, which produce economic pressure to provide minimally acceptable levels of MTM to suppress costs. Such a structure is likely to slow the rate of adoption of a quality improvement approach for MTM program development.[28] CMS could consider basing its reimbursement model for MTM on continuous quality improvement (e.g., pay-for-performance) rather than on administrative cost,[28,29] in order to expand options and intensity for MTM services as determined by plan and enrollee needs.

To evolve from cost avoidance models to quality improvement models, we have several suggestions for consideration and discussion. First, the pharmacy profession could use its experiences in developing the MTM consensus definition[1-3] to collaborate with other stakeholders to build consensus models for provision, payment, and pay-for-performance evaluation of pharmacist-provided MTM. Professionwide models would contribute to a level playing field for practitioners and organizations and serve as a basis for monitoring and evaluating the effects of MTM on desired outcomes. Second, research could be conducted on developing evidentiary and analytical standards for monitoring and assessing MTM services and programs. Such standards are being developed around the world for evaluating the value provided by pharmaceutical products and associated services (e.g., National Institute for Health and Clinical Excellence, www.nice.org.uk/; Oregon Evidence-Based Practice Center, www.ohsu.edu/epc/about/index.htm). Similar approaches for developing consensus standards regarding relevant evidence and analytical methods that should be used for evaluating MTM services could be developed. Third, CMS, NQF, AHRQ, PQA, NCQA, and other standard-setting organizations are expected to continue to work on establishing quality measures that will be used to gauge MTM services and outcomes. Investments for research and demonstration projects for these measures will be needed to keep these initiatives moving forward in a credible, valid manner. Finally, to help overcome patient and physician resistance to pharmacist-provided MTM, national campaigns could be initiated to demonstrate pharmacist capabilities with these groups. In addition, MTM marketing toolkits could be developed for both providers and payers of these services and used to promote MTM to patients and physicians at the local level.[30,31]

Each of these suggestions will take years to develop. However, we believe that such inquiry and work would create incentives for payers to more commonly adopt continuous quality improvement models rather than cost avoidance models when implementing MTM programs for their clients.

Limitations

The findings of this study should be interpreted in light of the study's limitations. First, we applied a pharmacy profession consensus definition for MTM. Other definitions or perspectives for MTM services could lead to alternate findings. Second, we used a purposive sampling technique in which we sought to survey individuals who either were likely to have had direct involvement with paying for MTM services or to have had responsibility for individuals who paid for MTM services. This approach allowed for "informed opinions" from "engaged key opinion leaders" in our data collection, but the findings cannot be generalized to the overall MTM payer population in the United States. Third, respondents who reportedly offered pharmacist-provided MTM were asked questions specific to those services. However, based on their responses and comments, we believe that their answers provide information about all of their MTM programs and not just pharmacist-provided MTM. Finally, use of an online survey provided both time and cost advantages. However, this survey method suffers from poor response rates. To help overcome this limitation, we also used telephone interviews to gain further insight for interpreting our findings, but our findings are based on relatively small samples and are exploratory in nature. They should not be used for description or prediction in the broader MTM payer population.

Conclusion

The results of this study showed that payers for MTM services varied widely on how they implemented and monitored their organization's MTM programs. They associated value of these programs with cost avoidance/minimization, improved member satisfaction, improved member medication adherence, and quality indicators (e.g., Healthcare Effectiveness Data and Information Set, NCQA). We uncovered evidence that, for 2008, some MTM payer organizations plan to expand their use of face-to-face pharmacist–patient interaction. During 2008, plans may have greater opportunity to measure outcomes in a longitudinal fashion and make adjustments to MTM provision strategies. Some evidence for this was suggested in respondent comments to our survey, but future validation is needed before reaching a firm conclusion. Based on our findings, we proposed suggestions for future consideration such as (1) further development of professionwide models for MTM, (2) conduct of research regarding evidentiary and analytical standards for monitoring MTM services, (3) establishment of standards and quality measures to gauge MTM services and outcomes, and (4) creation of MTM marketing toolkits to improve patient and physician understanding and acceptance of pharmacist-provided MTM services.

References

1. Bluml BM. Definition of medication therapy management: development of professionwide consensus. J Am Pharm Assoc. 2005;45:566–72.

2. American Pharmacists Association, National Association of Chain Drug Stores Foundation. Medication therapy management in community pharmacy practice: core elements on an MTM service (version 1.0). J Am Pharm Assoc. 2005;45:573–9.

3. American Pharmacists Association, National Association of Chain Drug Stores Foundation. Medication therapy management in pharmacy practice: core elements on a MTM service model (version 2.0). J Am Pharm Assoc. In press.

4. Smith SR, Clancy CM. Medication therapy management programs: Forming a new cornerstone for quality and safety in Medicare. Am J Med Qual. 2006;21:276–9.

5. McGivney MS, Meyer SM, Duncan-Hewitt W, et al. Medication therapy management: its relationship to patient counseling, disease management, and pharmaceutical care. J Am Pharm Assoc. 2007;47:620–8.

6. Isetts BJ, Buffington DE, Pharmacist Services Technical Advisory Coalition. CPT code-change proposal: national data on pharmacists' medication therapy management services. Am J Health Syst Pharm. 2007;64:1642–6.

7. American Medical Association. Current Procedural Terminology: CPT 2007. Professional Edition. Chicago: American Medical Association; 2007.

8. Thompson CA. National billing codes announced for pharmacists' clinical services. Am J Health Syst Pharm. 2005;62:1640–2.

9. Thompson CA. Pharmacists' CPT codes become permanent. Am J Health Syst Pharm. 2007;64:2410–2.

10. Garret D, Bluml B. Patient self-management program for diabetes: first-year clinical, humanistic, and economic outcomes. J Am Pharm Assoc. 2005;45:130–7.

11. Cranor CW, Bunting BA, Christensen DB. The Asheville Project: long-term clinical and economic outcomes of a community pharmacy diabetes care program. J Am Pharm Assoc. 2003;43:173–90.

12. Chrischilles EA, Carter BL, Lund BC, et al. Evaluation of the Iowa Medicaid pharmaceutical case management program. J Am Pharm Assoc. 2004;44:337–49.

13. Bunting BA, Cranor CW. The Asheville Project: long-term clinical, humanistic, and economic outcomes of a community-based medication therapy management program for asthma. J Am Pharm Assoc. 2003;46:133–47.

14. Carter BL, Chrischilles EA, Scholz D, et al. Extent of services provided by pharmacists in the Iowa Medicaid pharmaceutical case management program. J Am Pharm Assoc. 2003;43:24–33.

15. Isetts BJ. Evaluating effectiveness of the Minnesota Medication Therapy Management Care Program. Accessed at www.dhs.state.mn.us/main/groups/business_partners/documents/pub/dhs16_140283.pdf, December 14, 2007.

16. Doucette WR, Kreling DH, Schommer JC, et al. Evaluation of community pharmacy service mix: evidence from the 2004 National Pharmacist Workforce Survey. J Am Pharm Assoc. 2006;46:348–55.

17. Touchette DR, Burns AL, Bough MA, Blackburn JC. Survey of medication therapy management programs under Medicare Part D. J Am Pharm Assoc. 2006;46:683–91.

18. Touchette DR, Burns AL, Bough MA, Blackburn JC. Effective Health Care Research Reports: survey of Medicare Part D plans' medication therapy management programs. Accessed at http://effectivehealthcare.ahrq.gov/repFiles/Medication_Therapy_Management_Programs.pdf, February 1, 2008.

19. Guthrie RM. The effects of postal and telephone reminders on compliance with pravastatin therapy in a national registry: results of the first myocardial infarction risk reduction program. Clin Ther. 2001;23:970–80.

20. Elliott RA, Barber N, Clifford S, et al. The cost effectiveness of a telephone-based pharmacy advisory service to improve adherence to newly prescribed medicines. Pharm World Sci. 2008;30:17–23.

21. Rickles NM, Svarstad BL, Statz-Paynter JL, et al. Pharmacist telemonitoring of antidepressant use: effects on pharmacist-patient collaboration. J Am Pharm Assoc. 2005;45:344–53.

22. Tutty S, Simon G, Ludman E. Telephone counseling as an adjunct to antidepressant treatment in the primary care system: a pilot study. Eff Clin Pract. 2000;3:170–8.

23. Schommer JC, Planas LG, Johnson KA, Doucette WR. Pharmacist-provided medication therapy management (part 1): provider perspectives in 2007. J Am Pharm Assoc. 2008;48:e-6–e45.

24. The Lewin Group. Medication therapy management services: a critical review. J Am Pharm Assoc. 2005;45:580–7.

25. Zingone MM, Malcolm KE, McCormick SW, Bledsoe KR. Analysis of pharmacist charges for medication therapy management services in an outpatient setting. Am J Health Syst Pharm. 2007;64:1827–31.

26. Doucette WR, Witry MJ, Alkhateeb F, et al. Attitudes of Medicare beneficiaries toward pharmacist-provided medication therapy management activities as part of the Medicare Part D benefit. J Am Pharm Assoc. 2007;47:758–62.

27. Buffington DE. Pharmacist Current Procedural Terminology codes and medication therapy management. Am J Health Syst Pharm. 2006;63:1008–10.

28. Berwick DM. Continuous improvement as an ideal in health care. N Engl J Med. 1989;320:53–6.

29. Nau DP, Kliethermes MA, McCabe S. Quality measurement: time to get serious. J Am Pharm Assoc. 2006;46:668–79.

30. Holdford DA. Marketing for pharmacists. Washington, D.C.: American Pharmacists Association; 2003.

31. Holdford DA, Kennedy DT. The service blueprint as a tool for designing innovative pharmaceutical services. J Am Pharm Assoc. 1999;39:545–52.

SPECIAL FEATURE

The Diabetes Ten City Challenge: Interim clinical and humanistic outcomes of a multisite community pharmacy diabetes care program

Toni Fera, Benjamin M. Bluml, William M. Ellis, Cynthia W. Schaller, and Daniel G. Garrett

Abstract

Objective: To assess clinical and humanistic outcomes 1 year after initiating the Diabetes Ten City Challenge (DTCC), a multisite community pharmacy health management program for patients with diabetes.

Design: Interim observational analysis of deidentified aggregate data from participating employer clients.

Setting: 29 employers at 10 distinct geographic sites contracting for patient care services with pharmacy providers in the community setting.

Participants: 914 patients with diabetes covered by self-insured employers' health plans who received 3 or more months of pharmacist care and had an initial glycosylated hemoglobin (A1C) measurement. Community-based pharmacists were trained in a diabetes certificate program and reimbursed for clinical services.

Interventions: Community-based pharmacists provided patient care services using scheduled consultations, clinical goal setting, a validated patient self-management program tool, and health status monitoring within a collaborative care management model.

Main outcome measures: Changes in key direct and surrogate outcomes, including glycosylated hemoglobin (A1C), low-density lipoprotein (LDL) cholesterol,, blood pressure measurements, and body mass index; influenza vaccinations; foot examinations; eye examinations; numbers of patients with goals for nutrition, exercise, and weight; and patient satisfaction.

Results: At initial visit compared with 1 year, mean A1C decreased from 7.6% to 7.2%, mean LDL cholesterol decreased from 96 to 93 mg/dL, and mean systolic blood pressure decreased from 131 to 129 mm Hg. Increases were seen for influenza vaccination rate (from 43% to 61%), eye examination rate (from 60% to 77%), and foot examination rate (from 38% to 68%) for the initial visit to the end of the analysis period. For all patients in DTCC, those who perceived that their overall diabetes care was very good to excellent increased from 39% to 87%. Overall, 97.5% reported being very satisfied or satisfied with the diabetes care provided by pharmacists.

Conclusion: Employers demonstrated a willingness to offer a voluntary health benefit to employees and their dependents with diabetes that uses pharmacists to help participants achieve self-management goals. Patients participating in the first year of DTCC had measurable improvement in clinical indicators of diabetes management, higher rates of self-management goal setting, and increased satisfaction with diabetes care. Based on results of previous studies, these positive trends are expected to drive a corresponding decline in projected total direct patient medical costs.

Keywords: Diabetes Ten City Challenge, Patient Self-Management Program, pharmaceutical care, diabetes, disease management, chronic disease, quality of life, health care costs, health outcomes, health benefits, collaborative practice, Asheville Project.

J Am Pharm Assoc. 2008;48:181–190.
doi: 10.1331/JAPhA.2008.07166

Received December 18, 2007, and in revised form February 7, 2008. Accepted for publication February 12, 2008.

Toni Fera, PharmD, is Director, Patient Self-Management Programs; Benjamin M. Bluml, BPharm, is Vice President for Research; William M. Ellis, BPharm, MS, is Chief Executive Officer; Cynthia W. Schaller, MBA, is Director of Operations; and Daniel G. Garrett, BPharm, MS, FASHP, is Senior Director, Medication Adherence Programs, American Pharmacists Association (APhA) Foundation, Washington, D.C.

Correspondence: Toni Fera, PharmD, APhA Foundation 1100 15th Street, NW, Suite 400, Washington, D.C., 20005. Fax: 202-638-3793. E-mail: tfera@aphanet.org

Disclosure: Other than employment by the APhA Foundation and development of the APhA Foundation's Web-based documentation system by Mr. Bluml, the authors declare no conflicts of interests or financial interests in any product or service mentioned in this article, including grants, gifts, stock holdings, or honoraria.

Funding: GlaxoSmithKline, Inc.

Acknowledgments: The Patient Self-Management Program is a Service Mark of the APhA Foundation.

According to the Centers for Disease Control and Prevention, diabetes affects 20.8 million people in the United States (7% of the total population).[1] By 2050, that total is projected to increase to 39 million people. Many of these individuals are part of the U.S. workforce and an important part of the country's economy. Diabetes costs the nation nearly $132 billion a year ($92 billion in direct medical costs). The National Diabetes Education Program (NDEP) states that employees involved in their own self-management typically have better outcomes. Individuals who are active self-managers, in addition to their working to improve glycemic control, experience fewer complications from comorbidities such as stroke, heart disease, and renal disease. They are also more productive at home and at work. In its White Paper, "Making a Difference: The Business Community Takes on Diabetes," NDEP issues a call to action to employers "to improve diabetes care and education (because that) will help workers remain productive, decrease diabetes-related complications, and reduce associated costs over time. A

dedicated effort and financial investment at the senior management level are essential to achieving these goals."[2]

Researchers have also shown that decreased adherence to treatment regimens leads to increased hospitalizations and mortality in patients with diabetes, thereby increasing the costs associated with this disease in both human and economic terms.[3] Previously published research, such as that conducted by the American Pharmacists Association (APhA) Foundation and researchers in the Asheville Project, has discussed the important role of patients in self-managing their disease.[4-8] This research has shown that when patients become effective self-managers, with the support of a pharmacist coach, considerable improvements in clinical care are achievable while decreasing total health care costs.

In light of the success achieved by the APhA Foundation's Patient Self-Management Program and other clinical care programs that include pharmacists, keen interest has arisen for testing the scalability of the patient self-management/pharmacist coach model in diverse communities. Successful implementation of such a model on a broad scale would have the capacity to transform the health care system by improving outcomes and controlling costs. In 2005, the APhA Foundation, with support from GlaxoSmithKline, set out to test the scalability of this model in 10 unique locations across the country, through the Diabetes Ten City Challenge (DTCC). The ongoing project includes components that are hallmarks of Foundation projects and programs, including aligned incentives, collaborative care, and a validated patient self-management credentialing process for diabetes. DTCC established a voluntary health benefit for employees and dependents who are deemed eligible under the employers' benefit, provided incentives through waived copayments for antidiabetic medications and related supplies, and helped people manage their diabetes with support from a pharmacist coach in collaboration with physicians and diabetes educators.

The findings presented in this article include clinical and humanistic results from the first year of implementation of DTCC.

At a Glance

Synopsis: In its initial year of operation, the Diabetes Ten City Challenge demonstrated improvements in mean glycosylated hemoglobin (from 7.6% to 7.2%), low-density lipoprotein cholesterol (from 96 to 93 mg/dL), and systolic blood pressure (from 131 to 129 mm Hg). A total of 29 self-insured employers contracted for patient care services in this collaborative health management program, with community pharmacists coaching 914 patients with diabetes on effective self-management strategies to improve medication adherence. The percentage of patients with current influenza vaccinations increased from 43% to 61%, current eye examinations from 60% to 77%, and current foot examinations from 38% to 68%. Patients with self-management goals for nutrition, exercise, and weight increased from 22% to 66%, from 24% to 72%, and from 23% to 64%, respectively.

Analysis: The U.S. Centers for Disease Control and Prevention estimates that, of the approximately $2 trillion spent by public and private sectors on health care in 2005, more than 75% went toward treatment of chronic disease. The Partnership to Fight Chronic Disease reports that chronic diseases such as diabetes, if left unchecked, have the potential to bankrupt our health care system. The indirect costs of chronic disease, resulting from factors such as absenteeism and reduced on-the-job productivity far outweigh the cost of treatments. By investing in aligned incentives and keeping patients with diabetes healthy, productive, and on the job, employers can expect to see considerable moderation of increases in overall health care costs over the long term.

Objectives

DTCC is designed to establish a voluntary health benefit for employers in 10 distinct geographic areas of the United States, with an enrollment goal of approximately 125 patients at each site for a minimum duration of 12 months. The program objectives are

- To implement an employer-funded, collaborative health management program using community-based pharmacist coaching, evidence-based diabetes care guidelines, and self-management strategies designed to keep patients with diabetes healthy and productive.
- To implement the patient self-management training and assessment credential that equips patients with the knowledge, skills, and performance-monitoring priorities needed to actively participate in managing their diabetes.

■ To assess participant satisfaction with overall diabetes care and pharmacist care provided in the program.

Methods

Setting

DTCC was offered as a voluntary benefit by employers at 10 distinct geographic sites that included both individual employers and coalitions of employers. Employers were recruited on a rolling basis, so most employers started at different times (Table 1). DTCC locations were selected for their diversity in terms of size, demographics, and geography, in order to test the model in a variety of circumstances.

The program was offered in community independent pharmacies, in community chain pharmacies, in ambulatory care clinics, and at on-site workplace locations if designated by the employer. The sites included the following characteristics.

■ Private area for patient consultation
■ Management support freeing pharmacists for patient care activities
■ Access to Internet for recording and tracking patient care interventions
■ Availability of pharmacist coach with demonstrated communication skills and specialized training or certification in diabetes management

The model was designed to allow sufficient flexibility to accommodate the different practice settings represented in the program, the specific demographics of the patient population served, and practice arrangements made within local and/or regional health care market places, including contracts with pharmacist networks to provide patient care services.

Intervention

The practice model implemented for DTCC is designed as a collaborative care model that emphasizes the roles of the employer, physician, pharmacist, and patient. The employer/payer agreed to invest in incentives for patients and pharmacist providers. At a minimum, these incentives included waived copayments for antidiabetic medications and related supplies. Some employers added other incentives as a way to integrate the program into their existing plan offerings. Examples included counting participation toward wellness points, waiving copayments for diabetes-related medications, diabetes education classes, and/or laboratory test copayments. The employer recruited patients into the program through various announcement methods, including direct mailings, e-mail blasts, newsletters, and live orientation sessions. All patients were required to enter into a program participation agreement, which included information about how the program works, their responsibility as a participant in the program, their right to confidentiality, how data would be reported to the employer, and their right to withdraw from the program at any time. In addition, the participants completed an enrollment form, including authorization to release medical information. This consent was provided to

Table 1. Diabetes Ten City Challenge sites

Charleston, S.C.
Chicago
Colorado Springs, Colo.
Cumberland, Md.
Honolulu, Hawaii
Milwaukee, Wis.
Northwest Georgia
Pittsburgh, Pa.
Los Angeles
Tampa Bay, Fla.

pharmacists so that they could obtain relevant laboratory and other information from other health care providers. Patients were also asked to complete a baseline diabetes care satisfaction survey and medical history form. They were instructed to complete the medical history form and bring it with them on the first visit with their pharmacist. Once enrolled in the program, the patient was assigned a unique identifier. Eligible participants selected their first- and second-choice pharmacist coach and/or location from a local pharmacy network directory. The enrollment period and program duration agreed to at each site was a minimum of 12 months.

Physicians were informed of participant enrollment and encouraged to share their care plan with the pharmacist, who reinforced that plan with participants. Pharmacists communicated with physicians after every visit, as necessary, and referred patients as needed to their physician (e.g., for referrals, laboratory test recommendations, or medication-related problems identified), dietitian (e.g., for intensive nutrition education), or diabetes education centers (e.g., for additional education support).

Pharmacists were assigned to a participant through their network coordinator. Once assigned, participant enrollment materials were transferred to the pharmacist, who contacted the patient to set up their first appointment. During regularly scheduled visits, pharmacists applied a prescribed process of care that focused on clinical assessments and progress toward clinical goals, established self-management goals specific to each patient, and included working with other health care providers to recommend adjustments in patient treatment plans. Pharmacists who participated in the program were required to complete an Accreditation Council for Pharmacy Education–accredited diabetes certificate training program or its equivalent, such as certification by the Board of Pharmaceutical Specialties as a pharmacotherapy specialist with experience in diabetes management. Pharmacists were instructed to follow American Diabetes Association (ADA) guidelines unless otherwise specified by the physician. Pharmacists collected subjective and objective assessment information, both self-reported and laboratory conducted. Assessment data were then entered into the APhA Foundation's Web-based documentation system.

Pharmacists were reimbursed by employers for patient visits according to fee schedules negotiated by the local pharmacy network.

Process of care

To ensure consistent application of the care model, the pharmacists were required to attend additional training on the Patient Self-Management Program for Diabetes process of care (Figure 1), documentation forms, Patient Self-Management Credential for Diabetes, and the documentation system. Patients worked with their pharmacist through a structured series of visits that focused on knowledge, skills, and performance, and patients were "scored" as either beginner, proficient, or advanced in these three domains. These assessments were designed to help the providers understand the area(s) in which each patient needed additional education and the diabetes care standards upon which each patient needed to improve. The overall goal of the credential is to serve as an empowerment tool and to assist in standardizing care goals for all patients.

At the first visit (or series of visits), the pharmacist assessed the patient's knowledge about their diabetes, reviewed the program requirements, and reviewed any existing patient goals and his or her medical history. The pharmacist, after meeting with the patient and identifying their primary physician, sent an introduction letter informing the physician of the patient's participation in the program and a progress note. (In some instances, the introduction letter was sent by the employer or network.)

Ongoing visits focused on clinical and self-management credential assessments and progress on related goals. Laboratory tests were periodically performed at the physician's office, at the designated lab, or by point-of-care testing. Key laboratory indicators and patient goals were documented on a trifold documentation form that provided the basis for ongoing monitoring and communication between patients and health care providers. Patients were provided with a copy of this form for reference between visits. The clinical data and visit documentation were also entered via the APhA Foundation's Web-based system.

Over the course of the enrollment period, pharmacists worked through the self-management credential domains with patients. Visits were scheduled by appointment, usually once a month for the first 3 months, then at least quarterly or more often if deemed necessary by the pharmacist. Pharmacists coached patients and worked with them to set goals. Pharmacists maintained ongoing communication with patients, their physicians, diabetes educators, and other specialist providers involved in the patient's care. Patients were actively involved in their therapy, treatment plans, goal setting, and performance monitoring.

Design

This report is an observational analysis of deidentified aggregate data collated from initial reports developed for par-ticipating employers. Program participants were employees or other eligible beneficiaries with diabetes who volunteered to participate in the program at no charge, agreed to regular meetings with matched pharmacists, and were eligible for designated incentives provided for participation. As described above, the providers were community-based pharmacists who received certificate training in diabetes care or equivalent.

Inclusion criteria and data measurement

Patients at the 10 different sites were enrolled into the program. See Table 1 for a listing of sites. Patients who had an initial glycosylated hemoglobin (A1C) recorded and at least 3 months of pharmacist care were included in clinical data analysis, resulting in aggregated data for 914 patients. Clinical laboratory data were obtained from the physician, laboratory, or point-of-care testing.

Behavioral goal-setting rates and achievement for patient self-management of nutrition, exercise, and weight were based on patient self-reports and documented by the pharmacists during each patient visit and are reported for the patients meeting inclusion criteria. Knowledge, skills, and performance assessments were administered by pharmacists for patients in a manner consistent with the psychometrically validated credential. (Note: The Patient Self-Management Credential for Diabetes is an externally validated tool developed by the APhA Foundation.) Subjective and objective data were submitted via the Foundation's Web-based documentation system.

Patient satisfaction was recorded on surveys using two instruments that were previously developed and used.[5] (Note: David P. Nau, PhD, Assistant Professor, College of Pharmacy, University of Kentucky, developed the patient satisfaction surveys for the program.) One survey on overall satisfaction with diabetes care was completed at baseline as part of the enrollment packet, and, approximately 6 months after enrollment at a follow-up patient visit, the survey was repeated. Another survey was administered after approximately 6 months of enrollment to measure satisfaction with care from the pharmacist. Completion of the survey was optional and the responder anonymous; therefore, we are not able to match the surveys to the aggregate population.

Timeline

Patient enrollment began in January 2006 and continued at each site dependent on employer-specific enrollment timetables. The ending point for data in this initial evaluation was September 30, 2007.

Outcome definitions

Clinical outcome measures included recognized standards for diabetes care and those used in the "State of Health Care Quality: 2006" report from the National Committee for Quality Assurance (NCQA).[9] The following clinical indicators were measured: A1C, low-density lipoprotein (LDL) cholesterol, systolic blood pres-

DIABETES TEN CITY CHALLENGE **SPECIAL FEATURE**

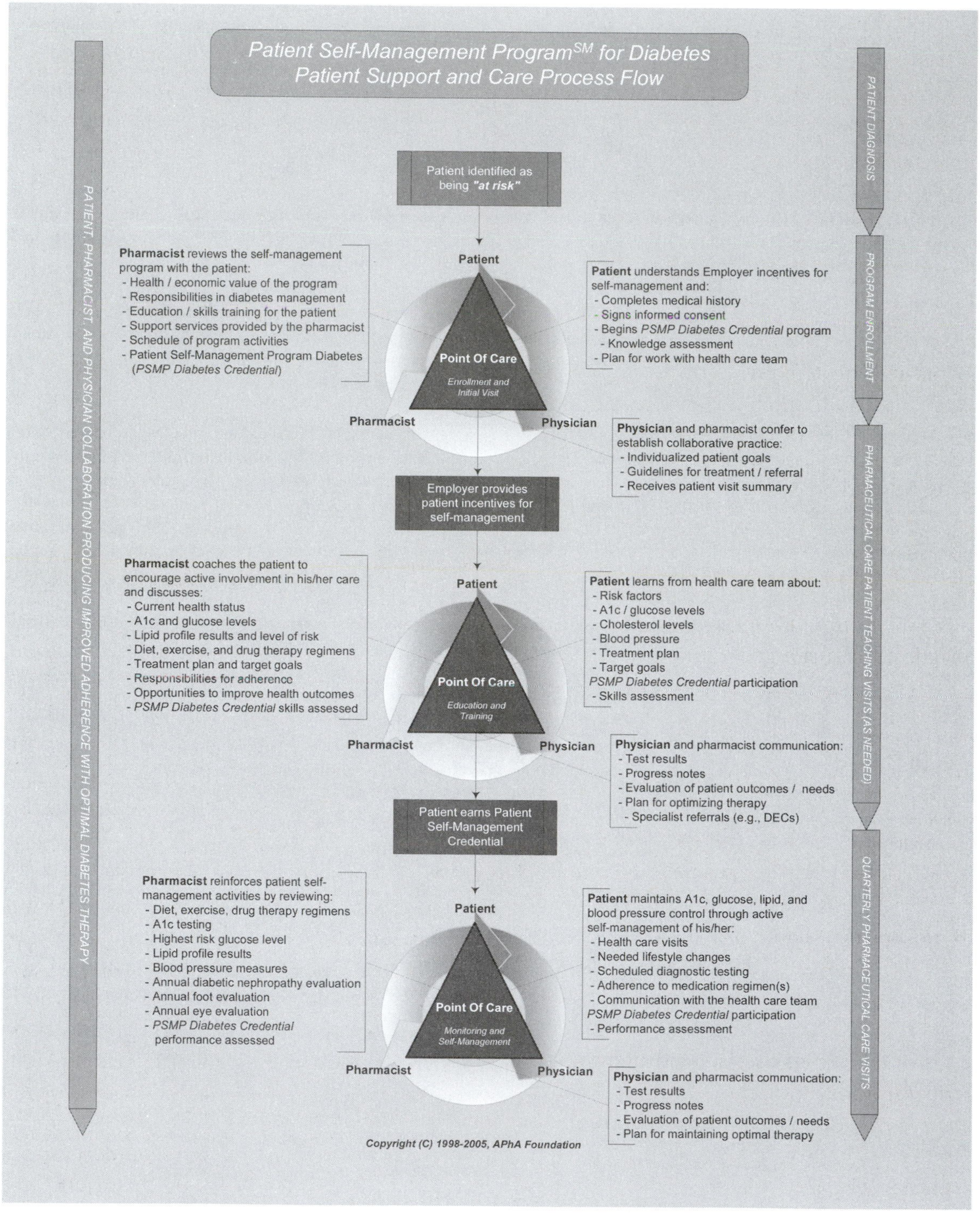

Figure 1. Patient Self-Management Program for Diabetes patient support and care process flow

Abbreviations used: A1C, glycosylated hemoglobin; DEC, diabetes educator; PSMP, Patient Self-Management Program.

Journal of the American Pharmacists Association www.pharmacist.com MAR/APR 2008 • 48:2 • JAPhA • 185 sure, diastolic blood pressure, current influenza vaccination, current foot examination, and current eye examination.

Patient satisfaction with overall diabetes care was measured on a 10-point Likert-type scale, and patient satisfaction with pharmacist care was measured on a 5-point Likert-type scale.

Knowledge, skills, and performance assessments were evaluated based on the Patient Self-Management Credential standards. Each patient was assigned an achievement level of beginner, proficient, or advanced for each assessment domain.

Data sources

Aggregated, deidentified data were collated from employer reports that included the designated measures for general demographics, clinical, behavioral, and patient satisfaction data. These data were recorded in the Web-based documentation system by the pharmacists after each patient visit. This Web-based resource was designed based on the electronic health data management principles previously outlined by the APhA Foundation.[10] Patient satisfaction survey data were sent by the employer (upon enrollment) or by participants (at follow-up) directly to the APhA Foundation for data entry.

Data analysis

Data were combined from all sites to create one aggregate cohort. The analysis compared initial and follow-up outcomes that were collected during the course of the patient care visits.

Results

Patient population characteristics

As previously described, 914 patients met the inclusion criteria and received pharmacist care for 3 or more months, with an average of 4.6 pharmacist visits per patient. The mean (± SD) duration of enrollment was 10.2 ± 3.7 months. The combined population consisted of 49% women and 51% men, with an average age of 53.4 years. Of patients, 72% were 50 years of age or older. Patient ethnicity was as follows: 77% white, 13% black, 4% Hispanic, 2% Asian, 1% Native American, 1% Pacific Islander, 1% other, and 1% not specified. Education distribution was as follows: 2% eighth grade or less, 3% some high school, 30% high school graduates, 31% some college, 22% college graduates, 8% postgraduate education, and 4% not specified. These characteristics are summarized in Figure 2.

Clinical outcomes

Using the two-tailed Student's t test for paired data, statistically significant improvements were found for the enrolled patients using beginning and ending A1C, LDL cholesterol, and systolic and diastolic blood pressure measures (Table 2). In the primary clinical indicator for diabetes, mean A1C decreased from 7.6% to 7.2% (a 5.2% reduction) and a 21% increase in ADA goal achievement of A1C less than 7% occurred. Mean LDL cholesterol decreased from 96.3 to 93.3 mg/dL, with an increase in

National Cholesterol Education Program Adult Treatment Panel III goal (LDL <100 mg/dL) achievement from 43.8% to 57.7%, an improvement of 32%.[9,11] In this group, people who had an LDL measurement increased from 77% to 88%. Mean systolic blood pressure decreased from 131.3 to 128.7 mm Hg, with a 15.7% increase in the goal (130 mm Hg) recommended in the Seventh Report of the Joint National Committee on Prevention, Detection, Evaluation, and Treatment of High Blood Pressure (JNC 7).[12] Mean diastolic blood pressure decreased from 79.3 to 77.3 mm Hg, with a 9.2% increase in JNC 7 goal achievement (80 mm Hg).

Diabetes care indicator outcomes

Table 3 summarizes the improvements in the diabetes process-of-care indicators compared with the Health Plan Employer Data and Information Set (HEDIS) indicators for NCQA commercially accredited health plans. DTCC participant results were notably higher than the HEDIS measures achieved by current health plans.[9] The percentage of patients with current influenza vaccination increased from 43% to 61%, current eye examinations from 60% to 77%, and current foot examinations from 38% to 68%.

Patient self-management goal outcomes

At the beginning of the program, only 22%, 24%, and 23% of patients had individual self-management goals for nutrition, exercise, and weight, respectively. These percentages increased to 66% for nutrition, 72% for exercise, and 64% for weight at the ending visit.

Patient Self-Management Credential assessment

The Patient Self-Management Credential knowledge and skills assessment was used initially so that members of the health care team could identify potential knowledge and diabetes management skill gaps. Patients were expected to progress over time and improve their scores across all three domains. At the end of the reporting period, aggregate knowledge achievement scores were 4% beginner, 40% proficient, 48% advanced, and 2% not yet scored. The skills assessment was used during the first several visits to evaluate patient skill levels within six different categories. Aggregate skill achievement scores at the end of the reporting period were 11% beginner, 35% proficient, 32% advanced, and 32% not yet scored. The performance assessment was used periodically after the other two so that patients and providers could identify potential opportunities for ongoing performance improvement. Aggregate performance achievement scores were 12% beginner, 26% proficient, and 22% advanced. In this group, as a result of the limited time some patients had been in DTCC, 40% had not been scored for performance achievement at the time this article was prepared.

Patient satisfaction outcomes

Subjective responses at baseline and follow-up were evaluated for all program participants who submitted surveys. The

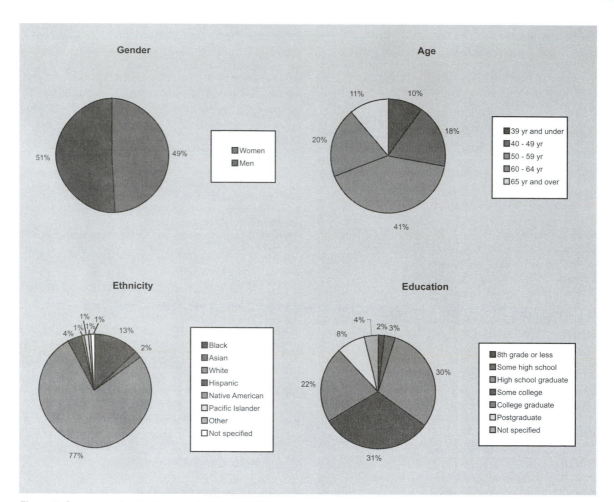

Figure 2. Summary of patient characteristics, DTCC

Abbreviation used: DTCC, Diabetes Ten City Challenge.

Table 2. Clinical indicator measures for patients in DTCC

Parameter (no. patients)	Beginning measure Mean ± SD	Ending measure Mean ± SD	Change Mean ± SD	Duration (months) Mean ± SD	P[a]
A1C, % (914)	7.6 ± 1.7	7.2 ± 1.4	−0.4 ± 1.2	10.2 ± 3.7	<0.001
LDL-C, mg/dL (815)	96.3 ± 31.5	93.3 ± 31.7	−3.8 ± 25.4	10.2 ± 3.7	<0.001
SBP, mm Hg (806)	131.3 ± 15.7	128.7 ± 15.6	−2.5 ± 15.9	10.2 ± 3.7	<0.001
DBP, mm Hg (806)	79.3 ± 10.1	77.3 ± 9.2	−2.3 ± 10	10.2 ± 3.7	<0.001

Abbreviations used: A1C, glycosylated hemoglobin; DBP, diastolic blood pressure; DTCC, Diabetes Ten City Challenge; LDL-C, low-density lipoprotein cholesterol; SBP, systolic blood pressure.

[a]P value calculated by applying a two-tailed Student's t test for paired data to the mean ± SD change data.

SPECIAL FEATURE DIABETES TEN CITY CHALLENGE

Table 3. Comparison of DTCC and HEDIS process measures

HEDIS commercial indicator	HEDIS 2006 commercially accredited plans % Patients	DTCC (10.2 months) % Patients
Tested for A1C	87.5	100[a]
Good A1C control (A1C ≤9%)	70.3	91.2
Tested for lipid profile	92.3	89.2
LDL-C ≤100 mg/dL	43.8	57.7
Current eye examinations	54.8	76.9
Immunized against influenza	36.3[b]	61.5

Abbreviations used: A1C, glycosylated hemoglobin; DTCC, Diabetes Ten City Challenge; HEDIS, Health Plan Employer Data and Information Set; LDL-C, low-density lipoprotein cholesterol; DTCC, Diabetes Ten City Challenge.

[a]Inclusion criteria.

[b]All adults.

participants were asked to rate their overall satisfaction with diabetes care on a scale of 1 to 10 (1, worst possible care; 10, best possible care). Satisfaction with pharmacist care was evaluated on a 5-point Likert-type scale (1, very dissatisfied; 5, very satisfied). The surveys have been previously used,[5] and results are reported in Figure 3. For all patients in DTCC, those who perceived that their overall diabetes care was a 9 or 10 (excellent) increased from 39% to 87%. Of patients, 97.5% reported being very satisfied or satisfied with the diabetes care provided by the pharmacists.

Discussion

The overall goal of DTCC is to transform how the health care system manages chronic disease, by investing in aligned incentives and helping people self-manage their condition with the help of a pharmacist coach and a team of health care professionals. DTCC scales previous models developed in the Asheville Project and by the APhA Foundation and demonstrates that this model could be implemented in the diverse health care markets exemplified by the participating public and private employers in 10 geographic regions.

The clinical and humanistic outcome measurements and metrics presented in this report are those established as key indicators of the program's effectiveness. By implementing this standardized model, employers in a variety of markets can improve health outcomes for their health plan beneficiaries with diabetes. The system also provides employers with meaningful results to use in making data-driven health care and business decisions.

The key findings supported the employers' objectives for the program and included the following:

■ Diabetes control improved during the 1-year of care, and mean A1C values were reduced from 7.6% to 7.2% for the entire enrolled population in the first year of the program, approaching the goal for A1C set by ADA (<7.0%).

■ Significant improvements have occurred in other key indicators of diabetes care, such as influenza vaccinations, recorded blood pressure, lipid profiles, and percentage of patients receiving foot and eye examinations, as outlined above.

■ For most indicator categories, results have exceeded those of the HEDIS outcomes for commercially accredited plans.

■ More than 97% of patients reported that they were either very satisfied or satisfied with the care provided by pharmacists in the program.

■ In the next reporting phase of the program, employers will be able to evaluate the economic impact of the program across the spectrum of total health care costs.

Health benefit design

Consistent with the findings of prior APhA Foundation and Asheville Project studies, the clinical and humanistic outcomes for the first year of DTCC support the idea of a new employee benefit model for the management of chronic disease.

The Partnership to Fight Chronic Disease projects that, left unchecked, chronic diseases such as diabetes will negatively affect the U.S. economy and the nationwide employment base, with the very real potential to bankrupt the health care system in this country.[13] Mays et al.[14] point out that insurers and employers have responded to the burden of chronic disease by increasing their investment in disease management programs to help contain costs. However, the authors also note that a disconnect exists between disease management efforts to enhance adherence to treatment regimens and the higher patient cost sharing that can occur, which ultimately will be an impediment to patient involvement in disease management programs.

Within DTCC, the health benefit design offered to employees and their beneficiaries endeavors to align the incentives for all parties involved. Features of this employee health benefit include the following:

■ Voluntary nature: Workers and their families must opt in to the program with the understanding that their individual clinical results will not be disclosed to the employer. The voluntary nature of the benefit starts the process of the patient choosing to address their disease in a proactive manner.

■ Waived copayments: The program asks employers to waive copayments for antidiabetic and related medications as an incentive for patients to enroll and stay in the program. As previously reported, this economic incentive can be the decisive factor in enrollment.[14] Out-of-pocket patient savings have been published at $300 per patient per year; however, this can vary based on benefit design.[5] The figure of $300 can serve as an incentive to not only enroll but also stay in the program because the waived copayments can be dropped if the patient is not keeping regular appointments with the pharmacist coach.

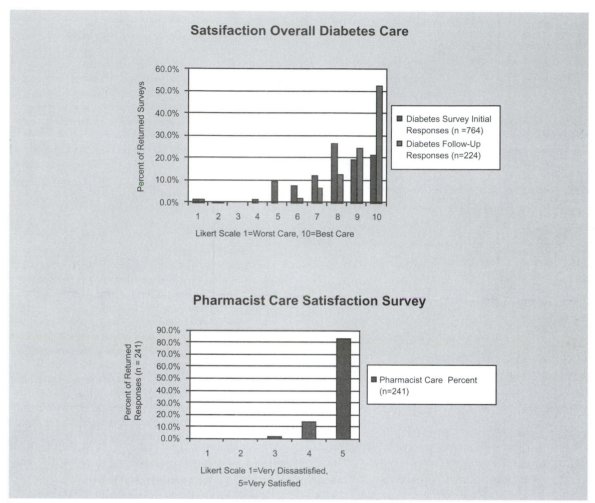

Figure 3. Participant satisfaction surveys, DTCC

Abbreviation used: DTCC, Diabetes Ten City Challenge.

■ Face-to-face contact: Patients have reported that the face-to-face contact with a pharmacist and the other health care providers in this model helped them to be more accountable and supported in their efforts to self-manage their disease.[8]

■ Pharmacist and other health care provider services: The pharmacist's time with the patient is compensated by the employer, thereby allowing this important aspect of the program to be sustained. In addition, the APhA Foundation recommends that the services of a diabetes education center also be made available by the employer to help reinforce the behaviors needed to successfully self-manage diabetes.

■ Physicians receive regular communication from the pharmacist on their patients, which helps create a collaborative practice model and improve overall care.

■ Employer return: Employers expect to receive savings on overall health care costs and the ability to offer a benefit with which participants are highly satisfied.

DTCC also shows that self-insured employers are interested in piloting new employee benefits that align the incentives for all parties in an attempt to mitigate the potentially catastrophic effect that chronic disease has on America's workforce. Recently, the Milken Institute reported that the total lost economic output related to diabetes was $105 billion.[15] Employers such as those in DTCC realize that the indirect impact of chronic disease—including absenteeism and reduced on-the-job productivity—far outweigh the cost of treatments. We believe that DTCC validates that this collaborative practice model can be replicated in diverse geographic locations among both public- and private-sector employers.

SPECIAL FEATURE DIABETES TEN CITY CHALLENGE

Limitations

This is an observational interim report, and the outcomes analysis was intended from the outset to meet the needs of employers in improving the health of their workforce and their dependents with diabetes. In addition, the different starting dates for the participating employers has limited the data set for this interim report.

Conclusion

This interim DTCC report shows that the collaborative practice model using community-based pharmacist coaching, evidence-based diabetes care guidelines, and self-management strategies can play a key role in helping patients to successfully manage chronic disease. Patients participating in the first year of the program had measurable improvement in clinical indicators of diabetes management, higher rates of self-management goal setting, and increased satisfaction with diabetes care. In addition, 97.5% of patient survey respondents indicated that they were satisfied or very satisfied with pharmacist care.

References

1. Centers for Disease Control and Prevention. Division of Laboratory Sciences: diabetes. Accessed at www.cdc.gov/nceh/dls/diabetes.htm, December 10, 2007.
2. The National Diabetes Education Program. Making a difference: the business community takes on diabetes. Accessed at http://ndep.nih.gov/resources/business/index.htm, December 11, 2007.
3. Ho PM, Rumsfeld JS, Masoudi FA, et al. Medication nonadherence increases hospitalization and mortality among patients with diabetes mellitus. Arch Intern Med. 2006;166:1836–41.
4. Bluml BM, McKenney JM, Cziraky MJ. Pharmaceutical care services and results in Project ImPACT: Hyperlipidemia. J Am Pharm Assoc. 2000;40:157–65.
5. Bluml BM, Garrett DG. Patient self-management program for diabetes: first-year clinical, humanistic, and economic outcomes. J Am Pharm Assoc. 2005;45:130–7.
6. Cranor CW, Christensen DB. The Asheville Project: short-term outcomes of a community pharmacy diabetes care program. J Am Pharm Assoc. 2003;43:149–59.
7. Cranor CW, Bunting BA, Christensen DB. The Asheville Project: long-term clinical and economic outcomes in a community pharmacy diabetes care program. J Am Pharm Assoc. 2003;43:173–84.
8. Garrett DG, Martin LA. The Asheville Project: participants' perceptions of factors contributing to the success of a Patient Self-Management Program for Diabetes. J Am Pharm Assoc. 2003;43:185–90.
9. National Committee for Quality Assurance. The state of health care quality 2006. Accessed at www.ncqa.org/tabid/447/Default.aspx, December 12, 2007.
10. Bluml BM, Crooks GM. Designing solutions for securing patient privacy: meeting the demands of health care in the 21st century. J Am Pharm Assoc. 1999;39:402–7.
11. National Heart, Lung, and Blood Institute. Detection, evaluation, and treatment of high cholesterol in adults (Adult Treatment Panel III). Accessed at www.nhlbi.nih.gov/guidelines/cholesterol/atp3xsum.pdf December 10, 2007.
12. Chobanian AV, Bakris GL, Black HR, et al. The Seventh Report of the Joint National Committee on Prevention, Detection, Evaluation, and Treatment of High Blood Pressure: the JNC-7 report. JAMA. 2003;289:2560–72.
13. Partnership To Fight Chronic Disease. A vision for a healthier future: the implications. Accessed at www.fightchronicdisease.org/implications/index.cfm, December 10, 2007.
14. Mays GP, Au M, Claxton G. Convergence and dissonance : evolution in private-sector approaches to disease management and care coordination. Health Aff (Millwood). 2007;26:1683–91.
15. DeVol R, Bedroussian A. An unhealthy America: the economic burden of chronic disease: charting a new course to save lives and increase productivity and economic growth. Santa Monica, Calif.: Milken Institute; 2007.

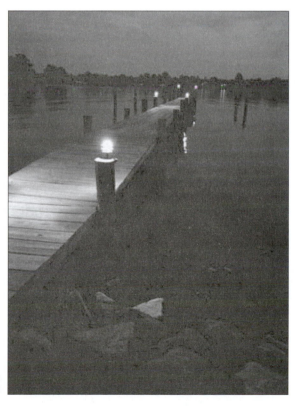

Dock on Chesapeake Bay • Maryland's Eastern Shore August 2007 • Stuart T. Haines, PharmD, FCCP, FASHP

COMMENTARY

Medication therapy management: Its relationship to patient counseling, disease management, and pharmaceutical care

Melissa Somma McGivney, Susan M. Meyer, Wendy Duncan–Hewitt, Deanne L. Hall, Jean-Venable R. Goode, and Randall B. Smith

Abstract

Objective: To delineate the relationship, including similarities and differences, between medication therapy management (MTM) and contemporary pharmacist-provided services, including patient counseling, disease management, and pharmaceutical care, to facilitate the continued evolution of commonly used language and a standard of practice across geographic areas and practice environments.

Summary: Incorporation of MTM services into the array of Medicare-funded services affords an opportunity for pharmacists to develop direct patient care services in the community. Defining the role of MTM within the scope of pharmacist-provided patient care activities, including patient counseling, disease management, and all currently provided pharmacy services is essential to the delineation of a viable and sustainable practice model for pharmacists. The definitions of each of these services are offered, as well as comparisons and contrasts of the individual services. In addition to Medicare-eligible patients, MTM services are appropriate for anyone with medication-related needs. MTM is offered as an all-encompassing model that incorporates the philosophy of pharmaceutical care, techniques of patient counseling, and disease management in an environment that facilitates the direct collaboration of patients, pharmacists, and other health professionals.

Conclusion: Defining the role of MTM within the current patient care models, including patient counseling, disease management, and all who provide pharmacy services, is essential in delineating a viable and sustainable practice model for pharmacists.

Keywords: Medication therapy management, pharmaceutical care, patient counseling, disease management.

J Am Pharm Assoc. 2007;47:620–628.
doi: 10.1331/JAPhA.2007.06129

Received for publication November 10, 2006, and in revised form February 12, 2007. Accepted for publication May 30, 2007.

Melissa Somma McGivney, PharmD, CDE, is Assistant Professor, and **Susan M. Meyer, PhD,** is Professor and Associate Dean for Education, School of Pharmacy, University of Pittsburgh, Pittsburgh. **Wendy Duncan–Hewitt, PhD,** is Dean of Pharmacy, St. Louis College of Pharmacy, St. Louis. **Deanne L. Hall, PharmD, CDE,** is Assistant Professor, School of Pharmacy, University of Pittsburgh, Pittsburgh. **Jean-Venable R. Goode, PharmD, BCPS, FAPhA,** is Associate Professor, School of Pharmacy, Virginia Commonwealth University, Richmond. **Randall B. Smith, PhD,** is Professor and Senior Associate Dean, School of Pharmacy, University of Pittsburgh, Pittsburgh.

Correspondence: Melissa Somma McGivney, PharmD, CDE, School of Pharmacy, University of Pittsburgh, 721 Salk Hall, 3501 Terrace St., Pittsburgh, PA 15261. Fax: 412-624-8175. E-mail: somma@pitt.edu

Disclosure: Dr. Somma McGivney is a faculty consultant to the Rite Aid Corporation for the development of medication therapy management (MTM) services and has received honoraria for her work on advisory panels for the American Pharmacists Association (APhA)/American Society of Consultant Pharmacists MTM Certificate Training Course and the APhA/National Association of Chain Drug Stores Medication Therapy Management Continuing Education Training. Dr. Meyer is the principal investigator on a grant designed to provide MTM training to faculty and preceptors. Dr. Goode has received honoraria for her work as an APhA Immunization Trainer. Drs. Hall and Smith have received an educational grant for their work in designing a diabetes education training course for pharmacists.

Acknowledgments: To Teresa McKaveney and Erik Rueter of the University of Pittsburgh School of Pharmacy for assistance in preparing this manuscript.

PLACING MTM IN PHARMACY'S HISTORICAL CONTEXT **COMMENTARY**

The profession of pharmacy has been integral to the delivery of drug therapy to patients since its inception, yet pharmacists commonly have been dissociated from the use, evaluation, and monitoring of drug therapy. The widely cited reports of the Institute of Medicine (IOM)[1–4] articulate an increased awareness of a lack of continuity of care and associated challenges for the provision of health care in the United States. Society has experienced an increase in adverse drug reactions and drug costs, which has prompted a call for an enhanced role for pharmacists in ensuring effective drug use and patient safety. Recently, the U.S. government has begun to formulate a plan for the Medicare population through the passage of the Medicare Modernization Act of 2003 and the Medicare Prescription Medication Benefit (Part D), and this incorporates medication therapy management (MTM) services.

The advent of these changes in health care services has raised important questions for patients, pharmacists, other health care professionals, and payers. How do the functions and activities of MTM differ from current pharmacy services? How is MTM similar to or different from patient counseling and disease management? How are these patient care services related to pharmaceutical care?

Incorporation of MTM services into the array of Medicare-funded services affords an opportunity for pharmacists to develop direct patient care services in the community. The first step toward successfully developing MTM services is to attain an understanding of where MTM fits into the scope of contemporary pharmacy services. This commentary serves to delineate the relationship of MTM to pharmaceutical care, patient counseling, and disease management and suggests a way to envision how each fits into the scope of a pharmacist's patient care activities (Figure 1). A glossary of key terms commonly used by pharmacists when referring to various patient care services is provided in Appendix 1, as it may be useful in developing a uniform understanding by practitioners, patients, and payers.

Defining MTM services

MTM has been defined by the pharmacy profession as "a distinct service or group of services that optimize therapeutic outcomes for individual patients [that] are independent of, but can occur in conjunction with, the provision of a drug product."[5] Specific desired outcomes of MTM are appropriate drug use, enhanced patient understanding of appropriate drug use, increased patient adherence with prescribed drug therapies, reduced risk of adverse events associated with drugs, and reduced need for other costly medical services.[5] The Centers for Medicare & Medicaid Services describes MTM as a mechanism to ensure that "medications prescribed for targeted beneficiaries are appropriately used to optimize therapeutic outcomes and reduce the risk of adverse events."[6] The American Pharmacists Association and the National Association of Chain Drug Stores Foundation established "core elements" of an MTM service, including medication therapy review, personal medication record, medication action plan, intervention and/or referral, and documentation and follow-up.[7] These core elements provide a mechanism to accomplish the comprehensive goal of MTM, which is to focus on and create solutions for patient-specific drug therapy problems and collaborate with other health care professionals. The core elements provide the foundation of an MTM service that allows more robust services to be built based on the specific patient needs of a given community.

Pharmaceutical care

In 1990, Hepler and Strand[8] defined a new way to look at the responsibilities of the pharmacist and pharmacy services, applying the term "pharmaceutical care" to this new concept of pharmacists' services. Over the course of more than a decade, pharmacists have worked to develop pharmaceutical care practices. Many examples of these practices have been published in the literature, suggesting that the inclusion of a pharmacist in the evaluation of a patient's drug therapy regimen improves outcomes.[9–13] However, several practice-management barriers have prohibited the widespread adoption and implementation

At a Glance

Synopsis: The Medicare Modernization Act of 2003 and Medicare Part D have raised important questions for patients, pharmacists, other health practitioners, and payers, including how medication therapy management (MTM) differs from pharmaceutical care, patient counseling, and disease management. MTM can be viewed as a comprehensive framework for all drug-focused patient care service components of the practice of the pharmacist. MTM is driven by the philosophy of pharmaceutical care, which calls for the pharmacist to take responsibility and accountability for the drug-related needs of the patient. Patient counseling, in accordance with the Omnibus Budget Reconciliation Act of 1990, is the expected service provided by pharmacists to ensure that patients have the information they need to use a specific drug product properly. Disease management programs provide patients with the tools they need to manage a specific disease, often through population-based approaches.

Analysis: Clear definitions of pharmacist-provided services become increasingly important as MTM programs evolve and payer groups become more aware of the benefits associated with safe and efficacious drug use. The professionwide success of effective MTM provision requires not only the willingness of individual pharmacists to master a number of behaviors and techniques, but also acceptance by pharmacy networks, pharmacy organizations, the medical community, the federal government, payer groups, and patients.

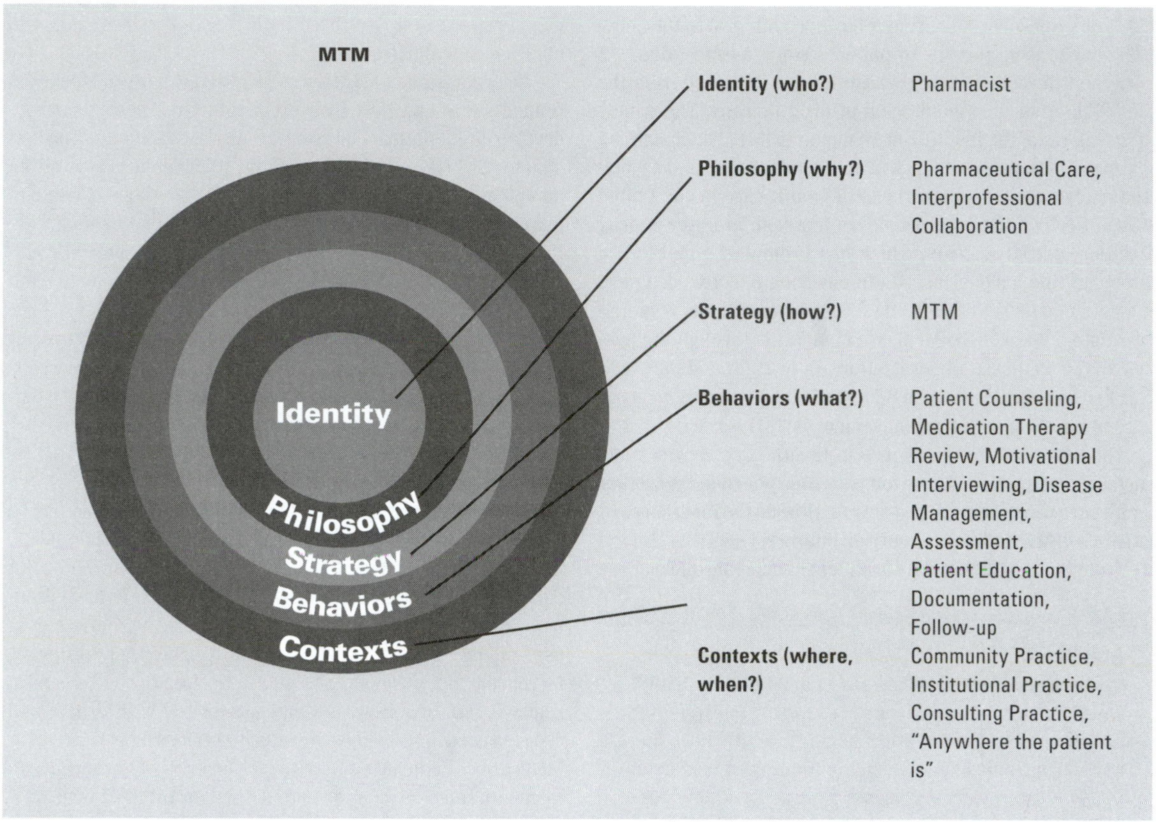

Figure 1. Relationship of MTM to disease management, patient counseling, and pharmaceutical care: A framework for all pharmacy practice

Abbreviation used: MTM, medication therapy management.

of pharmaceutical care practices in the community. The physical organization and workflow of community pharmacies, the shortage of pharmacists and other resources, and the lack of a standard payment mechanism for pharmacist–patient care services and targeted pharmacist–patient care training are examples of these barriers.

An updated definition describes pharmaceutical care as "a patient-centered practice in which the practitioner assumes responsibility for a patient's drug-related needs and is held accountable for this commitment."[14] Pharmaceutical care meets the IOM challenge to the whole medical community to provide patient-centered care. The IOM 2001 report, *Crossing the Quality Chasm: A New Health System for the 21st Century*,[2] called for health care systems that respect patients' values, preferences, and expressed needs; coordinate and integrate care across boundaries of the system; provide the information, communication, and education that people need and want; and guarantee physical comfort, emotional support, and the involvement of family and friends.

The philosophy of pharmaceutical care focuses on the responsibility of the pharmacist to meet all of the patient's drug-related needs, be held accountable for meeting those needs, and assist the patient in achieving his or her medical goals through collaboration with other health professionals. Another question often arises as to the relationship between pharmaceutical care and clinical pharmacy. Hepler[15] described the similarities and differences in detail, suggesting the importance of the incorporation of clinical pharmacy practice into the practice of pharmaceutical care. MTM, as intended in the Medicare Prescription Medication Benefit, can be viewed as a strategy, including payment for services rendered, to incorporate the philosophy of pharmaceutical care into everyday pharmacy practice for a defined patient population.

Patient counseling

Various iterations of the definition of patient counseling appear in the literature, but two guidelines are most commonly cited. According to the patient counseling standards in the

Omnibus Budget Reconciliation Act of 1990 (OBRA '90), pharmacists are expected to offer an explanation of the purpose of the prescribed drug; proper administration, including length of therapy, special directions for use, proper storage, and refill instructions; information on common adverse effects, potential interactions, and contraindications to the use of the drug; and guidance on steps to take given specific outcomes.[16] The Indian Health Service model uses a series of questions to determine a patient's understanding of his or her drugs, including the following[17]:

■ What did your prescriber tell you the medication is for?
■ How did your prescriber tell you to take the medication?
■ What did your prescriber tell you to expect?

In 2004, more than 3.2 billion prescriptions were dispensed in 55,375 community pharmacies.[18] According to a 2004 study, on average, only 63% of people received any verbal information about drug therapy from their pharmacists, despite the OBRA '90 guideline.[19] OBRA '90 mandated the "offer" to counsel Medicare recipients,[16] but even when an offer is given, a simple refusal from the patient halts the counseling service. Thus, despite the high volume of prescriptions dispensed, patients are not routinely receiving individualized information about their drug therapies.

Based on the OBRA '90 and Indian Health Service models, patient counseling alone does not constitute pharmaceutical care; rather, it is a tool included in the provision of pharmaceutical care. From the payer's perspective, patient counseling is drug product focused and generally involves one-way (pharmacist to patient or caregiver) transmission of information. Despite the casual use of the term *patient counseling* to mean more than this, payer groups and the literature support this simple view of patient counseling. This is an important distinction when considering the scope of MTM to encompass more than just patient counseling.

Patient counseling begins with, and focuses on, providing information related to the immediately prescribed drug, with the final responsibility for following the instructions belonging to the patient. The only documentation required is a "yes" or "no" checked on a form next to the patient's signature to indicate whether he or she accepted the offer to provide this information. Follow-up is not required, and no formal compensation mechanism is in place beyond the dispensing fee.[16,20]

Disease management

Disease management programs were developed and widely adopted in the 1990s, largely due to the establishment of health maintenance organizations. At about the same time, pharmacists began to implement strategies to apply the philosophy of pharmaceutical care to practice. The Disease Management Association of America defines *disease management* as "a system of coordinated health care interventions and communications for populations with conditions in which patient self-care efforts are significant."[21] Disease management programs have

been developed to ensure that population guidelines are followed. These programs are interprofessional in nature and may be provided by a wide variety of health care professionals, including physicians, nurses, nutritionists, and pharmacists. Disease management focuses on a specific disease, providing patients with the tools and knowledge they need to assume some responsibility for their own care. Multiple health professionals can participate in the management of one patient to achieve his or her health care goals.

Disease management programs meet a variety of patient drug and disease-specific needs. Programs developed by pharmacists include anticoagulation, hypertension, dyslipidemia, asthma, diabetes, and others.[9] These programs have facilitated considerable improvement in the patient's ability to meet his or her disease-oriented goals. Payment for disease management services is usually through payer contracts, yet these payment mechanisms are not distinct to any one profession. Pharmacists often have had difficulty obtaining adequate compensation for managing a patient's drug-related needs because the time is often shared with other health professionals. Table 1 further illustrates the characteristics of disease management and offers a comparison to patient counseling. Disease management goes considerably beyond patient counseling by addressing the patient's drug and nondrug therapy, as well as lifestyle modifications associated with a specific disease. However, disease management by definition does not address the patient's entire drug regimen.

Distinguishing MTM from other pharmacist-provided services

Using the definitions referenced in this article, the distinctions among patient counseling, disease management, and MTM are presented in Table 1. MTM goes beyond patient counseling associated with the dispensing of a single product or the education and management of a specific disease. The focus of MTM is on the individual patient, with the intention of optimizing the patient's drug regimen to best achieve appropriate therapeutic goals for that patient. To best understand the patient's experience with the regimen, the pharmacist must enter into a dialogue with the patient about expectations and current results from their drug regimen. The pharmacist must gather pertinent patient history to understand the scope of the patient's health needs. If drug therapy problems are identified, the pharmacist works together with the patient and the patient's health care practitioners to create a solution. Documentation of the consultation provides a basis for follow-up between the patient and the pharmacist to determine the outcome of the devised plan and further optimize the therapy, if needed. The pharmacist's documentation also serves as a means of communication among health professionals and justification for services provided, and is required by the payer, along with follow-up, to receive compensation for the service.

MTM services offer an opportunity for a patient to engage with his or her pharmacist in a more meaningful and

COMMENTARY PLACING MTM IN PHARMACY'S HISTORICAL CONTEXT

Table 1. Similarities and differences among pharmacist-provided patient counseling, disease management, and MTM

Aspects of service	Patient counseling	Disease management	MTM
Focus	Drug product information	Disease management and use of population guidelines	Patient drug therapy regimen
Practitioner–patient communication	One way	Two way	Two way
Documentation	"Offer to counsel" documentation required	Documentation in patient care record required	Documentation in patient care record required
Practitioner follow-up	Not required	Required	Required
Practitioner	Pharmacist or other qualified health care practitioner	Physician, nurse, pharmacist, dietitian, or other	Pharmacist or other qualified health care practitioner

Abbreviations used: MTM, medication therapy management.

effective way. The pharmacist takes the responsibility to prevent or identify and resolve drug therapy problems that arise by using a variety of strategies, including comprehensive medication therapy review, discussion with and education of the patient and/or caregiver, discussion and intervention with other health professionals, and possible referral to other health professionals and pharmacist specialists, as needed. MTM focuses on the whole patient, drug therapy use, and the recognition of a specific patient's drug therapy needs. It integrates the philosophy and practice of pharmaceutical care and elements of disease management through the pharmacist's provision of personalized drug-related information and interventions suited to individual patient needs.

Distinguishing financial factors

Distinguishing between MTM and other services provided by pharmacists becomes essential when considering their financial impact. Dispensing services are reimbursed individually by drug product, with an associated standard dispensing fee that remains the same regardless of whether a pharmacist provides counseling. Patient counseling is an expected, not reimbursable, service connected with dispensing. To receive payment for disease management services, the pharmacist or pharmacy enters into a contract with a payer group (e.g., employer, health maintenance organization) and the compensation rates are negotiated by individual contract. The competition for these contracts among pharmacists and other health practitioners, such as nursing groups, is strong.

MTM is a distinct service that involves pharmacist review of all of the patient's drug therapies and diseases; documentation and follow-up are included. Individual contracts between the pharmacist or pharmacy are made with a payer group. Along with the Medicare Prescription Medication Benefit, Current Procedural Terminology (CPT) codes have been developed to provide a standard means of payment for MTM services. The current CPT codes are time based and considered category III codes, meaning they are in a "test and trial" period. Elevating these codes to category I status will provide higher visibility to payer groups and lead to an increased likelihood of their use for payment of services. A petition for this change is pending with

the American Medical Association CPT Panel, with a decision imminent.[22]

Suggested compensation rates can include payment by level of complexity and time, similar to systems for billing for physician services.[23] In contrast with patient counseling, both disease management and MTM offer a potential opportunity for growth of pharmacist-provided services by creating mechanisms for new revenue. The Minnesota Department of Health Services offers a distinguishing example of how the number and complexity of drug therapy problems can be delineated in MTM services.[24] Other payment models have been developed through businesses supporting pharmacist services.[25,26]

MTM: Framework for all pharmacist-provided care

MTM can be viewed as a comprehensive framework for all drug-focused patient care service components of the practice of the pharmacist. Figure 1 provides a pictorial description of the relationship among the pharmacist-provided services described in this report. The pharmacist is the ideal health care professional to provide MTM services, based on his or her knowledge of drug therapy and accessibility to patients, especially in the community. The strategy of interprofessional collaboration provides a requisite connection with all other aspects of a patient's care.

MTM is driven by the philosophy of pharmaceutical care, which calls for the pharmacist to take responsibility and accountability for the drug-related needs of the patient. MTM offers a variety of strategies to meet patient-specific drug therapy needs. A series of techniques and behaviors are required to perform MTM, including patient counseling, motivational interviewing, patient assessment, patient education, documentation, follow-up, and interprofessional collaboration. A specific setting is not required to conduct MTM, but this service may be performed anywhere the pharmacist and patient can conduct a medication evaluation in a comfortable, private area. MTM settings may include, but are not limited to, community pharmacy practice, ambulatory clinics, institutional pharmacy practice, consulting practice, and other community facilities where a private area is available for a pharmacist to meet with a patient.

As MTM programs continue to evolve and payer groups begin to realize the benefits associated with patients achieving optimal and safe use of drug therapies, a clear distinction among the growing number of pharmacist-provided services will become increasingly important. Making differences clear will allow the services to grow and marketing to be conducted in a clear manner. MTM is an all-inclusive review of a patient's entire drug regimen and a mechanism to refer and connect with other health professionals based on the needs of the individual patient. Patient counseling is a tool used to ensure that patients have the information they need to use a specific drug product properly. Disease management is a mechanism to ensure patients have the education and resources needed to manage a particular disease. Simply stated, patient counseling is drug specific, disease management is specific to one disease in a given patient, and drug therapy management is patient centered, comprehensive, and focused on a patient's broad drug therapy needs. The commonality among these services is the ability of the pharmacist to provide them and the direct interaction between the pharmacist and the patient. MTM can be provided as a service to a subset of patients identified by a payer group, such as patients with diabetes, as long as the focus of the interventions includes a comprehensive review of the patient's entire drug regimen in accordance with the components of the MTM core elements.

The overall success of MTM depends on a multitude of factors, including acceptance by the profession (including individual pharmacists, pharmacy networks, and pharmacy organizations), the medical community, patients, payer groups, and the federal government. Defining the role of MTM in relation to other pharmacist–patient care models, including patient counseling, disease management, and all pharmacy services currently provided, is essential to the establishment of a viable and sustainable practice model for pharmacists.

References

1. Institute of Medicine. To err is human: building a safer health system. Washington, D.C.: National Academy Press; 2001.

2. Institute of Medicine. Crossing the quality chasm: a new health system for the 21st century. Washington, D.C.: National Academy Press, 2001.

3. Institute of Medicine. In: Greiner AC, Knebel E, eds. Health professional education: a bridge to quality. Washington, D.C.: National Academy Press; 2003:1–3.

4. Institute of Medicine. Aspden P, Wolcott J, Bootman JL, Cronenwett LR, eds. Preventing medication errors: quality chasm series. Washington, D.C.: National Academy Press; 2006.

5. Bluml BM. Definition of medication therapy management: development of professionwide consensus. J Am Pharm Assoc. 2005;45:566–72.

6. Centers for Medicaid & Medicare Services. Higher quality care through Medicare's modernization benefits. Accessed at www.cms.hhs.gov/PrescriptionDrugCovContra/08.asp, August 15, 2007.

7. American Pharmacists Association, National Association of Chain Drug Stores Foundation. Medication therapy management in community pharmacy practice: core elements of an MTM service (version 1.0). J Am Pharm Assoc. 2005;45:573–9.

8. Hepler CD, Strand L. Opportunities and responsibilities in pharmaceutical care. Am J Hosp Pharm. 1990;47:533–43.

9. Knapp KK, Okamoto MP, Black BL. ASHP survey of ambulatory care pharmacy practice in health systems: 2004. Am J Health Syst Pharm. 2004;62:274–84.

10. Chrischilles EA, Carter BL, Lund BC, et al. Evaluation of the Iowa Medicaid Pharmaceutical Care Management Program. J Am Pharm Assoc. 2004;44:337–49.

11. Cranor CW, Bunting BA, Christensen DB. The Asheville Project: long-term clinical and economic outcomes of a community pharmacy diabetes care program. J Am Pharm Assoc. 2003;43:173–84.

12. Ellis SL, Carter BL, Malone DC, et al. Clinical and economic impact of ambulatory care clinical pharmacists in management of dyslipidemia in older adults: the IMPROVE Study. Pharmacotherapy. 2000;20:1508–16.

13. Schumock GT, Butler MG, Meek PD, et al. Evidence of the economic benefit of clinical pharmacy services: 1996–2000. Pharmacotherapy. 2003;23:113–32.

14. Cipolle RJ, Strand LM, Morley PC. Pharmaceutical care practice: the clinician's guide. 2nd ed. New York: McGraw-Hill; 2004.

15. Hepler CD. Clinical pharmacy, pharmaceutical care, and the quality of drug therapy. Pharmacotherapy. 2004;24:1491–8.

16. The Omnibus Budget Reconciliation Act of 1990. Pub. L. no. 101–508, 104 Stat 1388, § 4401.

17. Lee AJ, Borham A, Korman NE, et al. Staff development in pharmacist-conducted patient education and counseling. Am J Health Syst Pharm. 1998;55:1792–8.

18. National Association of Chain Drug Stores Foundation. The chain pharmacy industry profile 2005. Washington, D.C.: National Association of Chain Drug Stores Foundation; 2005:11,45.

19. Svarstad BL, Bultman DC, Mount JK. Patient counseling provided in community pharmacies: effects of state regulation, pharmacist age, and busyness. J Am Pharm Assoc. 2004;44:22–9.

20. Puumalainen I. Development of instruments to measure the quality of patient counseling: doctoral dissertation. Accessed at www.uku.fi/vaitokset/2005/isbn951-27-0401-3.pdf, September 13, 2006.

21. Disease Management Association of America. Disease State Management Definition. Accessed at www.dmaa.org/dm_definition.asp, March 30, 2006.

22. Isetts BJ, Buffington DE. CPT code-change proposal: National data on pharmacists' medication therapy management services. J Am Pharm Assoc. 2007;47:491–5.

23. The Lewin Group. Medication therapy management services: a critical review. J Am Pharm Assoc. 2005;45:580–7.

24. Minnesota Department of Human Services. MHCP enrolled providers: pharmacies: medication therapy management. Accessed at www.dhs.state.mn.us/main/groups/business_partners/documents/pub/dhs_id_054232.hcsp, September 13, 2006.

25. Outcomes Pharmaceutical Health Care. Outcomes Encounter Program. Accessed at www.getoutcomes.com, October 24, 2006.

26. Mirixia. Partnering with pharmacists, personalizing patient care. Accessed at www.communitymtm.com, October 24, 2006.

Appendix 1. Glossary of terms commonly used by pharmacists when referring to various patient care services

Collaboration
A mutually beneficial and well-defined relationship entered into by two or more individuals or organizations to achieve a common goal through shared understanding of the issues, open communication, mutual trust, and tolerance of differing points of view. This includes a provider–provider relationship within or across disciplines in order to maximize areas of expertise, as well as patient–provider relationship through a combination of the medical care model and patient-empowerment approach to medical care.[1–3]

Community-based care (practice)
A planned, coordinated, ongoing effort operated by a community or for a community that characteristically includes multiple interventions intended to improve the health status of the community.[1]

Compensation
Payment for a service that reflects both reimbursement for the cost of an item or service and the value added by the provider.[4]

Comprehensive consultation
In medication therapy management, this term connotes a face-to-face consultative session between a pharmacist and the patient and/or caregiver in which all the patient's medication and health-related concerns are assessed. A plan is created with the patient and other health care providers. The plan is communicated with the patient verbally and in writing and with the other health care providers verbally, as appropriate, and in writing. Complete documentation and follow-up are required. The session occurs in an area that affords privacy for the patient and usually lasts 15 to 60 minutes, and collaboration with other health care professionals involved in the patient's care is expected.

Comprehensive medication therapy review
A session between patient and/or caregiver and pharmacist in which all of the patient's medications (prescription, nonprescription, and dietary supplements such as herbal products and vitamins/minerals) are evaluated to ensure the patient is taking the medications correctly, therapy is appropriate, and medication-related problems are avoided. The pharmacist provides education and information to improve the patient's self-management of medications. This review aids in identifying new medication-related problems that may require intervention and follow-up.[5,6]

Disease management
A system of coordinated health care interventions and communications for populations with conditions in which patient self-care efforts are important. The goal is to manage and improve the health status for patients with chronic conditions that depend on appropriate pharmaceutical care for proper maintenance.[7,8]

Documentation
The detailed description of a patient–provider or provider–provider interaction. Documentation serves as a record for stating relevant participants, evidence, assumptions, rationale, and analytical methods used in evaluating patient progress and quality of care or outcomes for individuals and populations. Also functions as a means of communication among providers and analysis for billing purposes.[6,9]

Drug-related needs
Any issue perceived by a patient or provider concerning a medication. Includes an appropriate indication, medical benefit, efficacy, appropriate dosage, lack of adverse reactions, and the patient's ability to take the medication appropriately.[14]

Drug therapy problems
Event or circumstance that involves a patient's medication treatment that actually, or potentially, interferes with the achievement of the optimal outcome. Drug therapy problems are classified under seven headings: unnecessary drug therapy, need for additional drug therapy, ineffective drug, subtherapeutic dosage, adverse drug reaction (including drug interactions), overdosage, and nonadherence.[11,12,14]

Follow-up
To add continuing care to monitor an established health-related need or to assess for future needs; follow-up is considered and essential component of the patient care process.[13]

Institutional-based care (practice)
Health care provided in a structured setting in which the patient resides overnight.

Appendix 1. Glossary of terms commonly used by pharmacists when referring to various patient care services (continued)

Interprofessional collaboration
The cooperation between health care decision makers from different disciplines, who assess and plan care in a interdependent, complimentary, and coordinated manner. Decision making to obtain optimal patient outcomes occurs in a joint fashion, and members feel empowered and assume leadership on the appropriate issues, depending on the patient needs and their expertise.

Intervention
A directive or consultative communication (written or verbal) between health care providers, or patient and provider, that alters or enhances the care plan. Pharmacist interventions serve to resolve or prevent medication therapy—related problems and can occur as part of any pharmacy service, including dispensing of medication.[6]

Medication action plan
Documented decisions created collaboratively between the patient, pharmacist, and/or physician or other health professionals to assist the patient in improving medication self-management and enhancing continuity of care between health care providers. Includes patient identifier and date of birth, pharmacist identifier, physician identifier, date, medication-related issue, proposed action, person responsible for the action, and result of the action and date taken.[6]

Medication therapy management
Services or programs furnished by a qualified pharmacist to an eligible beneficiary, individually or on behalf of a pharmacy provider, which are designated to ensure that medications are used appropriately by such individual, enhance the individual's understanding of the appropriate use of medications, increase the individual's adherence with prescription medication regimens, reduce the risk of potential adverse events associated with medications, and reduce the need for other costly medical services through better management of medication therapy.[14,15]

Medication therapy review
See comprehensive medication therapy review.

Motivational interviewing
A directive, client-centered counseling style for eliciting behavior change by helping clients explore and resolve ambivalence.[16]

Patient care planning
A systematic process for assessing a patient's health-related problems and needs, setting patient-specific goals, performing interventions, and evaluating results.[17]

Patient-centered care
Applies to the approach to medical care in which the practitioner respects the patient's needs, wants, and preferences before his/her own. This approach requires the practitioner to treat the patient as a partner in care planning and the ultimate decision maker. The practitioner must individualize population-centered care and/or best-practice guidelines through the consideration of the patient's health-related and cultural beliefs and values. This process involves coordination across boundaries of the health system in order to provide the information, communication, and education that are desired. A practitioner is to guarantee emotional and physical support and include the involvement of family and friends.[13,18,19]

Patient counseling
Providing product-specific advice to a patient regarding medications, health-related devices, concerns, or disease states. It is a tool used for providing pharmaceutical care but is not considered pharmaceutical care in and of itself. The patient is accountable for carrying out the information discussed, not the practitioner.[20,21]

Patient education
The process of teaching a patient and or/caregiver information about a related medication, product, device, or health care topic. This may be a monologue or dialogue and may require patient participation. Education is differentiated from counseling by inclusion of an evaluative component to assess the patient's level of understanding.

Personal medication record
A portable record generated during a comprehensive medication review. This allows the patient to voluntarily share their medication information with other health care providers to enhance continuity of care. It includes the following components: patient name/identifier; medication name and strength; intended use, directions for use, precautionary information, and start and stop date; pharmacist contact information; prescriber's contact information; and the date the record was originally created and updated.[5]

COMMENTARY PLACING MTM IN PHARMACY'S HISTORICAL CONTEXT

Appendix 1. Glossary of terms commonly used by pharmacists when referring to various patient care services (continued)

Pharmaceutical care

The provision of patient-centered practice in which the practitioner assumes responsibility for a patient's medication-related needs and is held accountable for this commitment for the purpose of achieving definite outcomes through designing, implementing, or monitoring of a therapeutic plan. Medication therapy management is a structure in which to provide pharmaceutical care.[12,13]

Population-centered care

Applies to the approach to medical care for specific groups identified by a common demographic characteristic, risk factors, or disease states. The focus is on the general guidelines for the whole as opposed to the individual patient.[1]

Practice guidelines

A systematic review written by experts in their respective fields that provides the best prevention and treatment information at the time for a given health-related issue. These may be adapted by insurers as a best-practice monitor for participating providers.

Referral

The request for additional services from another health care provider outside of one's own scope of practice.[6,9]

Standards of care

The level at which a practitioner is expected to provide patient care. This includes behavioral and clinical expectations that are usually set forth by a governing body or expert panel.[13]

References

1. Peters KE, Elster AB. Roadmaps for clinical practice: a primer on population-based medicine. Chicago: American Medical Association; 2002.
2. Anderson RM. Patient empowerment and the traditional medical model: a case of irreconcilable differences. Diabetes Care. 1995;18:412–5.
3. National Center for Children exposed to violence. Resource center: glossary of terms. Accessed at www.nccev.org/resources/terms.html, November 8, 2006.
4. Snella KA, Trewyn RR, Hansen LB, Bradberry JC. Pharmacist compensation for cognitive services: focus on the physician office and community pharmacy. Pharmacotherapy. 2004;24:372–88.
5. American Pharmacists Association, National Association of Chain Drug Stores Foundation. Medication therapy management in community pharmacy practice: core elements of an MTM service. Version 1.0. J Am Pharm Assoc. 2005;45:573–9.
6. Academy of Managed Care Pharmacy. Glossary of managed care terms. Alexandria, Va.: Academy of Managed Care Pharmacy; 2004.
7. Disease Management Association of America. Disease State Management Definition. Accessed at www.dmaa.org/dm_definition.asp, March 30, 2006.
8. Tufts Center for the Study of Drug Development. Information services glossary of terms. Accessed at http://csdd.tufts.edu/InfoServices/Glossary.asp, November 8, 2006.
9. Academy of Managed Care Pharmacy Consensus Document. Sound medication therapy management programs. Alexandria, Va.: Academy of Managed Care Pharmacy; 2006.
10. Bislew HD, Sorensen TD. Use of focus groups as a tool to enhance a pharmaceutical care practice. J Am Pharm Assoc. 2003;43:424–33.
11. Johnson JA, Bootman JL. Drug-related morbidity and mortality: a cost-of-illness model. Arch Intern Med. 1995;155:1949–56.
12. Hepler CD, Strand L. Opportunities and responsibilities in pharmaceutical care. Am J Hosp Pharm. 1990;47:533–43.
13. Cipolle RJ, Strand LM, Morley PC. Pharmaceutical care practice: the clinician's guide. 2nd ed. New York: McGraw-Hill; 2004.
14. Bluml BM. Definition of medication therapy management: development of professionwide consensus. J Am Pharm Assoc. 2005;45:566–72.
15. Centers for Medicaid & Medicare Services. Higher quality care through Medicare's modernization benefits. Accessed at www.cms.hhs.gov/PrescriptionDrugCovContra/08.asp, August 15, 2007.
16. Doherty Y, James P, Roberts S. Stage of change counseling. In: Snoek FJ, Skinner TC, eds. Psychology in diabetes care. Chichester, U.K.: John Wiley & Sons; 2000:99–139.
17. National Association of Pharmacy Registry Authorities. Developing a pharmaceutical care plan. Accessed at www.napra.ca/pdfs/practice/developing.pdf, November 8, 2006.
18. Committee on Quality of Health Care in America, Institute of Medicine. Crossing the quality chasm: a new health system for the 21st century. Washington, D.C.: National Academy Press; 2001.
19. American Academy of Orthopedic Surgeons. Patient-centered care. Accessed at www2.aaos.org/aaos/archives/bulletin/feb05/acdnws5.asp, November 8, 2006.
20. The Omnibus Budget Reconciliation Act of 1990. Pub. L. no. 101–508, 104. Stat 1388, § 4401.
21. Lee AJ, Borham A, Korman NE, et al. Staff development in pharmacist-conducted patient education and counseling. Am J Health Syst Pharm 1998;55:1792–8.

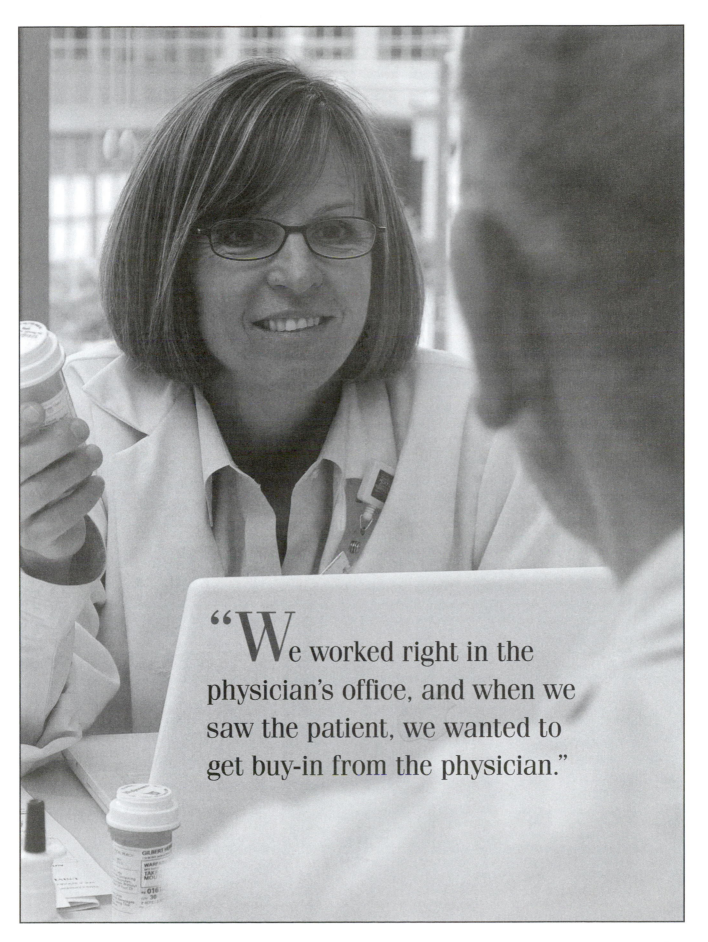

"We worked right in the physician's office, and when we saw the patient, we wanted to get buy-in from the physician."

Stebbins integrates MTM Core Elements into office-based practice

Helping physicians and patients navigate complexities of health care system, California pharmacist charts new paths for profession

W hen a headhunter called in 1996 to pitch a pharmacist position to Marilyn Stebbins, PharmD, her initial reaction was not exactly positive. In fact, she recalls thinking, "That sounds like one of the worst jobs I've ever imagined!" A 120-physician group practice in her hometown of Sacramento, Calif., was looking for a pharmacist who could police the group's prescribers and keep them on a drug budget. "Balancing my checkbook was hard enough," Stebbins now jokes. "How was I supposed to keep 120 physicians within budget?"

The position was later broadened to include development of a clinical rotation site from Stebbins' alma mater, the University of California, San Francisco (UCSF), which increased her interest. Finally, after 8 months and a few appeals from her school of pharmacy professors, Stebbins took the bait, and she's never looked back. For more than a decade now, she has been able to leverage the financial focus of the group—and related monetary concerns of many of her patients—to develop a full-fledged medication therapy management (MTM) practice that is engaged in all the clinical, humanistic, and economic outcomes of pharmacotherapy. In the process, she has both learned from and contributed to the profession's MTM Core Elements, including the second version being released this month

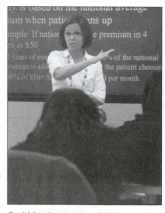

Stebbins lectures on Medicare Part D at the UCSF School of Pharmacy.

by APhA and other national pharmacy organizations (see related article beginning on page 64).

Cutting teeth at VA

Born the sixth of nine children in the Hedges family, Stebbins was influenced by her dad, a family practice physician, and her mom, a nurse. After finishing high school, Stebbins was off to the University of California (UC) at San Diego, where her intent was to follow her father's footsteps into a medical career. About midway through her coursework for a bachelor's degree in biochemistry, Stebbins figured out that she didn't really want to be a physician. "I didn't know why I had this sudden change," she recalls, "but I found I enjoyed my French literature minor a great deal more than biochemistry!"

As Stebbins pondered what to do, fate intervened, and a family member who was a pharmacist told her of his experiences in the profession and described a vision of where pharmacy was headed. She began volunteering at a Department of Veterans Affairs (VA) facility and working in a community pharmacy, and she soon found herself in pharmacy school at UCSF. After graduating in 1988, she moved back to Sacramento and completed a pharmacy practice residency at UC Davis. Her goal was a career in acute care and intensive care medicine.

But again, fate had other ideas, and Stebbins' first position was as an ambulatory pharmacist in the VA outpatient clinics in Sacramento. The 7 and a half years she spent there turned out to be great training for her—learning what is possible in a unified health system

coverstory

in which information was beginning to be shared among professionals in geographically dispersed points of care. Her professional development at VA was influenced by Joe Gee, the pharmacy director at the time, and Julio Lopez, then the drug information pharmacist and now the director of pharmacy at that VA facility.

Balancing sense with cents

After moving to Catholic Healthcare West Medical Foundation's Mercy Medical Group (CHW) in 1996, Stebbins' initial efforts were directed at developing physician profiles as a means of giving feedback on prescribing patterns and their impact on the cost of patient care. She started with oral medications and later moved into injectable drugs to help physicians lower costs, and she also began to show prescribers how they could reduce medication errors. Students began rotating through the site in UCSF's new Pathways program, and by 2000, Stebbins was also precepting a pharmacy resident each year.

In 2000, a major shift in the Sacramento health care marketplace brought Stebbins' VA experience to bear in the CHW environment. The town's three major payers with whom CHW worked (the fourth was Kaiser) eliminated beneficiaries' brand-name drug benefit. CHW administration asked, "Marilyn, didn't you used to work in clinics at VA? They didn't use a lot of brand names, did they?" She was asked to set up a process for advising patients on how they could have the lowest out-of-pocket costs for medications under the new rules.

The result was the Pharmacists Review to Increase Cost-Effectiveness (PRICE) clinic, in which Stebbins, one other pharmacist (initially), the resident (later two residents working part-time), and student pharmacists met with patients at CHW's five clinics around the metropolitan area, helped switch them to generic medications that were covered under the plans, and minimized the costs of necessary brand-name products through pill splitting, mail service pharmacy, and any other tactic the pharmacists could think of.

"My main job at CHW had always been to get physicians to prescribe cost-effectively," Stebbins shared with *Pharmacy Today*. "Very interestingly, the best tactic I could ever have employed was starting the PRICE clinic. We chose not to make changes under a collaborative practice agreement—we did not want to make these changes on our own. Instead, we worked right in the physician's office, and when we saw the patient, we wanted to get buy-in from the physician. That way, the patient would go home with an understanding that the plan was the plan, and the physician had signed off on it. At the same time, the physician was educated as to what we were going to do. For the first 6 months, we did all the interventions—therapeutic interchanges, pill splitting, mail order, you name it. But by then, the physicians had learned all the tricks. It was the best academic detailing I ever could have done. The physicians learned through their own patients what they should have been doing all along. We then moved very heavily into patient-assistance programs."

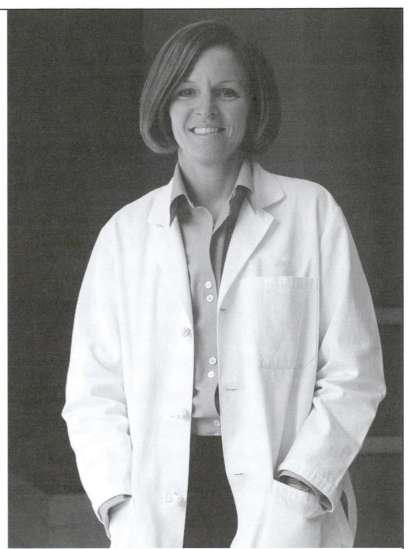

Stebbins wondered how student pharmacists could implement MAPs and PMRs during their practice experiences in community pharmacies where patient-specific data were not as plentiful as in the physician office.

This page intentionally left blank—originally an advertisement.

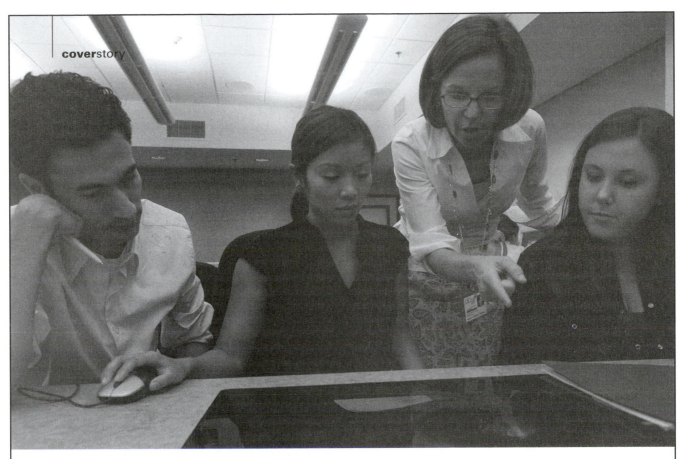

coverstory

In the **Partners in D** program, Stebbins works with student pharmacists in the delivery of peer-to-peer education to medical, nursing, osteopathic, physician assistant, and other health profession students. Here, Stebbins instructs UCSF student pharmacists (left to right) Troy Drysdale, Sharon Tran, and Kristy Hanson.

Looking for a template for MTM

By 2004, Stebbins and her coworker and colleague Tim Cutler knew that Medicare Part D was coming, and they began to hear in 2005 that patient-assistance programs would be eliminated for Medicare patients. This was a major concern because by then they had 2,500 patients receiving medications through these programs.

Stebbins was soon jetting off to Washington, D.C., to learn what was happening with Medicare Part D and the MTM ramp-up at the national level. She learned that the MTM Core Elements—especially the medication action plan (MAP) and the personal medication record (PMR)—meshed very well with what she was already doing at CHW clinics. Drawing on the process of care defined in the first set of MTM Core Elements, Stebbins refined the services she and colleagues were offering in Sacramento to meet the emerging national standards for just what constituted MTM.

Because of the emphasis her group had placed on patient-assistance programs, Stebbins and Cutler spearheaded educational efforts to get CHW patients ready for Medicare Part D. When it came to drawing Medicare beneficiaries into informational sessions about the prescription drug benefit, Stebbins found that one thing worked: Talk about money. "MTM is a very hard sell to people who don't know what they don't know," she explained. "But the dollar is a pretty great incentive. One of the biggest problems we found early on was that patients were fearful about telling their doctors that they weren't taking their medica-

tions because of costs, because they didn't want the doctors to be disappointed in them. But they had no trouble at all telling us. So if they saw a flyer on how to save money, they showed up. Our hook to get them in the door is cost savings. Once we get them in the door, though, our services constitute a full-fledged MTM program that addresses clinical, economic, and quality-of-life concerns."

"We were trying to implement the core elements in our clinics during this time, and in a very busy clinic, I can tell you that can be difficult," Stebbins shared. "These were all things we had been doing, but we hadn't captured them in our data. We changed all our forms and started trying to figure out how to capture this. We spent 2006 refining our forms, as we wanted our interventions to reflect the core elements of MTM and the definition of MTM as approved by the 11 pharmacy organizations."

Efforts pay off

In the 2 calendar years since Part D took effect, CHW pharmacists' results have been impressive. Among 320 patients seen in the PRICE clinic in 2007, five interventions per patient have been made on average, and not just simple ones, Stebbins explained. Patients were taking, on average, eight medications and had four chronic diseases. As a result of these pharmacist interventions, patients realized an average out-of-pocket savings of $165 per month.

In addition, Stebbins added, California is a strong pay-for-performance state, and the PRICE clinic patients do well when such metrics are applied. Studies are under way now to define the differences in surrogate markers such as glycosylated hemo-globin (A1C) levels and the percentage of patients at target goals and how high users of medications are faring under the MTM services offered at CHW.

One thing Stebbins and her colleagues soon realized was that they were in an ideal situation: They were in the clinics and in physician offices, all of which offered a very data-rich environment. As UCSF refines advanced pharmacy practice experiences

cine, Stebbins applied for and received a $3.7 million grant from the Amgen Foundation in late 2006. Partners in D (www.part-nersind.com) is a 3-and-a-half-year program designed to create a California-wide educational system and collaborative outreach network for student pharmacists and pharmacy faculty members at the state's seven schools and colleges of pharmacy.

The first leg of the grant is getting Medicare Part D education to underserved and vulnerable populations across California.

"MTM is a very hard sell to people who don't know what they don't know."

in community pharmacies, Stebbins thought about how much less information about patients was available in those settings, which are a data-poor environment. How, she wondered, could student pharmacists implement MAPs and PMRs during their practice experiences in community pharmacies in an effective way that was not just Part D related?

Spreading the message statewide
Working with UCSF's Helene Levens Lipton, PhD, a professor of health policy in the School of Pharmacy and a core faculty member in the Institute for Health Policy Studies in the School of Medi-

To accomplish this, three faculty from each California pharmacy school were trained last August and given a turnkey program based on the Medicare Part D elective course offered at UCSF, Stebbins told *Today*. The faculty use the program in their own schools, and the student pharmacists in turn take the program directly to the patients. "Students take computers with broadband cards into neighborhoods that don't have Internet access," noted Stebbins. "Our students are very diverse, speaking many languages, so at UCSF we are able to provide information in seven different languages. They go out equipped to get people into prescription drug plans, with no ties to any pharmacy."

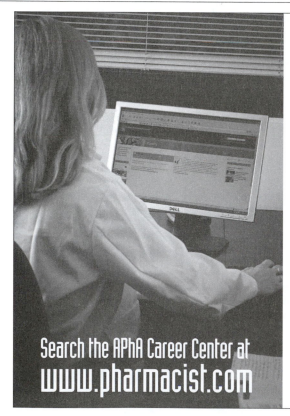
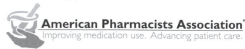

coverstory

The second leg of the grant involves peer-to-peer education. Stebbins and Lipton are working with student pharmacists to spread the MTM message to medical, nursing, osteopathic, physician assistant, and other health profession students and medical residents at UCSF and soon at nearby Stanford University and UC Davis. "Four students are selected per year to be our ambassadors to these other schools," she said. "As faculty, we help them develop the lectures on Medicare Part D and its policy implications that are pertinent to their audiences. We are now ingrained in the health policy curriculum in the medical and nursing schools at UCSF, and they go out and give lectures from the various stakeholder perspectives—patient, provider, and payer. The evaluations of the lectures are phenomenal. I wish as a faculty member that I had evaluations like those our students are getting. This has really stirred the pot at UCSF; the medical school is now looking for ways its students can teach students in the pharmacy school." This program will be the focus of the next train-the-trainer program for the seven California schools of pharmacy in August 2008.

The third leg of this grant explores an answer to the community pharmacy questions Stebbins had posed about getting the needed MTM data to student pharmacists in community pharmacy practice experiences. She recalled, "For the last year, we have been piloting at our Sacramento site a format and a template that our fourth-year students can use to provide MTM in their advanced community pharmacy practice experiences. This year, we will go live with this program for student pharmacists entering rotations at UCSF. The following year, we will have a train-the-trainer session for all seven California schools of pharmacy. By applying these skills and knowledge of MTM, the student pharmacists can provide value to the community pharmacy and value to the patient."

On the horizon

A self-described "night owl," Stebbins' current schedule is tiring just to listen to: She doesn't sleep much, she's a soccer mom to her 13-year-old daughter Lindsay, her husband Charlie is a professor of cardiovascular medicine at UC Davis, and she runs 5 or 6 days each week and tries to swim a couple more. Her Bluetooth headset is heavily used as she drives her hybrid between the (now) eight CHW Sacramento-area clinics and west on I-80 and across the Bay Bridge to lecture at UCSF up to one or two times a week.

The result is a complicated life, but one in which Stebbins finds a great deal of personal and professional satisfaction. What sounded like "an awful job" many years ago actually turned out to be the perfect combination of need, challenge, opportunity, and, ultimately, results. Stebbins has excelled in this whirlwind environment of change. As she told *Today*, "When I walked in the door, they had no idea what I did at VA or any concept of pharmacists having practices. I had four heads because I was the 'drug police,' but a few years later, the physicians in the group said, 'Fix this problem and start this clinic, and do whatever you have to do to do it.' It's all about trust, and figuring out what a pharmacist can do."

—**L. Michael Posey, BPharm**

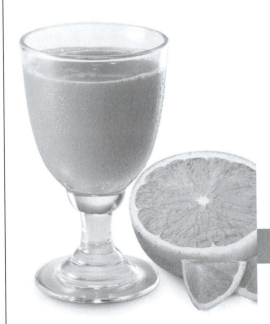

RESEARCH

New pharmacist supply projections: Lower separation rates and increased graduates boost supply estimates

Katherine K. Knapp and James M. Cultice

Abstract

Objective: To revise the 2000 Bureau of Health Professions Pharmacist Supply Model based on new data.

Design: Stock-flow model.

Setting: United States.

Participants: A 2004 estimate of active pharmacists reported by the Bureau of Labor Statistics was used to derive the base count for the 2007 supply model.

Interventions: Starting with a 2004 base of active pharmacists, new graduates are added to the supply annually and losses resulting from death and retirement are subtracted.

Main outcome measures: Age- and gender-based pharmacist supply estimates, 2004–2020

Results: Increased U.S. pharmacist supply estimates (236,227 in 2007 to 304,986 in 2020) indicate that pharmacists will remain the third largest professional health group behind nurses and physicians. Increases were driven by longer persistence in the workforce (59%), increased numbers of U.S. graduates (35%), and increases from international pharmacy graduates (IPGs) achieving U.S. licensure (6%). Since more pharmacists are expected to be working part time the full-time equivalent (FTE) supply will be reduced by about 15%. The mean age of pharmacists was projected to decline from 47 to 43 by 2020. Because of unequal distribution across age groups, large pharmacist cohorts approaching retirement age will result in fewer pharmacists available to replace them. The ratio of pharmacists to the over-65 population is expected to decrease after 2011 and continue to fall beyond 2020; this is likely a reflection of baby boomers passing through older age cohorts.

Conclusion: The revised estimated active U.S. pharmacist head count in 2006 is 232,597, with equivalent FTEs totaling approximately 198,000. The substantial increase over the 2000 pharmacist supply model estimates is primarily attributable to pharmacists remaining in the workforce longer and educational expansion. U.S. licensed IPGs account for less than 6% of overall increases. The pharmacist workforce is projected to become younger on average by about 4 years by 2020. Coincident demands for more physicians and nurses over the same period and shortages in all three professions stipulate that active steps be taken, including continued monitoring of work trends among pharmacists and other health professionals.

Keywords: Pharmacists, workforce, supply model, baby boomers, physicians, retired pharmacists, gender.

J Am Pharm Assoc. 2007;47:463–470.
doi: 10.1331/JAPhA.2007.07003

Received January 9, 2007, and in revised form March 30, 2007. Accepted for publication April 24, 2007.

Katherine K. Knapp, PhD, is Professor and Dean, College of Pharmacy, Touro University, Vallejo, Calif. **James M. Cultice, BS,** is Operations Research Analyst, Bureau of Health Professions, Health Resources and Services Administration, U.S. Department of Health and Human Services, Rockville, Md.

Correspondence: Katherine K. Knapp, PhD, College of Pharmacy, Touro University, 1310 Johnson Ln., Mare Island, Vallejo, CA 94592. Fax: 707-638-5226. E-mail: kknapp@touro.edu

Disclosure: The authors declare no conflicts of interests or financial interests in any product or service mentioned in this article, including grants, employment, gifts, stock holdings, or honoraria. The views expressed in this article are strictly those of the authors. No official endorsement by the Department of Health and Human Services or any of its components should be inferred.

Acknowledgments: To Surrey Walton, PhD, Associate Professor, College of Pharmacy, University of Illinois at Chicago, for his assistance on this project.

RESEARCH NEW PHARMACIST SUPPLY ESTIMATES

The federal government's 2000 National Pharmacist Workforce Survey of the supply and demand for pharmacists found clear evidence of a shortage of pharmacists and an increase in prescription volume that outpaced the growth in supply of pharmacists.[1] Since then, while the shortage appears to have been moderated by declines in the ambulatory prescription growth rate and changes in pharmacy practice involving wider use of pharmacist technicians and technology, concern remains over the adequacy of the future supply to meet expected demand.[2] The numbers of pharmacists working part time has been increasing, even while pharmacists appear to be staying in the workforce longer.[3] The workload on the individual pharmacist continues to increase, with more time spent in dispensing and administrative duties, usurping the time available for counseling and clinical activities.[4] In addition, while the vacancy rate in community pharmacies has declined since the government's 2000 study, the downward trend appears to have reversed in the past year toward a more severe national shortage level.[5]

With more than 230,000 pharmacists currently in practice, pharmacy is the third largest health profession in the United States behind nurses (2.4 million) and physicians (830,000).[6] All three of these health professions have reported a supply shortage relative to the demand for services.[1,7,8] Unless key factors affecting the balance between supply and demand change considerably, the continued aging of the baby boomer cohort in the U.S. population is likely to sustain or exacerbate existing health care personnel shortages in the near future.

The Bureau of Health Professions (BHPr) Pharmacist Supply Model estimates the size, age, and gender distribution of the active pharmacist workforce in the United States.[9] The model is revised periodically to reflect new or changed source data and has been expanded to estimate the full-time equivalent (FTE) supply, as well as head counts. The present study examines the current and future supply of pharmacists through trends in numbers of new graduates entering the workforce, new schools being built and expansion of existing programs, annual hours worked, age and gender distribution of the pharmacist population, and losses through death and retirement.

Model revision at this time is relevant because events related to the pharmacist shortage could affect key variables used to project the supply of pharmacists. A prime example is age-related separation rates, which reflect the proportion of men and women pharmacists who stop working as pharmacists at each year of age. Under shortage conditions, job-related stress, which tends to increase the likelihood of leaving pharmacy work, and rising salaries, which tend to decrease the likelihood of leaving pharmacy work, were coexistent and may have resulted in new work participation patterns and intrinsically related separation rates. The 2000 Census, which included an expanded work-related sample survey, provided an opportunity to tap into pharmacist work patterns during the peak of the shortage. The current study uses these data to calculate a new set of separation rates. We also used the National Pharmacist Workforce Surveys for 2000 and 2004, which reported pharmacy work participation rates, to corroborate our findings.[3,10]

Another reason for revision is the post-2000 expansion of pharmacy's educational enterprise through the formation of new schools and the expansion of existing programs—a trend that was not adequately foreseen in the 2000 supply model. The 2000 supply model assumed the addition of three new schools with approximately 95 graduates per year during each decade going forward and no expansion of existing programs. In reality, many more new programs have been launched since 2000 than the last model revision predicted. Of note, American Association of Colleges of Pharmacy and Accreditation Council for Pharmacy Education data show that the expansion of existing programs is making, now and in the near future, a much greater contribution to the number of new pharmacy graduates than graduates from new schools and colleges of pharmacy (personal communication, Peter Vlasses, PharmD, BCPS, Accreditation Council for Pharmacy Education, Chicago). Distributive education, with the formation of satellite campuses and classes offered on the Internet, has also contributed to training more pharmacists. The

At a Glance

Synopsis: U.S. pharmacist supply estimates of 236,227 in 2007 and 304,986 in 2020 were determined using a stock-flow model based on a 2004 estimate of active pharmacists reported by the Bureau of Labor Statistics. Pharmacists will remain the third largest professional health group behind nurses and physicians. The increase over a previous supply model estimate was attributed to pharmacists remaining in the workforce longer and educational expansion. The model predicted that the pharmacist workforce will become increasingly younger (by about 4 years by 2020) and female (more than 62% women pharmacists by 2020). Reductions in ratios of pharmacists per 100,000 over-65 population from 2011 onward and continuing past 2020 are expected as the large baby boomer population cohort moves into retirement age.

Analysis: *Factors affecting pharmacist supply include new graduates entering the workforce, the creation of new schools of pharmacy and expansion of existing programs, annual hours of employment, the age and gender distribution, and losses through death and retirement. The increasing age of the U.S. baby boomer cohort is likely to further exacerbate existing health care personnel shortages in the near future. The loss of experienced pharmacists could accelerate the rate at which younger pharmacists are moved into positions that demand greater responsibility. Ongoing monitoring of work patterns and maintaining pharmacist supply with attention to leadership issues are of utmost importance.*

2007 supply model reflects updated U.S. graduate projections.

International pharmacy graduates (IPGs) who achieve U.S. pharmacist licensure are another source of supply. The 2007 supply model includes new IPG estimates based on recent data from the Foreign Pharmacy Graduate Equivalency Examination (FPGEE) and the North American Pharmacist Licensure Examination (NAPLEX).

Modeling the pharmacist supply has been critically important to the pharmacist workforce research effort because no strategies for dynamic supply determination currently exist. The most recent past pharmacist census, which was based on state licensure data and reported in 1994, produced supply estimates that closely matched those of the BHPr at that time.[11] Annual estimates from the Bureau of Labor Statistics (BLS) have, on the other hand, varied significantly from year to year, probably as a result of the small numbers of pharmacists in randomly selected population samples. The BHPr supply model is therefore an important touchstone for pharmacist workforce research and planning.

Objective

Our objective was to elucidate key findings from the 2007 supply model. Based on new data, we sought to further refine the head count estimates generated by the 2007 supply model using FTE participation rates by gender to project estimates of the available pharmacist workforce over time.

Methods

The base count for the 2007 supply model is drawn from a 2004 estimate of active pharmacists reported by BLS. The total count is distributed into 50 age groups by gender using data from the 2004 National Pharmacist Workforce Survey.[10] The model projects these numbers forward in time by (1) adding, each year, the projected number of new entrants and (2) subtracting, each year, the projected number of both base-year pharmacists and new entrants who will die or retire. At any point in time, the composite of base-year pharmacists and new entrants who have neither died nor retired constitutes the active pharmacist supply. The 2004 National Pharmacist Workforce Survey found that men worked 91% and women 81% of a 40-hour workweek, together averaging 84% of an FTE workweek.[3] We applied these factors by gender to estimate the projected FTE pharmacist supply.

Separation factors for men and women, composed of estimated deaths and retirements for ages 24 through 74 years, are based on Current Population Survey (CPS) data collected in a 5% sample of the 2000 Census population (approximately 10,000 surveys). The rates are based on the experiences of pharmacists in the sample. By comparison, separation rates in the 2000 supply model were based on 5-year averages of pharmacist work participation. The model was constructed to "retire" all pharmacists by age 75; therefore, we excluded all pharmacists 75 or older when making the projections.

The model includes estimates of IPGs and U.S. graduates. The National Association of Boards of Pharmacy provided data on pharmacists educated outside the United States who achieved U.S. licensure, specifically the number of pharmacists who had successfully completed both the FPGEE and the NAPLEX. National Association of Boards of Pharmacy data were available only for 2003 through August 2006. IPGs achieving U.S. licensure numbered 470 in 2003, 875 in 2004, 763 in 2005, and 883 in 2006. Data for 2006 were prorated to a full year based on actual data through August 2006. The mean for the 4 years was 738 new U.S. licensees per year. The U.S.-licensed IPG variable was modeled as a constant, as in the 2000 supply model, with the conservative estimate of 600 IPGs per year based on the limited global resource of eligible IPGs and shortages in countries other than the United States providing competition for these pharmacists.[12] U.S. graduate estimates were based on the assumption that the maturation of new schools and the expansion of existing U.S. PharmD programs would result in an additional 100 graduates each year; this is roughly equivalent to one new school starting to graduate pharmacists each year.

The relative contributions of separation rates, U.S. graduates, and IPGs toward the increase in predicted numbers of pharmacists in 2020 were calculated by using the updated model while first substituting the separation rates used in the earlier model and then substituting both the earlier separation rates and earlier U.S. and IPG graduate trends with the new separation rates and updated post-2004 graduates. Differences in year-to-year projections resulting from the new separation rates and updated trends in U.S. graduates and IPGs were then calculated for each year from 2005 through 2020 and the relative contributions averaged across the projection period.

We developed two alternative supply projections based on different retirement patterns. A basic series used the same separation rates as the 2007 Supply Model. We developed a low series that reflects retirement 2 years earlier and a high series that reflects retirement 2 years later.

To investigate the impact of supply changes in the 2007 supply model relative to population, we calculated pharmacist-to-population ratios for the total U.S. population and the population older than 65 years. The rationale for investigating the over-65 ratio is that the elderly are the largest per capita consumers of prescription medications, which have been shown to be a significant predictor of demand as reflected by pharmacy positions.[13]

Results

The supply model projected about 236,000 active pharmacists by 2007, and this increases to almost 305,000 by 2020 (Table 1). The projected supply of active pharmacists for the years 2010, 2015, and 2020 is 14%, 20%, and 27% higher, respectively, than estimates from the 2000 supply model. The model predicts that men and women pharmacists will be equal in number sometime during 2006 or 2007 and that the work-

RESEARCH NEW PHARMACIST SUPPLY ESTIMATES

Table 1. Estimated number of men, women, and total pharmacists, 2004–2020

Years	U.S. pharmacy graduates No.	U.S.-licensed IPGs No.	Total active men pharmacists No.	Total active women pharmacists No.	Women pharmacists %	Total active pharmacists No.
2004			125,199	101,201	45	226,400
2005	8,600	600	123,998	105,923	46	229,921
2006	9,204	600	121,142	111,455	48	232,597
2007	9,857	600	118,953	117,274	50	236,227
2008	10,256	600	117,448	123,098	51	240,546
2009	10,356	600	116,201	128,891	53	245,092
2010	10,456	600	115,322	134,633	54	249,955
2011	10,555	600	114,626	140,375	55	255,001
2012	10,655	600	114,133	146,042	56	260,175
2013	10,756	600	113,748	151,668	57	265,416
2014	10,856	600	113,498	157,236	58	270,734
2015	10,955	600	113,411	162,746	59	276,157
2016	11,055	600	113,465	168,262	60	281,727
2017	11,156	600	113,716	173,723	60	287,439
2018	11,256	600	114,048	179,156	61	293,204
2019	11,355	600	114,581	184,504	62	299,085
2020	11,455	600	115,206	189,780	62	304,986

Abbreviation used: IPGs, international pharmacy graduates.

force will become increasingly female, with more than 62% women pharmacists by 2020. Projections of U.S. graduates exceed 2000 supply model estimates by 546 (7%) in 2005, 2,323 (29%) in 2010, 2,662 (32%) in 2015, and 3,003 (36%) in 2020. IPG estimates exceed 2000 supply model estimates by 286 (91%) each year.

Table 2 shows a partial list of the relative contributions of the three variables to increased supply estimates. Revised separation rates had the largest impact, accounting for 59.5% on average (range, 81.2% in 2005 to 46.6% in 2020). The increase in U.S. graduates had the next largest impact, accounting for 34.8% on average (range, 12.3%–47.6%). IPGs, based on an estimated 600 achieving licensure annually, accounted for 5.7% (range, 6.5%–5.8%).

Based on the dominance of revised separation rates in increasing workforce estimates, we modeled the two rate sets. Figure 1 depicts the rate of workforce depletion over time using a hypothetical 100,000-person workforce and the two sets of

Table 2. Relative contributions of the supply model's source data in accounting for the increase in projections

Years	U.S. graduates %	IPGs %	Separation rates %	Total %
2005	12.3	6.5	81.2	100.0
2010	32.7	5.5	61.8	100.0
2015	34.4	5.5	60.1	100.0
2020	47.6	5.8	46.6	100.0
Means, 2005–2020	34.8	5.7	59.5	100.0

Abbreviation used: IPGs, international pharmacy graduates.

separation rates: the BLS-derived rates used in the 2000 supply model and the CPS rates used in the 2007 supply model. By design, all pharmacists were considered retired by age 75. Figure 1 illustrates that the newer rates used in the 2007 supply model result in a slower depletion of the active workforce. The greatest differences in persistence patterns were among older cohorts of pharmacists. The age at which 50% of the

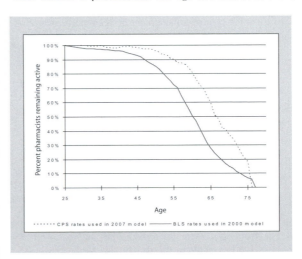

Figure 1. Separation rate–driven models of percent pharmacists remaining in the workforce from 25 to 75 years of age: Comparison of 2007 supply model versus 2000 supply model

Abbreviations used: BLS, Bureau of Labor Statistics; CPS, Current Population Survey.

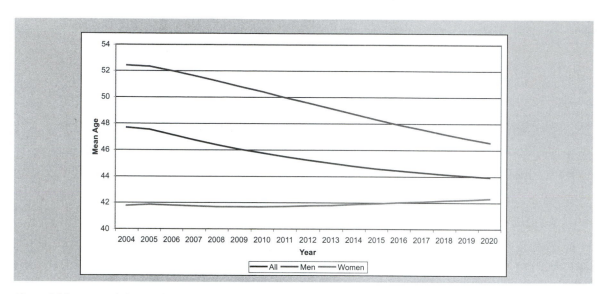

Figure 2. Mean age of pharmacists: 2004, projected to 2020

workforce was no longer active increased from 62 years in the 2000 supply model to 64 years in the 2007 supply model. Among older pharmacists, the rate of leaving the workforce was very similar for men and women pharmacists, suggesting that both men and women pharmacists were working more in their later years (data not shown). As noted earlier, these changes in the workforce depletion rate (or reciprocally participation) were the primary reason for increased supply estimates, accounting for about 59% of supply estimate increases in the 2007 supply model. Their effect on overall increase in supply decreases substantially over time (from 81% to 47%).

Figure 2 shows mean pharmacist age by gender to 2020. Larger-sized cohorts in younger age groups exert a downward influence on the mean age of the overall workforce and on men pharmacists through 2020—despite both men and women pharmacists remaining in the workforce for more years. The model portrays an overall drop in the mean age of all pharmacists from 47 to 43 years and for men pharmacists from 52 to 46 years from 2004 to 2020. Over the same period, the mean age for women pharmacists remains at 42 years.

Figure 3 shows the age distribution of pharmacists in 2006. The distribution is irregular. We note relatively higher counts from ages 48 to 55, which correlate with a period of educational expansion in the late 1970s and early 1980s. Lower counts are observed from ages 39 to 47, corresponding approximately to the decline in graduates in the mid-1980s.[1] Graduate counts grew again in the 1990s, but the national implementation of an entry-level PharmD program in the early 2000s caused a reduction in graduates. The youngest age cohorts have been increasing as a result of a new phase of educational expansion beginning in 2000.

Figure 4 shows the comparison of head counts and FTEs. As

noted earlier, gender-based differences in work patterns result in an increasing gap between head count projections and FTE projections as the ratio of women to men pharmacists increases. The gap between head count and FTE is 34,489 in 2005 and increases to 45,748 by 2020. The overall head count–to–FTE supply reduction is approximately 15%.

Figure 5 depicts alternative series for supply estimates. The basic series was drawn from CPS data as reported earlier. The maximum impact is an increase or decrease in head count of about 10,000 pharmacists in 2020.

Figure 6 illustrates ratios of pharmacists to population groups. The pharmacist–to–100,000-population ratio rises from 77 in 2004 to 91 in 2020. The pharmacist–to–100,000-over-65-population, however, starts at 625 in 2004, remains steady through 2011, decreases to 575 by 2020, and continues to decrease to 508 in 2030, rebounding slowly thereafter despite the sizable growth in the pharmacist supply shown by the model.

Discussion

The principal finding of the 2007 supply model was an unexpected supply estimate increase. Increased work participation, particularly by older pharmacists, accounted for, on average, 59% of the head count increase. Corroborative data from the 2000 and 2004 National Pharmacist Workforce Surveys also found that more near-elderly pharmacists have continued to remain active in the workforce, albeit on a part-time basis.[10] The same report observed that their remaining active may have mitigated the severity of the pharmacist shortage. Historical events that could have encouraged increased persistence in the workforce over the last decade include the rise in wages that occurred in the late 1990s as the pharmacist shortage became

RESEARCH NEW PHARMACIST SUPPLY ESTIMATES

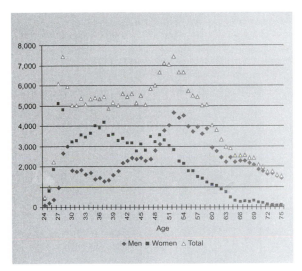

Figure 3. Active pharmacists by age: 2006

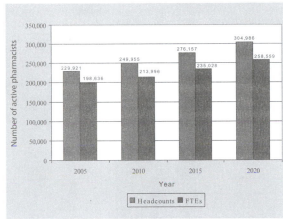

Figure 4. Projected supply of pharmacists by head count and FTEs: 5-year intervals, 2005–2020

Abbreviation used: FTE, full-time equivalent.

severe[14]; the 2000 stock market downturn that affected retirement savings significantly[15]; the rise in demand for pharmacists that made jobs plentiful, including part-time work, which is often attractive to older pharmacists[3]; and increased opportunities for clinical involvement and technology advances during the 1990s that resulted in professional job satisfaction and the motivation to continue working.[1]

Whether these new work patterns will persist or be adopted by younger pharmacists as they move closer to retirement age is impossible to predict. For this reason, frequent reassessment of work patterns will continue to be an important adjunct to supply modeling.

The educational expansion in pharmacy that began in the 1990s and continues unabated, accounting for about 35% of the increased supply, has resulted in a workforce that is projected to grow younger on average despite older pharmacists remaining employed. Generally, physician and nursing workforces are assumed to be growing older on average.[16,17] Recently, however, a call for educational expansion in the medical profession could result in a similar downward age trend for physicians.[8,18]

The effect of a younger pharmacist workforce has not been determined; however, in the face of shortages in other health professions, the presence of a growing, young workforce trained using today's more clinically oriented practice standards and technology advances is a positive factor for the prospect of meeting health care delivery needs through the end of the baby boomer era.

The fall in ratios of pharmacists per 100,000 over-65 population, beginning in 2011 and falling to 575 by 2020 and 508 in 2030 before rebounding slowly thereafter, despite the sizable growth in the pharmacist supply shown by the model, illustrates the challenge to pharmacy as the large baby boomer population moves through the senior age cohorts. This effect is likely to

occur with other health care workers as well, compounding the difficulty in providing health care services during this era. An equally important question for future research is how the balance between supply and demand will shift once the size of the baby boomer cohort begins to decrease.

A 2002 study suggested the need for additional pharmacists by the second and third decade of the 21st century.[19] The study did not anticipate the increased work participation of older pharmacists and educational expansion that have occurred. The new supply projections considerably lessen but do not eliminate the 157,000-pharmacist deficit projected for 2020, especially when reductions related to FTE participation are taken into account.

The unevenness of age distribution (Figure 3) poses a potential problem in the near future as the pharmacists currently in the 48- to 55-year age group, a relatively large cohort, begin to retire and turn over responsibilities to the current 39- to 47-year age group, which is much smaller in number. Sufficiency, not only in terms of numbers but also in terms of leadership and management potential and experience, may be questionable. Younger pharmacists may need to be moved more quickly into positions with higher levels of responsibility. This potential problem should draw the attention of pharmacist employers early enough to plan for its eventuality.

Limitations

The substantial change in workforce participation behavior over a retrospective 10-year period, as reflected by separation rate changes, suggests using caution when making longer-term supply predictions. Future changes in the economy and other factors could result in new shifts in workforce behaviors. In addition, the supply model assumes that the trend toward a predominantly female workforce will continue based on the current preponderance of women among student pharmacists. This dis-

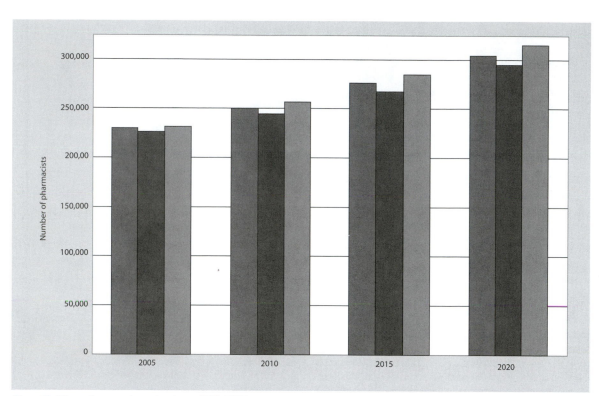

Figure 5. Alternative supply projections: 2005–2020

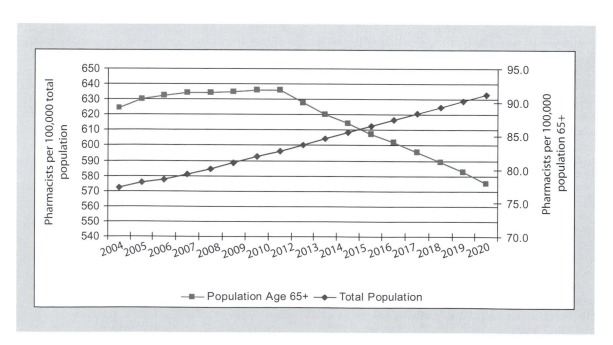

Figure 6. Ratios of pharmacists to U.S. population groups

tribution could possibly shift in the opposite direction. Finally, educational expansion has not proven to be predictable and is therefore difficult to model. The uncertainties in these three areas argue for continued research on work patterns and other supply issues to monitor whether model revision is indicated.

Conclusion

The revised estimated active U.S. pharmacist head count in 2006 is 232,597, with equivalent FTEs totaling approximately 198,000. The substantial increase over the 2000 pharmacist supply model estimates is primarily attributable to pharmacists remaining in the workforce longer and educational expansion. U.S.-licensed IPGs account for fewer than 6% of overall increases. The pharmacist workforce is projected to become younger on average by about 4 years by 2020. A trend toward part-time work reduces the effective pharmacist workforce by about 15%. Although the ratio of pharmacists to the general population will increase through 2020, the ratio of pharmacists to the over-65 population will decrease after 2011 and continue to do so past 2020 as the baby boomers move through their senior years. Historical fluctuations in graduates could create a shortfall of experienced, senior pharmacists during the early phase of the baby boomer retirement era. Coincident demands for more physicians and nurses over the same period and shortages in all three professions stipulate that active steps be taken, including continued monitoring of work trends among pharmacists and other health professionals.

References

1. Health Resources and Services Administration. The pharmacist workforce: a study of the supply and demand for pharmacists. Rockville, Md.: Health Resources and Services Administration; 2000.
2. Knapp KK, Quist RM, Walton SM, Miller LM. Update on the pharmacist shortage: national and state data through 2003. Am J Health Syst Pharm. 2005;62:492–9.
3. Mott DA, Doucette WR, Gaither CA, et al. Pharmacist participation in the workforce: 1990, 2000, and 2004. J Am Pharm Assoc. 2006;46:322–30.
4. Schommer JC, Pedersen CA, Gaither CA, et al. Pharmacists' desired and actual times in work activities: evidence of gaps from the 2004 National Pharmacist Workforce Study. J Am Pharm Assoc. 2006;46:340–7.
5. Knapp KK. Significant trends in the pharmacist shortage 2006. Presented at the National Association of Chain Drug Stores Pharmacy and Technology Conference, San Diego, Calif., August 28, 2006.
6. Hecker DE. Occupational employment projections to 2014. Accessed at www.bls.gov/opub/mlr/2005/11/contents.htm, February 3, 2007.
7. National Center for Health Workforce Analysis, Bureau of Health Professions. Projected supply, demand, and shortages of registered nurses: 2000–2020. Rockville, Md.: Health Resources and Services Administration; 2002.
8. Cooper RA, Getzen TE, McKee HJ, Laud P. Economic and demographic trends signal an impending physician shortage. Health Aff (Millwood). 2002;21:140–54.
9. Gershon SK, Cultice JM, Knapp KK. How many pharmacists are in our future? The Bureau of Health Professions projects supply to 2020. J Am Pharm Assoc. 2000;40:757–64.
10. Mott DA, Doucette WR, Gaither CA, et al. National Pharmacist Workforce Survey: 2004. Accessed at http://aacp.org/Docs/MainNavigation/Resources/7295_final-fullworkforcereport.pdf, February 3, 2007.
11. Vector Research. Pharmacy Manpower Project: state and national survey reports. Ann Arbor, Mich.: Vector Research; 1994.
12. International Pharmaceutical Federation. Global pharmacy workforce and migration report: 2006. Accessed at www.fip.org/files/fip/HR/FIP%20Global%20Pharmacy%20and%20Migration%20report%2007042006.PDF, February 3, 2007.
13. Walton SM, Cooksey JA, Knapp KK, et al. Analysis of pharmacist and pharmacist-extender workforce in 1998–2000: assessing predictors and differences across states. J Am Pharm Assoc. 2004;44:673–83.
14. Mott DA, Doucette WR, Gaither CA, et al. National Pharmacist Workforce Survey: 2006. Accessed at www.aacp.org/site/page.asp?VID=1&CID=1056&DID=6195 February 3, 2007.
15. Weller C. What the crash means for your retirement. Accessed at www.epinet.org/Issuebriefs/ib156/ib156.pdf, February 3, 2007.
16. Dower C, O'Neil E. Health workforce in California: 2002. Accessed at www.futurehealth.ucsf.edu/pdf_files/CD%20Sacramento %2010-29.ppt#21, February 3, 2007.
17. National Center for Health Workforce Analysis. Changing demographics and the implications for physicians, nurses and other health workers. Accessed at http://bhpr.hrsa.gov/healthworkforce/reports/changedemo/summary.htm, February 3, 2007.
18. Salsberg E. Is a physician shortage looming: issues, evidence, and implications. Washington, D.C.: Center for Workforce Studies, Association of American Medical Colleges; 2005.
19. Knapp DA. Professionally determined need for pharmacy services in 2020. Am J Pharm Educ. 2002;66:421–9.

RESEARCH

Examination of state-level changes in the pharmacist labor market using Census data

Surrey M. Walton, Katherine K. Knapp, Laura Miller, and Glen T. Schumock

Abstract

Objective: To examine long-term changes in the U.S. pharmacist labor market across states.

Design: Retrospective cohort study.

Setting: The United States as a whole and individual states in 1990 and 2000.

Participants: Pharmacists and pharmacy school graduates from Census data and previous research, respectively.

Intervention: Retrospective analysis of 5% Public Use Microdata Samples data on pharmacists from the 1990 and 2000 U.S. Census surveys, information on migration among states between 1995 and 2000, and previous research on pharmacy school graduates.

Main outcome measures: Changes in pharmacist counts and wages, as well as migration of pharmacists across states and pharmacy school graduates by state.

Results: From 1990 to 2000, the ratio of pharmacists to 100,000 population increased from 70 to 76, but 13 states experienced declines in this datum, and overall changes in pharmacist counts varied considerably among states. The average wage, expressed in 2000 U.S. dollars, for pharmacists increased from $26.58 per hour to $33.80 per hour (17%), while the average wages of nonpharmacist college graduates increased from $26.37 to only $28.76 (9%). Wage changes varied across states.

Conclusion: According to the Census, the number of pharmacists per 100,000 population varied substantially across states. This variance in supply across states is not converging or easily explained. Overall, the shortage had a clear impact on the pharmacist labor market, yet this effect was not consistent across states.

Keywords: Pharmacists, workforce, migration, salaries, Census.

J Am Pharm Assoc. 2007;47:348–357.

doi: 10.1331/JAPhA.2007.06081

Received July 11, 2006, and in revised form October 5, 2006. Accepted for publication October 9, 2006.

Surrey M. Walton, PhD, is Associate Professor, Department of Pharmacy Administration, College of Pharmacy, University of Illinois at Chicago. **Katherine K. Knapp, PhD,** is Professor and Dean, College of Pharmacy, Touro University, Vallejo, Calif. **Laura Miller, PhD,** is Senior Economist, National Association of Chain Drug Stores, Alexandria, Va. **Glen T. Schumock, PharmD, MBA, FCCP,** is Associate Professor, Department of Pharmacy Practice, University of Illinois at Chicago.

Correspondence: Surrey M. Walton, PhD, Department of Pharmacy Administration (M/C 871), College of Pharmacy, University of Illinois at Chicago, 833 S. Wood St., Rm. 241, Chicago, IL 60612. Fax: 312-996-0868. E-mail: walton@uic.edu

Disclosure: The authors declare no conflicts of interest or financial interests in any products or services mentioned in this article, including grants, employment, gifts, stock holdings, or honoraria.

Funding: Supported by the Health Resources and Services Administration, Bureau of Health Professions (grant U79 HP 00002 1 U76 MB 10004-01), through the Midwest Center for Health Workforce Studies.

Acknowledgments: To Kathleen Odell, University of Illinois at Chicago, for assistance with the data analysis.

Previous presentations: International Health Economics Association Annual Meeting, Barcelona, Spain, July 10–13, 2005.

STATE LEVEL CHANGES IN PHARMACIST LABOR MARKET **RESEARCH**

Available evidence indicates that, since 1998, there has been a national shortage in the labor market for pharmacists and that the shortage continues to be substantial.[1–5] Employers in most states continue to report difficulties in filling pharmacist positions, and a national survey reported an upturn in vacancies during the past year.[5] The development of longitudinal datasets has enabled some tracking of trends before and during the shortage, including changing pharmacist workforce characteristics and work patterns; however, little is known about long-term supply changes across states.[4–7]

Along with trends across time, state-level research is

At a Glance

Synopsis: The 5% Public Use Microdata Samples data on pharmacists from the 1990 and 2000 U.S. Census surveys and data from the authors' previous research on pharmacy school graduates were used to evaluate nationwide and state-level changes in the pharmacist labor market. On the national level, the ratio of pharmacists to 100,000 population increased from 70 to 76, but 13 states experienced declines, and wide variations were observed from state to state. In terms of pharmacy school graduates, New York produced the greatest number, while Alaska, Delaware, Hawaii, Maine, Nevada, New Hampshire, and Vermont had no pharmacy graduates in the 1990s. An overall reduction in pharmacist supply was suggested in several states by the observation of increased relative wages combined with fewer pharmacists per 100,000 population. Younger pharmacists (age 24–35 years) migrated more frequently than older pharmacists, and Florida had the greatest inflow of migrating pharmacists. Generally for the United States, a constrained supply is illustrated by the observation of a 17% increase in average wages for pharmacists from 1990 to 2000—nearly double that for college-educated Americans overall.

Analysis: *Specific reasons for the state-to-state variance in pharmacist supply are not easily identified. Florida, for example, underwent a relatively large increase in pharmacist supply despite having one of the strictest licensure policies in the country. California, and western states in general, continued to have lower numbers of pharmacists per population, but it is unclear whether pharmacists in the West are more productive, such that fewer are needed per population, or whether overall fewer services are being provided. Changes in technology, such as mail-service delivery, may help to explain why certain states had small positive or even negative changes in numbers of pharmacists during the period of study. Further research examining the productivity of pharmacists across states and differences in the general provision of services is needed.*

important because pharmacy practice is regulated at the state level and, historically, there have been large differences in pharmacists per population across states.[8] Efforts to describe and better understand factors that influence state-level differences in the labor market for pharmacists have recently been undertaken. For example, a recent analysis examined differences across states in terms of filled pharmacist positions relative to the population.[9] Analyses assessing differences in market conditions for pharmacists across four specific states have also been published.[10,11] Vacancy rates, difficulty in filling positions, and more recently a direct survey measure of the severity of the pharmacist shortage are examples of available measures related to the pharmacist shortage at the state level.[3] However, state-level data and analyses regarding the pharmacist workforce remain scarce. Furthermore, the most current and comprehensive predictive supply model provides estimates at the national rather than state level.[7]

Economic principles suggest that employers in states affected by the shortage would tend to raise wages and subsequently attract pharmacists from lower-wage states. Therefore, migration and long-term changes in pharmacist salaries are fundamental to understanding the shortage at the state level. Reports of periodic salary surveys have appeared along with anecdotal evidence of salary and bonuses during the shortage period, though most of these reports do not control for pharmacist age and education level, and very few offer comparisons between pharmacist salaries and salaries of other groups.[12,13] Overall, little examination has been made of salary changes across time at the national and state level.

In addition to migration, the number of new graduates from pharmacy programs is an important source of supply change that varies considerably across states. A recent study showed large differences in the number of pharmacy school graduates across states, even when adjusted for population.[14] Currently, many states are undergoing pharmacy education program expansion in an effort to increase graduates and hence ameliorate the shortage.

Objectives

The purpose of this study was to examine long-term changes in the U.S. pharmacist labor market across states. Specifically, our three objectives were to

1. Analyze in-state pharmacy school graduates, state-level migration of pharmacists between 1995 and 2000, and changes in the number of pharmacists by state between 1990 and 2000;
2. Examine pharmacist migration patterns by age; and
3. Measure long-term changes in the wages of pharmacists and variation in wages across states.

Conceptual framework

Considering a variety of possible sources of change in the supply of pharmacists is important when looking at labor market dynamics. The main sources of change examined in this study included increased pharmacy school graduates, increased net migration of pharmacists, and increased pharmacists returning from other professions or from being unemployed or retired. The relative size of supply changes and the relative contribution of migration, pharmacy school graduates, and in-state market supply changes in any particular state can be expected to vary based on numerous factors related to the costs and benefits of living in any particular state, as well as state-level policies related to pharmacy and state-level investments in the supply of pharmacists.

Wage rates in general are important indicators for market changes, and these can be compared among similarly skilled workers to help identify factors driving market changes. In this scenario, wages are viewed as an incentive to work in pharmacy and as an indicator of the demand for pharmacist services. Underlying this analysis of long-term trends in the pharmacist market is the emergence of the mainly demand-driven national market shortage of pharmacists in the middle to late 1990s. A demand-driven market shortage occurs when demand increases are larger than available supply, exerting upward pressure on wages. In general, a simultaneous increase in relative wages and the number of pharmacists suggests a demand-driven market shortage of pharmacists.

If a pharmacists shortage had affected all states to similar degrees, then basic economic theory suggests that wages would rise over time in all states and that supply would respond in all states. However, the relationship between wages and supply changes is more difficult to predict if such a shortage does not occur in any particular state. For example, if the supply of pharmacists is shifting substantially in a particular state (perhaps because of an expanded pharmacy education program), higher numbers and, accordingly, relatively lower wages could result.

In addition to considering long-term changes in numbers and wages of pharmacists across states, part of this analysis was devoted to an examination of migration rates for pharmacists relative to the population across age ranges. Given that costs of moving tend to increase with age (location-specific investments create benefits that are difficult to uproot), one would expect migration to decline with age. Aside from such a general trend, again basic economic theory does not provide a clear prediction for pharmacist migration relative to the population. Because the skills required to be a pharmacist are more transferable than those associated with many other occupations, pharmacists may be expected to migrate at a comparably higher rate. However, if the tendency is for pharmacists to develop more site-specific skills (such as opening an individual practice with local clients), then they may be less inclined to migrate than other members of the workforce.

Methods
Data

The majority of the analyses in this study were based on the 5% Public Use Microdata Samples (PUMS) from the 1990 and

2000 U.S. Census surveys[15,16]; these data provide a new source of information about the pharmacist workforce at both the national and state levels. The PUMS data are individual level and include self-reported information on age, gender, educational attainment, race, occupation, salary, state of residence, and state of primary employment. The 2000 PUMS data also contain information on where the individual lived in 1995, allowing an analysis of worker migration across state lines—an important variable for tracking one possible response to a workforce shortage. Further, the PUMS data contain sampling frequency weights, which allow estimation of total counts by occupation at the state level. The sample size (n = 10,346 in 2000 and 8,502 in 1990), roughly 5% of all pharmacists, is substantially larger than other recent datasets used to study workforce issues at the national level. Most recent studies have not had a sufficient sample size to address state-level differences. Finally, PUMS data from the 2000 U.S. Census can be compared with equivalent data from the 1990 U.S. Census to provide insights into overall changes in the market for pharmacists over time.

PUMS data were used to estimate the following information at the state level: pharmacist counts in 1990 and 2000, pharmacist salaries in 1990 and 2000, and in-migration and out-migration between 1995 and 2000. The PUMS data were also used in some instances to compare pharmacist earnings with subsections of the nonpharmacist population that share similar observable characteristics (see below). In addition, as an important scaling factor, many of the descriptive analyses incorporated total state populations, which also come from the 1990 and 2000 U.S. Census, but are taken from published statistics rather than calculated from the 5% PUMS datasets.[17,18] To complement the Census data, information on the number of pharmacy school graduates per state was used from previous research.[14]

Sample selection and variable definitions

Pharmacists were selected from the 1990 and 2000 Census data based on self-reported occupation; this included both employed and unemployed individuals. Fields indicating age and number of years of schooling were also used in record selection. The analyses focused on pharmacists 21 years of age or older who had, at minimum, a bachelor's degree. Age and education selection criteria were intended to reduce measurement error from miscoded or misidentified occupation. To make comparisons with the general population in terms of wages, total PUMS data (i.e., the total population) were used with the same restrictions on age and education.

We accounted for pharmacists' state of residence. Migration was measured using the "migration state" field in the Census data, which indicates where a person lived up to 5 years before a given Census year. In cases where "migration state" was different from the current state of residence, the person was considered to have migrated. The Census also provided information on total earnings from salary as well as weeks worked and

STATE LEVEL CHANGES IN PHARMACIST LABOR MARKET **RESEARCH**

hours per week. In addition, the data included information on demographic characteristics related to wages, such as educational attainment, age, gender, and race. Because many factors related to location may affect salaries, pharmacist salaries at the state level were compared with salaries of college-educated nonpharmacists of working age. The comparison group is meant to approximate the opportunity cost of practicing pharmacy using market earnings of similarly skilled workers in other occupations. In all salary calculations, a minimum hourly wage of $6.00 was used to help minimize measurement error. For consistency, 1990 salary data were converted to 2000 dollars using an inflator (1990 values were multiplied by 1.32) from the Bureau of Labor Statistics.[19]

Analyses

Various descriptive analyses were conducted to characterize state-level differences in the number of pharmacists and sources of change in the number of pharmacists across states, as well as comparisons of the number of pharmacists to the overall population in a state. Rates of migration across age for all pharmacists were examined. Descriptive statistics were also calculated for inflation-adjusted wages of pharmacists relative to inflation-adjusted wages of college-educated nonpharmacist workers in general.

Results

The sample of pharmacists in the Census projects to a total pharmacist workforce of 217,408 in 2000. This estimated pharmacist population, based on weights from the Census sample, compares well with other estimates in the literature.[2,7,20,21]

Table 1 shows population counts and the percentage of the population older than 65 years by state. The vast majority of states experienced population growth. In addition, all states had a steady or slightly increasing percentage of the population that was older than 65 years. Table 2 shows the number of pharmacists per 100,000 population by state in 1990 and 2000. Nationally, the ratio of pharmacists to 100,000 population increased from 70 to 76, but 13 states experienced declines, and the overall change in pharmacist counts varied considerably among states.

Note that because these numbers are based on a 5% sample survey of the Census, large changes in these ratios could be an artifact of small sample variance in states with small total populations. Hence, the 10 states with the lowest total population in 1990 are indicated in Tables 1 through 4. Nonetheless, substantial variance in gains and losses was evident, even among states with relatively large populations, and not all states gained in terms of pharmacists. For example, Virginia and Ohio, two states with a relatively large population (top 15), had lower pharmacist-to-population ratios in 2000 than in 1990.

Table 3 shows cumulative pharmacy school graduates from 1990 to 1995, cumulative pharmacy school graduates from 1995 through 2000, net in-migration overall and for those younger than 30 years between 1995 and 2000, and changes in the number of pharmacists between 1990 and 2000. All values are adjusted by state populations in 1990. Alaska, Delaware, Hawaii, Maine, Nevada, New Hampshire, and Vermont did not produce any new pharmacy school graduates in the 1990s, and the District of Columbia, North Dakota, and Rhode Island produced the most pharmacy school graduates per population count. The state with the largest number of pharmacy school graduates was New York, and the state with the largest rate of net in-migration was Florida. Figure 1 shows the percentage change in the number of pharmacists per 100,000 population across the United States. Relatively high increases in the pharmacist numbers are observed fairly consistently across time in the western-most states and in the Southeast; however, as shown in Table 4, the sources of change in those areas appear to be different.

Figure 2 shows migration patterns across age-groups for all pharmacists 21 years of age or older, working pharmacists (those who reported that they were currently employed), and the comparison groups from the nonpharmacist population. The main finding is that younger pharmacists (age 24–35 years) migrated more frequently than older pharmacists and the population in general.

Comparative salary information across time for pharmacists and the general population revealed that, nationally, salaries grew significantly for pharmacists between 1990 and 2000 and that pharmacists earned substantially more than the general population of working, college-educated Americans. Specifically, the average wages (in 2000 U.S. dollars) for pharmacists increased from $26.58 per hour to $33.08 per hour (17% increase), while the average wages for all college graduates increased from $26.37 to $28.76 (9% increase). Table 4 shows wage changes by state.

Despite the general U.S. market clearly moving towards higher pharmacist salaries, the variation across states was substantial. In 32 states, a demand-driven shortage is evidenced by increases in relative wages and relative numbers of pharmacists. Reductions in both relative wages and pharmacist counts occurred in only two states (Wyoming and North Carolina). A reduction in supply is suggested by the increased relative wages along with fewer pharmacists per 100,000 population observed in a fair number of states.

Discussion

Consistent with past findings, the number of pharmacists and the number of pharmacists per 100,000 population across states varied substantially in 1990 and 2000, according to the Census. Further, this variance in supply across states does not seem to be converging or easily explained. For example, Florida experienced a relatively large growth in pharmacists and had relatively high numbers in net in-migration despite having one of the strictest licensure policies in the country. California produced small increases in pharmacy school graduates and had

RESEARCH STATE LEVEL CHANGES IN PHARMACIST LABOR MARKET

Table 1. Total state population and population older than 65 years

States	1990 total state population No.	2000 total state population No.	1990 population >65 years No. (%)	2000 population >65 years No. (%)
Alabama	4,040,389	4,447,100	486,038 (12)	576,503 (13)
Alaska[a]	550,043	626,932	19,840 (4)	34,776 (6)
Arizona	3,665,339	5,130,632	442,405 (12)	668,033 (13)
Arkansas	2,350,624	2,673,400	325,087 (14)	374,345 (14)
California	29,811,427	33,871,648	2,897,228 (10)	3,586,264 (11)
Colorado	3,294,473	4,301,261	302,241 (9)	417,066 (10)
Connecticut	3,287,116	3,405,565	410,258 (12)	471,379 (14)
Delaware[a]	666,168	783,600	73,486 (11)	101,440 (13)
District of Columbia[a]	606,900	572,059	71,026 (12)	69,933 (12)
Florida	12,938,071	15,982,378	2,209,854 (17)	2,806,660 (18)
Georgia	6,478,149	8,186,453	606,982 (9)	786,402 (10)
Hawaii	1,108,229	1,211,537	114,590 (10)	161,356 (13)
Idaho[a]	1,006,734	1,293,953	111,236 (11)	147,123 (11)
Illinois	11,430,602	12,419,293	1,331,616 (12)	1,492,697 (12)
Indiana	5,544,156	6,080,485	644,747 (12)	755,041 (12)
Iowa	2,776,831	2,926,324	399,188 (14)	436,464 (15)
Kansas	2,477,588	2,688,418	319,463 (13)	354,790 (13)
Kentucky	3,686,892	4,041,769	432,577 (12)	505,144 (12)
Louisiana	4,221,826	4,468,976	432,675 (10)	518,010 (12)
Maine	1,227,928	1,274,923	149,698 (12)	183,330 (14)
Maryland	4,780,753	5,296,486	477,323 (10)	597,048 (11)
Massachusetts	6,016,425	6,349,097	760,208 (13)	858,931 (14)
Michigan	9,295,287	9,938,444	1,025,274 (11)	1,217,439 (12)
Minnesota	4,375,665	4,919,479	508,679 (12)	593,962 (12)
Mississippi	2,575,475	2,844,658	297,690 (12)	345,891 (12)
Missouri	5,116,901	5,595,211	667,432 (13)	761,401 (14)
Montana[a]	799,065	902,195	99,200 (12)	119,855 (13)
Nebraska	1,578,417	1,711,263	209,145 (13)	232,242 (14)
Nevada	1,201,675	1,998,257	116,012 (10)	218,622 (11)
New Hampshire	1,109,252	1,235,786	116,200 (10)	148,106 (12)
New Jersey	7,747,750	8,414,350	953,612 (12)	1,110,795 (13)
New Mexico	1,515,069	1,819,046	149,499 (10)	212,102 (12)
New York	17,990,778	18,976,457	2,183,554 (12)	2,456,373 (13)
North Carolina	6,632,448	8,049,313	742,149 (11)	972,080 (12)
North Dakota[a]	638,800	642,200	85,740 (13)	94,539 (15)
Ohio	10,847,115	11,353,140	1,307,316 (12)	1,507,518 (13)
Oklahoma	3,145,576	3,450,654	392,249 (12)	454,607 (13)
Oregon	2,842,337	3,421,399	363,020 (13)	436,861 (13)
Pennsylvania	11,882,842	12,281,054	1,700,199 (14)	1,922,917 (16)
Rhode Island[a]	1,003,464	1,048,319	140,714 (14)	151,798 (14)
South Carolina	3,486,310	4,012,012	363,801 (10)	488,074 (12)
South Dakota[a]	696,004	754,844	96,588 (14)	108,813 (14)
Tennessee	4,877,203	5,689,283	571,203 (12)	706,134 (12)
Texas	16,986,335	20,851,820	1,577,958 (9)	2,066,585 (10)
Utah	1,722,850	2,233,169	139,269 (8)	191,653 (9)
Vermont[a]	562,758	608,827	59,184 (11)	76,091 (12)
Virginia	6,189,197	7,078,515	611,478 (10)	788,814 (11)
Washington	4,866,669	5,894,121	534,165 (11)	659,658 (11)
West Virginia	1,793,477	1,808,344	250,067 (14)	273,831 (15)
Wisconsin	4,891,954	5,363,675	609,914 (12)	703,843 (13)
Wyoming[a]	453,589	493,782	44,461 (10)	57,437 (12)
U.S. total/average	248,790,925	281,421,906	28,933,538 (12)	34,980,776 (13)
Population-weighted U.S. average (%)			12	12

[a]Denotes the 10 states with the lowest total population in 1990.

STATE LEVEL CHANGES IN PHARMACIST LABOR MARKET **RESEARCH**

Table 2. Resident pharmacists per 100,000 state population in 1990 and 2000

States	1990 resident pharmacists No.	2000 resident pharmacists No.	Change in resident pharmacists (1990–2000) %	1990 resident pharmacists per 100,000 population %	2000 resident pharmacists per 100,000 population %	Change in pharmacists per 100,000 population %
Alabama	3,243	4,247	31	80.3	95.5	19
Alaska[a]	255	190	−25	46.4	30.3	−35
Arizona	2,542	3,748	47	69.4	73.1	5
Arkansas	1,749	2,153	23	74.4	80.5	8
California	17,671	22,284	26	59.3	65.8	11
Colorado	2,598	2,863	10	78.9	66.6	−16
Connecticut	2,638	2,616	−1	80.3	76.8	−4
Delaware[a]	385	562	46	57.8	71.7	24
District of Columbia[a]	250	269	8	41.2	47.0	14
Florida	9,054	12,830	42	70.0	80.3	15
Georgia	4,893	7,367	51	75.5	90.0	19
Hawaii	497	900	81	44.8	74.3	66
Idaho[a]	988	799	−19	98.1	61.7	−37
Illinois	7,263	8,906	23	63.5	71.7	13
Indiana	4,316	5,642	31	77.8	92.8	19
Iowa	1,739	2,619	51	62.6	89.5	43
Kansas	2,085	2,327	12	84.2	86.6	3
Kentucky	2,967	3,368	14	80.5	83.3	4
Louisiana	3,399	4,226	24	80.5	94.6	17
Maine	515	628	22	41.9	49.3	17
Maryland	3,427	4,290	25	71.7	81.0	13
Massachusetts	4,786	5,500	15	79.5	86.6	9
Michigan	6,015	7,025	17	64.7	70.7	9
Minnesota	2,921	4,180	43	66.8	85.0	27
Mississippi	1,836	2,371	29	71.3	83.3	17
Missouri	3,331	3,713	11	65.1	66.4	2
Montana[a]	669	722	8	83.7	80.0	−4
Nebraska	1,462	1,327	−9	92.6	77.5	−16
Nevada	685	1,580	131	57.0	79.1	39
New Hampshire	673	802	19	60.7	64.9	7
New Jersey	6,445	7,772	21	83.2	92.4	11
New Mexico	858	1,275	49	56.6	70.1	24
New York	13,496	15,625	16	75.0	82.3	10
North Carolina	4,818	5,447	13	72.6	67.7	−7
North Dakota[a]	335	699	109	52.4	108.8	108
Ohio	8,516	8,817	4	78.5	77.7	−1
Oklahoma	2,551	3,168	24	81.1	91.8	13
Oregon	2,125	3,043	43	74.8	88.9	19
Pennsylvania	9,333	11,389	22	78.5	92.7	18
Rhode Island[a]	755	713	−6	75.2	68.0	−10
South Carolina	2,748	3,606	31	78.8	89.9	14
South Dakota[a]	614	695	13	88.2	92.1	4
Tennessee	3,696	4,988	35	75.8	87.7	16
Texas	10,677	13,610	27	62.9	65.3	4
Utah	1,333	1,104	−17	77.4	49.4	−36
Vermont[a]	418	335	−20	74.3	55.0	−26
Virginia	4,653	4,753	2	75.2	67.1	−11
Washington	2,979	4,475	50	61.2	75.9	24
West Virginia	1,148	1,506	31	64.0	83.3	30
Wisconsin	3,716	4,144	12	76.0	77.3	2
Wyoming[a]	225	190	−16	49.6	38.5	−22
U.S. total/average	176,291	217,408	24	70.4	76.0	9.6
Population-weighted U.S. average			23	70.9	77.3	9

[a]Denotes the 10 states with the lowest total population in 1990.

Table 3. Cumulative pharmacy school graduates, net migration, and change in counts of pharmacists by state, adjusted by 1990 total state population

States	Cumulative graduates (1990–1995) per 100,000 population	Cumulative graduates (1995–2000) per 100,000 population	Net in-migration of pharmacists (1995–2000) per 100,000 population	Net in-migration of pharmacists <30 (1995–2000) per 100,000 population	Change in resident pharmacists (1990–2000) per 100,000 population
Alabama	23	21	–1	–2	15
Alaska[a]	0	0	–20	–1	–16
Arizona	6	7	23	11	4
Arkansas	13	15	4	1	6
California	7	8	2	1	7
Colorado	13	19	17	7	–12
Connecticut	13	14	–2	–3	–3
Delaware[a]	0	0	–3	14	14
District of Columbia[a]	51	44	–10	7	6
Florida	8	10	11	3	10
Georgia	18	16	6	2	14
Hawaii	0	0	0	5	29
Idaho[a]	19	25	4	–4	–36
Illinois	5	11	–6	–1	8
Indiana	22	23	–4	–1	15
Iowa	31	34	–7	–6	27
Kansas	16	17	–1	3	2
Kentucky	14	10	2	2	3
Louisiana	30	30	–7	–7	14
Maine	0	0	5	4	7
Maryland	10	8	2	1	9
Massachusetts	26	29	0	0	7
Michigan	13	15	3	1	6
Minnesota	10	8	10	7	18
Mississippi	19	15	–3	–1	12
Missouri	18	20	–3	–3	1
Montana[a]	24	30	–16	–2	–4
Nebraska	39	46	–18	–5	–15
Nevada	0	0	41	10	22
New Hampshire	0	0	–3	9	4
New Jersey	8	8	3	2	9
New Mexico	19	24	–8	–2	13
New York	19	22	–5	–2	7
North Carolina	17	15	7	3	–5
North Dakota[a]	44	43	–42	–32	56
Ohio	18	20	–1	0	–1
Oklahoma	28	28	–8	–9	11
Oregon	15	20	16	6	14
Pennsylvania	25	26	–5	–4	14
Rhode Island[a]	45	44	–6	1	–7
South Carolina	20	17	–4	1	11
South Dakota[a]	40	32	–28	–25	4
Tennessee	7	8	6	7	12
Texas	10	9	6	4	2
Utah	13	13	4	0	–28
Vermont[a]	0	0	10	0	–19
Virginia	8	7	5	–2	–8
Washington	12	11	7	2	15
West Virginia	20	22	–14	–5	19
Wisconsin	11	11	2	–1	1
Wyoming[a]	43	25	–35	–9	–11
U.S. average	17	17	–1b	0	6
Population-adjusted U.S. average	14	15	1b	0	6

[a]Denotes the 10 states with the lowest total population in 1990.
[b]Non-zero averages for net immigration can be explained by in-migration from Puerto Rico and abroad.

STATE LEVEL CHANGES IN PHARMACIST LABOR MARKET **RESEARCH**

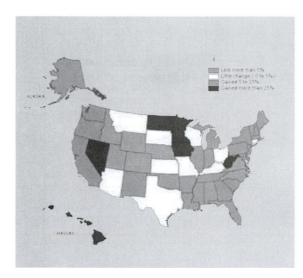

Figure 1. Percentage change (1990–2000) in U.S. resident pharmacists per 100,000 population

Table 4. Pharmacists hourly wage, 1990 and 2000, and percent change

States	1990 pharmacists hourly wage (converted to 2000 dollars)	2000 pharmacists hourly wage	Change in pharmacists hourly wage (1990–2000) %
Alabama	26.08	42.67	64
Alaska[a]	28.79	31.60	10
Arizona	24.33	34.97	44
Arkansas	22.71	29.36	29
California	47.86	37.66	−21
Colorado	22.47	42.13	87
Connecticut	27.99	33.16	18
Delaware[a]	46.65	28.26	−39
District of Columbia[a]	27.05	30.47	13
Florida	29.10	34.44	18
Georgia	25.44	32.01	26
Hawaii	25.51	33.25	30
Idaho[a]	22.71	27.37	21
Illinois	27.74	33.95	22
Indiana	26.25	32.59	24
Iowa	21.94	28.15	28
Kansas	26.83	29.40	10
Kentucky	25.30	33.57	33
Louisiana	22.16	29.86	35
Maine	22.58	29.69	31
Maryland	26.55	33.21	25
Massachusetts	25.96	30.17	16
Michigan	28.11	34.75	24
Minnesota	25.82	30.28	17
Mississippi	23.62	32.01	36
Missouri	23.85	28.99	22
Montana[a]	20.98	24.25	16
Nebraska	19.83	26.06	31
Nevada	30.40	33.18	9
New Hampshire	27.66	32.36	17
New Jersey	27.56	38.34	39
New Mexico	24.32	25.64	5
New York	26.92	34.25	27
North Carolina	31.65	31.48	−1
North Dakota[a]	22.39	28.10	25
Ohio	28.94	31.95	10
Oklahoma	21.35	30.12	41
Oregon	36.31	32.64	−10
Pennsylvania	26.10	31.88	22
Rhode Island[a]	24.24	55.78	130
South Carolina	28.31	31.24	10
South Dakota[a]	21.56	27.00	25
Tennessee	26.68	34.22	28
Texas	30.08	38.22	27
Utah	24.60	31.90	30
Vermont[a]	22.07	45.28	105
Virginia	26.11	31.45	20
Washington	26.16	32.72	25
West Virginia	24.75	32.63	32
Wisconsin	26.61	34.38	29
Wyoming[a]	26.81	21.20	−21
U.S. total/average	26.58	32.55	25
Population-weighted U.S. average	28.91	33.80	17

[a]Denotes the 10 states with the lowest total population in 1990.

modest in-migration (perhaps as a result of strict rules) but managed to achieve moderate growth in the number of pharmacists per 100,000 population. California and the western states in general still tend to have lower numbers of pharmacists per population. Hawaii and Iowa experienced substantial growth in the number of pharmacists per population, while Nebraska, Idaho, and Utah saw relatively large declines.

Specific reasons for the differing pharmacist totals are beyond the scope of the analyses but may result from variance in the underlying demand for pharmacist services or different delivery methods of pharmaceutical care across states. For example, relatively high pharmacist growth in Florida may be related to population growth, particularly among those older than 65 years. There may also have been changes in the demand for specific pharmacist services, such as counseling on specific products, that were not captured in the data used here. In contrast, technology changes such as mail-service delivery may explain why certain states had small positive or even negative changes in numbers of pharmacists during this period. Two important areas for future research are to examine the productivity of pharmacists across states and differences in the general provision of services across states. Are pharmacists in the West more productive, such that fewer are needed per population, or are they providing fewer services?

Younger pharmacists are more likely to migrate than older pharmacists and the population in general. This suggests that state policy regarding migration would tend to have the greatest effect on younger pharmacists. High levels of migration from a state by younger pharmacists does not necessarily mean lower overall supply if there are large numbers of pharmacy school graduates in a state. Overall, with the recent opening of new pharmacy schools and colleges and the expansion of

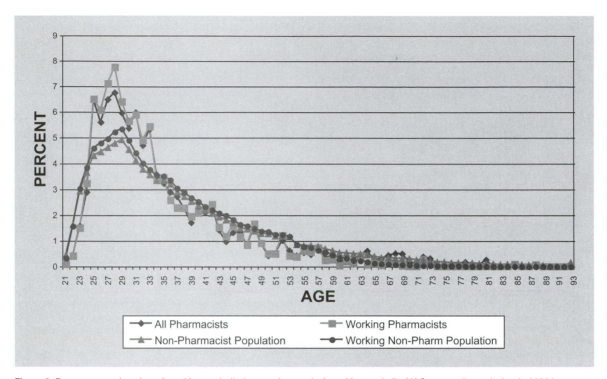

Figure 2. Percentage migration of working and all pharmacists and of working and all of U.S. general population in 2000 by age

existing programs, the total number of graduates per year has been increasing.[22] The relatively high migration levels for young pharmacy school graduates suggest that future dynamics in this labor market are important to track.

Despite increased numbers of pharmacists, the demand-driven shortage clearly has had a major impact on the market. Substantial increases in pharmacist wages relative to similarly educated workers were observed over the decade studied. However, not all states experienced large increases in wages and not all states saw an increase in the number of working pharmacists. These differences in market reactions are difficult to explain with available data. In general, employer surveys have shown similar levels of difficulty across states in filling pharmacist positions; this would suggest similar market pressures to increase wages on the part of all employers.[4] Why wage changes would not be similar across states is a question for future research. Basic characteristics of the population, such as age, wealth, and health status, as well as availability of technology, use of technicians, and local policy decisions related to pharmacists, can all have an impact on market equilibrium. The data discussed here provide important baseline information, but a definite need remains for more detailed data collection and synthesis, and a great deal more research to gain an understanding of what drives supply and demand in the market for pharmacists and the effect on the health of the population.

Limitations

The results of this research should be interpreted in the context of limitations in the analysis. In the Census data, pharmacists are identified based on self-reported occupation rather than licensure and/or employment records. Therefore, the totals reported here may differ from those using licensure information. In addition, totals by state are based on sampling weights from the 5% PUMS, which introduces inherent sampling-related error. This limitation may have greater relevance in states with small populations or limited numbers of pharmacists.

The analysis is based on the most recent Census (2000) data available. The Census is completed every 10 years, and the PUMS data are typically released around 4 years after the survey. Hence, these are the latest available data that examine the pharmacist market across states. Data from 2000 may not represent current levels of pharmacists. However, the distribution of pharmacists across states is unlikely to have changed substantially enough to negate the general findings, and many of the relationships examined (such as migration patterns across age and relationships between net migration and new pharmacy school graduates) would not be expected to change considerably over time.

The migration statistics are based on information on the state of residence 5 years previously. Hence, multiple state changes between 1995 and 2000 would not be counted in the migration analyses.

STATE LEVEL CHANGES IN PHARMACIST LABOR MARKET **RESEARCH**

Further, the pharmacy school graduate data and Census data are from separate sources that cannot be linked. Hence, the migration patterns of pharmacy school graduates are not able to be determined, and whether pharmacists migrated for work, school, or other reasons is unknown. Nevertheless, the data presented here provide a reasonable estimate of the migration patterns of pharmacists across age ranges.

Conclusion

As the United States moves towards greater reliance on the use of medications to manage medical conditions, understanding the pharmacist market will grow increasingly important. This report provides a variety of descriptive information about general supply levels and sources of change in the supply of pharmacists. The general variance seen across states in broad measures of supply, as well as underlying causes of the dynamics of supply, remains unexplained, and detailed, consistent data at the state level are scarce. Increased effort to measure and evaluate the labor market for pharmacists is needed, particularly on a longitudinal basis.

Clearly, ample room exists for future research to identify and measure structural factors related to pharmacist productivity (e.g., available technology, use of technicians, payment policies) and the underlying demand for pharmacist services (e.g., patient characteristics, insurance coverage, practice patterns of physicians). Finally, more effort should be made to establish data that can be used to identify and examine the effect of policy decisions surrounding the pharmacist labor market (e.g., licensure rules, laws regarding technicians, local tax incentives). Given the constraints imparted by the available data, a strong argument can be made for increased investment into tracking the pharmacist workforce.

References

1. Health Resources and Services Administration. The pharmacist workforce: a study of the supply and demand for pharmacists. Bethesda, Md.: Health Resources and Services Administration, U.S. Department of Health and Human Services; 2000.

2. Cooksey JA, Knapp KK, Walton SM, et al. Challenges to the pharmacist profession from escalating pharmaceutical demand. Health Aff (Millwood). 2002;21:165–73.

3. Knapp KK, Livesey JC. The Aggregate Demand Index: measuring the balance between pharmacist supply and demand. J Am Pharm Assoc. 2002;42:391–8

4. Knapp KK, Quist RM, Walton SM, Miller LM. Update on the pharmacist shortage: national and state data through 2003. Am J Health Syst Pharm. 2005;62:492–9.

5. Pharmacy Manpower Project. Aggregate Demand Index. Accessed at www.pharmacymanpower.com, March 1, 2006.

6. Mott DA. Pharmacist turnover, length of service, and reasons for leaving: 1983–1997. Am J Health Syst Pharm. 2000;57:975–84.

7. Gershon SK, Cultice JM, Knapp KK. How many pharmacists are in our future? The Bureau of Health Professions projects supply to 2020. J Am Pharm Assoc. 2000;40:757–64.

8. Vector Research, Inc. Pharmacy manpower project: state and national survey reports. Ann Arbor, Mich.: Vector Research, Inc.; 1994.

9. Walton SM, Cooksey JA, Knapp KK, et al. An analysis of pharmacists and the total pharmacist-related workforce from 1998–2000: assessing workforce predictors and differences across states. J Am Pharm Assoc. 2004;44:673–83.

10. Cline RR, Mott DA. Job matching in pharmacy labor markets: a study in four states. Pharm Res. 2000;17:1537–45.

11. Cline RR. Disequilibrium and human capital in pharmacy labor markets: evidence from four states. J Am Pharm Assoc. 2003;43:702–9.

12. Zgarrick D, Fjortoft N. Pharmacist compensation in Illinois. Part I: overall marketplace trends. KeePosted 2002;28(6):18–27.

13. Cardinale V. Are rising wages and generous benefits enough to attract pharmacists and keep them from roaming? Drug Top. Accessed at www.drugtopics.com/drugtopics/content/contentDetail.jsp?id=151425, March 1, 2006.

14. Cooksey JA, Walton SM, Stankewicz T, Knapp KK. Pharmacy school graduates by state and region: 1990–1999. J Am Pharm Assoc. 2003;43:463–9.

15. US Census Bureau. The Census of Population and Housing, 1990 [United States]: Public Use Microdata Sample: 5-Percent Sample.

16. US Census Bureau. The Census of Population and Housing, 2000 [United States]: Public Use Microdata Sample: 5-Percent Sample.

17. US Census Bureau. State population estimates and demographic components of population change: April 1, 1990 to July 1, 1999. ST-99-2. Accessed at www.census.gov/population/estimates/state/st-99-2.txt, March 1, 2006.

18. US Census Bureau. Population, housing units, area, and density (geographies ranked by total population): 2000. GCT-PH1-R. Accessed at http://factfinder.census.gov/servlet/GCTTable?_bm=y&-geo_id=01000US&-_box_head_nbr=GCT-PH1-R&-ds_name=DEC_2000_SF1_U&-redoLog=false&-format=US-9S&-mt_name=DEC_2000_SF1_U_GCTPH1R_US9S, March 1, 2006.

19. Bureau of Labor Statistics. Inflation calculator. Accessed at www.bls.gov/cpi/home.htm, March 1, 2006.

20. Pedersen CA, Doucette WR, Gaither CA, et al. Final report of the National Pharmacist Workforce Survey: 2000: Midwest Pharmacy Workforce Research Consortium. Accessed at www.aacp.org/, March 1, 2006.

21. Mott DA, Doucette WR, Gaither CA, et al. A ten-year trend analysis of pharmacist participation in the workforce. Am Pharm Educ. 2002;66:223–33.

22. Hussar DA. How many colleges of pharmacy is enough? J Am Pharm Assoc. 2005;45:428–30.

RESEARCH

Attitudes and interests of pharmacists regarding independent pharmacy ownership

Carolyn M. Brown, Roxanne Cantu, Zach Corbell, and Kristy Roberts

Abstract

Objective: To examine the beliefs, attitudes, and interests of Texas pharmacists at different career stages with respect to independent pharmacy ownership.

Design: Nonexperimental, cross-sectional study.

Setting: Texas in November–December 2004.

Participants: 180 practicing pharmacists.

Intervention: Mail survey.

Main outcome measures: Pharmacists' self-reported attitudes (ranging from –90, unfavorable, to +90, favorable) about and interest (–3, very unlikely, to +3, very likely) in independent pharmacy ownership.

Results: Pharmacists reported an overall favorable attitude toward independent pharmacy ownership (mean [± SD] 18.6 ± 28, range –63.0 to 90.0). Beliefs that ownership would increase their business autonomy, professional autonomy, and ability to establish patient loyalty made the largest contributions to overall attitude. Pharmacists' attitudes toward ownership differed by career stage ($F = 3.12$, $df = 2$, $P = 0.047$), with middle– (age 36–49 years) and early– (age ≤35 years) career-stage pharmacists reporting the most and least favorable attitudes, respectively. Pharmacists reported a low interest in pursuing ownership (–2.2 ± 1.6, –3.0 to +3.0). Financial rewards ($r = 0.26$, $P < 0.001$) and the need for business/managerial skills ($r = 0.25$, $P < 0.001$) were most highly correlated with pharmacists' interest in pursuing ownership. Multivariate findings indicated that pharmacists with a higher interest in pursuing ownership and those with advanced training certifications had significantly more favorable attitudes toward ownership than their counterparts. In addition, interest in pursuing pharmacy ownership was higher in pharmacists who offered compounding services, could obtain financial resources, practiced in rural locations, and had more favorable attitudes toward ownership.

Conclusion: Overall, pharmacists indicated favorable attitudes toward independent pharmacy ownership but low interest in pursuing ownership. Their attitudes differed based on career stage, and more favorable attitudes—grounded especially in beliefs about autonomy and patient loyalty—were associated with a greater interest in ownership. Strategies to stimulate pharmacy ownership should be varied and targeted to influence beliefs that are driving pharmacists' attitudes at various career stages.

Keywords: Attitudes, pharmacy ownership, community pharmacy, surveys, Texas.

J Am Pharm Assoc. 2007;47:174–180.

Received March 3, 2006, and in revised form July 10, 2006. Accepted for publication August 11, 2006.

Carolyn M. Brown, PhD, is Associate Professor; Roxanne Cantu, PharmD, is Graduate Student; Zach Corbell, PharmD, is Graduate Student; and Kristy Roberts, is Student Pharmacist, College of Pharmacy, University of Texas–Austin.

Correspondence: Carolyn Brown, PhD, College of Pharmacy, PHR–Pharmacy Admin., 2409 University Ave., 1 University Sta. A1930, University of Texas, Austin, TX 78712-0127. Fax: 512-471-8762. E-mail: cmbrown@mail.utexas.edu

Disclosure: The authors declare no conflicts of interests or financial interests in any product or service mentioned in this article, including grants, employment, gifts, stock holdings, or honoraria.

Funding: Supported by a grant from the National Community Pharmacists Association Foundation.

Acknowledgments: To Hazel Pipkin, Clinical Professor, University of Texas-Austin Pharmacy Administration, for advice and guidance. To the Texas pharmacists for participation in all phases of this study. To the University of Texas–Austin Pharmacy Administration graduate students and faculty for help with survey construction and data collection.

ATTITUDES TOWARD INDEPENDENT PHARMACY OWNERSHIP **RESEARCH**

Independent community pharmacies represent 41% of the retail prescription market and 42% of community pharmacies in the United States.[1] Being independent and entrepreneurial, pharmacy owners have often been the pioneers in the profession, offering new and innovative services to their patients. Now more than ever, prospective pharmacy owners realize that the opportunities for pharmaceutical care services are unlimited. Always identified by a more service-oriented environment, today's independent pharmacies are delivering expanded patient care services by offering disease management, implementing medication therapy management services under Medicare Part D, working with patients who need durable medical equipment, and adding compounding and other niche-market services around the country.[2] The professional aspects of independent practice are reported as more rewarding by pharmacists, and those practicing in this setting view their worklife issues more positively as well.[3]

A national study revealed that pharmacists who work in independent settings report lower levels of job ambiguity, role

conflict, role overload, and job stress, when compared with pharmacists who work in chain, mass merchandise, and hospital settings.[3] In addition, current research also supports the belief that pharmacists in independent practice settings consistently report higher levels of job satisfaction.[3] No previous studies have identified the beliefs, attitudes, and interests of pharmacists regarding independent pharmacy ownership that might contribute to these positive views on professional life. Identifying the beliefs driving pharmacists' attitudes toward ownership, both positive and negative, is important to maintaining the independent segment of community pharmacy practice. Stimulating interest in independent pharmacy ownership is contingent on identifying and targeting those beliefs that are driving interest in pursuing ownership.

Objectives

The objectives of this study were to (1) assess the attitudes toward pharmacy ownership of Texas pharmacists in different career stages, (2) identify which beliefs are the primary determinants of attitude toward pharmacy ownership among Texas pharmacists in different career stages, and (3) determine the level of interest in pharmacy ownership among Texas pharmacists in different career stages.

Methods

This cross-sectional study assessed pharmacists' attitudes and interest toward independent pharmacy ownership. A self-administered mail survey was sent to a random sample of pharmacists licensed and residing in Texas. Approval of the study design and survey instrument was granted by the University of Texas–Austin Institutional Review Board.

Pharmacist survey

Pilot interviews. Using the framework of marketing research on attitudes,[4] pilot interviews were conducted to identify salient beliefs about pharmacy ownership among currently practicing pharmacists and pharmacy owners in different career stages. This belief-based approach to attitude measurement was used to provide more insight into why participants held certain attitudes. Interviews were used to identify participants' beliefs, both positive and negative, about pharmacy ownership. These beliefs served as the basis for the initial draft of the survey instrument.

The three-section survey was designed to collect information on pharmacists' (1) likelihood of independent pharmacy ownership; (2) attitudes and beliefs toward independent pharmacy ownership; and (3) demographic, professional, and practice-setting characteristics (see Appendix 1 in the electronic version of this article, available online at www.japha.org). Both closed- and open-ended response formats were used. The following is a more detailed description of each of the survey sections.

Section I: Interest in independent pharmacy ownership. This section of the survey was designed to assess pharmacists'

At a Glance

Synopsis: Pharmacists' attitudes toward independent pharmacy ownership tended to be favorable, but interest in actually pursuing ownership was low, according to this survey of 180 Texas pharmacists. Beliefs that owning an independent pharmacy would increase business and professional autonomy and increase the ability to establish patient loyalty made the largest positive contribution to overall attitude, whereas believing that ownership would decrease power to negotiate contracts and price discounts made the strongest negative contribution. Mid-career pharmacists generally had more favorable attitudes toward ownership than did late- and early-career pharmacists. Beliefs about financial risk, time commitment, competitive markets, and business/managerial skills significantly influenced pharmacists' attitudes about and interest in community pharmacy ownership.

Analysis: Independent community pharmacists have reported lower levels of job ambiguity, role conflict, and job stress, compared with pharmacists working in chain, mass merchandise, and hospital settings. Independent pharmacy ownership offers increased potential to provide innovative and expansive patient care services in areas such as disease management, durable medical equipment, and compounding. While many pharmacists believe that ownership provides a favorable work environment, the actual pursuit of ownership is hindered by a number of perceived barriers, particularly money concerns. Financial advice and mentoring are two resources that can help assuage fears about and stimulate interest in pharmacy ownership.

interest in pursuing independent pharmacy ownership. Likelihood of pursuing pharmacy ownership was used to measure level of interest. Likelihood of pursuing ownership represents a stronger indicator of interest than a simple interest statement. This section consisted of one item requiring a response on a 7-point scale of "very unlikely" (–3) to "very likely" (+3).

Section II: Attitudes toward independent pharmacy ownership. This section of the survey was designed to assess pharmacists' beliefs and attitudes about independent pharmacy ownership. It measured pharmacists' perceived likelihood ("very unlikely" [–3] to "very likely" [+3]) and evaluation ("very bad" [–3] to "very good" [+3]) of 10 outcome beliefs of independent pharmacy ownership identified in the pilot study: business autonomy, professional autonomy, financial rewards, financial risks, patient loyalty, professional responsibility, time commitment, tax liability, competitive market, and business/managerial skills.

Pharmacists were asked how likely each of the 10 outcomes would be if they owned an independent pharmacy. The pharmacists were then asked to evaluate how good or bad each of the 10 outcomes would be if the outcome occurred. The overall attitude toward pharmacy ownership was determined by multiplying each belief strength by its corresponding outcome evaluation and then summing the products for the total set of salient beliefs (Att = $\Sigma e_i b_i$). The sum of the mean products of the likelihood and evaluative scores determined the overall attitude score. The possible range for the overall attitude score was –90 to +90, with higher numbers indicating a more favorable attitude toward independent pharmacy ownership.

Section III: Demographics and practice-setting information. This section of the survey was designed to assess pharmacists' demographic and practice-setting characteristics. Demographic items included age, gender, years licensed, current position, hours worked per week, advanced training, and membership in professional organizations. Practice characteristics included type of practice, geographic location, prescriptions dispensed per day, and patient care services offered. Information regarding pharmacists' ability to obtain the financial resources to own an independent pharmacy and their perceived resource needs for the pursuit of independent pharmacy ownership were also assessed.

The primary independent variable of this study was career stage. The career stage of respondents (early, middle, or late) was assessed based on the respondent's age. Pharmacists younger than 35 years of age were categorized as being in the early career stage, those 36–49 years of age in the mid-career stage, and those 50 years of age or older in the late career stage. This age-based method of defining career stage has been used in other studies.[5,6]

Pretest. The survey instrument was assessed for content and face validity by a group of practicing pharmacists. Modifications were made to the survey instrument based on the pretest group's comments and recommendations.

Study sample and data collection procedures

A random sample of 500 pharmacists was drawn from a list of pharmacists who are licensed and reside in Texas. The Texas State Board of Pharmacy provides this list via the Internet.

In November 2004, each of the randomly selected pharmacists was sent a cover letter explaining the purpose of the project and a self-addressed, postage-paid survey. Pharmacists were asked to return the completed survey within 2 weeks. Two weeks after the initial mailing, a reminder package was sent to the pharmacists. The survey was due 2 weeks after the second mailing. Surveys were collected over a 6-week period. All responses were anonymous.

Data analysis

Pharmacists' responses were analyzed both descriptively and inferentially. Correlation analysis, chi-square tests, t tests, and analysis of variance techniques were used to examine the associations among career-stage, demographic, and practice-site characteristics and pharmacists' interest in and attitudes toward pharmacy ownership. In addition, regression analyses were used to examine if career stage predicted interest and attitudes, after accounting for demographic, professional, and practice-site differences shown to be significant in the bivariate analyses. The a priori level of significance for all statistical computations was $P < 0.05$. Data were analyzed using SAS version 9.1 (SAS Institute, Cary, N.C.).

Results

A total of 500 pharmacists were mailed surveys, and 17 surveys were returned as undeliverable (Table 1). Of the 483 assumed delivered, 199 were returned, yielding a response rate of 41.2%. In all, 19 surveys were excluded because they were incomplete or completed by current owners or pharmacists who were retired and thus no longer practiced. This left 180 surveys that could be used in the analyses (usable response rate, 36.0%).

Respondent and practice setting characteristics

The demographic characteristics of respondents are shown in Table 1. Respondents were approximately evenly distributed between women (50.3%) and men (49.7%), with a mean (± SD) age of 44.8 ± 12.5 years. They had been licensed for an average of 19.1 ± 13.0 years. Most (83.4%) respondents worked full time (32 or more hours per week). Community chain pharmacy (36.9%) and urban settings (57.8%) were the most commonly reported work environments. Current position title of staff pharmacist (41.5%) accounted for the largest percentage of the sample. The mean number of prescriptions dispensed per day was 1,668.4 ± 6,853.4 and was skewed by responses from pharmacists practicing in mail-service facilities; therefore, the median value of 225.0 per day is more representative. Most respondents (41.1%) were classified as late career stage (50 years of age or older).

Table 1. Demographic and professional characteristics of responding pharmacists

Characteristics	No.	No. respondents (%)	Mean ± SD
Age (years)	176		44.8 ± 12.5 (range 24–82)
Years as a licensed pharmacist	176		19.1 ± 13.0 (range <1 to 55)
Gender	177		
Men		88 (49.7)	
Women		89 (50.3)	
Primary practice site[a]	176		
Community chain		65 (36.9)	
Institutional		40 (22.7)	
Community independent		18 (10.2)	
Consultant/ long-term care		10 (5.7)	
Community clinic		5 (2.8)	
Other[b]		38 (21.6)	
Primary practice area	173		
Urban		100 (57.8)	
Rural		51 (29.5)	
Suburban		22 (12.7)	
Current position title	176		
Staff pharmacist		73 (41.5)	
Manager/assistant manager		53 (30.1)	
Relief pharmacist		12 (6.8)	
Clinical pharmacist		12 (6.8)	
Other[c]		26 (14.8)	
Hours worked	175		
Full time (≥32 hours/week)		146 (83.4)	
Part time (<32 hours/week)		29 (16.6)	
Daily prescription workload at pharmacy site[d]	148		1,668.4 ± 6,853.4 (median 225.0)
Career stage	180		
Early (≤ 35 years of age)		55 (30.6)	
Middle (36–49 years of age)		51 (28.3)	
Late (≥ 50 years of age)		74 (41.1)	

[a]Sum of percentages do not equal 100% due to rounding.
[b]Other sites: mail service, pharmacy benefits management company/managed care, oncology, home infusion, and corporate.
[c]Other positions/titles were director and vice president.
[d]Mean number of prescriptions processed per day was inflated by large numbers from some respondents practicing at mail-service pharmacies.

Many respondents (44.9%) indicated that they engage in pharmaceutical care practices, defined in the survey instrument as assessment and monitoring of drug therapy problems (Table 2). The respondents also commonly (31.4%) held advanced training certifications. Most (67.8%) pharmacists indicated that they could obtain the financial resources necessary to buy out or start up an independent pharmacy, and a financial advisor was the most commonly cited resource (n = 124 respondents [70.5%]) that pharmacists considered helpful in pursuing independent pharmacy ownership. Other helpful resources included mentor/apprenticeship (44.3%), continuing education or postgraduate programs (41.5%), and certification programs (40.9%).

Attitudes toward independent pharmacy ownership

As shown in Table 3, the overall (summated) mean attitude score was 18.6 ± 28 (range, –63.0 to 90.0), indicating an overall favorable attitude toward independent pharmacy ownership. The mean product of the belief and outcome evaluation scores for the beliefs that owning an independent pharmacy would increase business autonomy (4.5 ± 3.7), increase professional autonomy

Table 2. Respondents' activities, certifications, and professional memberships (n = 180)

Activities	No. respondents (%)[a]
Patient care services	
Pharmaceutical care practice	79 (44.9)
Disease management	51 (29.0)
Compounding services	45 (25.6)
Health promotion services	34 (19.3)
Other[b]	23 (13.1)
Advanced training certifications	55 (31.4)
Current organizational memberships	
Texas Pharmacy Association	45 (25.6)
American Pharmacists Association	32 (18.2)
American Society of Health-System Pharmacists	29 (16.5)
Texas Society of Health-System Pharmacists	22 (12.5)
American Society of Consultant Pharmacists	10 (5.7)
National Community Pharmacists Association	9 (5.1)
Professional Compounding Centers of America	8 (4.6)
Other[c]	30 (17.1)

[a]Percentages sum to more than 100% because of multiple responses.
[b]Other services listed by respondents were patient assistance programs, pharmacokinetic monitoring/dosing and renal dosing, pharmacoeconomics, pain management, prior authorization, telephonic medication counseling, cholesterol and blood glucose testing, computer/software maintenance, specialty pharmacy (injectables), orientation talks to residents on prescription writing, homeopathy/nutrition/natural medicine, poison prevention, international normalized ratio monitoring.
[c]Other organizations were the American College of Clinical Pharmacy, Metroplex Society of Health-System Pharmacists, American Association of Diabetes Educators, and West Texas Pharmacy Association.

Chapter 11

Table 3. Products of belief and outcome evaluation scores (n = 180)

Items	Product mean ± SD[a]
Owning an independent pharmacy will increase my business autonomy (e.g., control of staffing and hours of operation).	4.5 ± 3.7
Owning an independent pharmacy will increase my professional autonomy (e.g., implementation of patient care services, such as compounding and disease management).	4.2 ± 3.6
Owning an independent pharmacy will be financially rewarding (e.g., income and investments).	2.2 ± 3.7
Owning an independent pharmacy will increase my financial risk as a pharmacist.	−1.1 ± 5.5
Owning an independent pharmacy will increase my ability to establish patient loyalty.	4.3 ± 3.6
Owning an independent pharmacy will increase my sense of professional responsibility as a pharmacist.	3.3 ± 4.1
Owning an independent pharmacy will require an increased time commitment to fulfill duties as a pharmacy owner.	0.2 ± 6.4
Owning an independent pharmacy will increase my tax liability.	−0.7 ± 5.2
Owning an independent pharmacy will decrease power to negotiate contracts and price discounts in a competitive market (e.g., wholesalers, insurance companies).	−1.4 ± 4.5
Owning an independent pharmacy will require an increase in my business and managerial skills.	3.1 ± 4.3
Overall attitude (sum of individual product calculations)	18.6 ± 28.0

[a]Overall attitude toward pharmacy ownership was determined by multiplying each belief strength by its corresponding outcome evaluation and then summing the products for the total set of salient beliefs (Att = $\Sigma e_i b_i$).

(4.2 ± 3.6), and increase the ability to establish customer/patient loyalty (4.3 ± 3.6) were all greater than 4. These beliefs made the largest positive contribution to overall attitude. The largest negative contribution to overall attitude was made by the belief that owning an independent pharmacy would decrease power to negotiate contracts and price discounts in a competitive market (−1.4 ± 4.5).

In the bivariate analyses, several demographic and setting characteristics were significantly related to pharmacists' attitudes toward independent pharmacy ownership. Age ($r = 0.18$,

$P = 0.02$) and years licensed ($r = 0.16$, $P = 0.04$) were positively related to attitude. Community independent pharmacists reported the most favorable attitude (44.2 ± 21.2) . Pharmacists who were men (23.9 ± 31.4), had advanced training (27.6 ± 28.8), or were members of National Community Pharmacists Association (50.0 ± 28.5) or Professional Compounding Centers of America (44.4 ± 31.2) had more favorable attitudes than their respective counterparts.

Controlling for all other variables in the model, multivariate analyses indicated that interest in pursuing independent pharmacy ownership and advanced training were significant predictors of attitude toward independent pharmacy ownership ($F = 4.03$, $df = 11$, $P < 0.0001$). Pharmacists who were more interested in independent pharmacy ownership and had advanced training reported more favorable attitudes toward independent pharmacy ownership than their counterparts. Career stage was not a significant predictor of attitudes when other variables were taken into account.

Interest in independent pharmacy ownership

The mean interest in pursuing independent pharmacy ownership was −2.2 ± 1.6 (range, −3.0 to +3.0), indicating a low likelihood of pursuing independent pharmacy ownership. Table 4 shows the correlation of each salient belief measure with pharmacists' interest in pursuing independent pharmacy ownership. The salient belief measures for financial rewards ($r = 0.23$, $P < 0.01$) and business/managerial skills ($r = 0.23$, $P < 0.01$) showed the highest correlation with pharmacists' interest in pursuing ownership. Beliefs concerning business autonomy, patient loyalty, responsibility, tax liability, and competitive market were not significantly correlated with pharmacists' interest in pursuing ownership.

Several characteristics were significantly correlated with interest in pursuing independent pharmacy ownership. Community independent pharmacists were most likely (−1.1 ± 2.5)

Table 4. Correlations of salient beliefs and overall attitude with interest in pursuing independent ownership (n = 180)

Beliefs	Correlations (r)	P values
Business autonomy	0.15	0.05
Professional autonomy	0.17	0.02[a]
Financial rewards	0.23	< 0.01[a]
Financial risks	0.17	0.02[a]
Customer loyalty	0.15	0.05
Responsibility	0.14	0.06
Time commitment	0.20	0.01[a]
Tax liability	0.13	0.09
Competitive market	0.10	0.20
Business/managerial skills	0.23	< 0.01[a]
Attitude	0.26	< 0.001[a]

[a]Statistically significant at $P < 0.05$.

to pursue ownership. Pharmacists who practiced in rural settings (-1.4 ± 2.3), who offered compounding services (-1.5 ± 2.2), and who reported having the ability to obtain financial resources (-2.0 ± 1.8) were more likely to pursue ownership than their respective counterparts.

Controlling for all other variables in the model, multivariate analyses indicated that attitude, geographic location of practice site, the ability to obtain financial resources, and involvement in compounding activities were significant predictors of interest in independent pharmacy ownership ($F = 4.10$, $df = 10$, $P < 0.0001$). Pharmacists who had a more favorable attitude, practiced in rural locations, could obtain financial resources, and were involved with compounding activities were more interested in pursuing independent pharmacy ownership than their counterparts.

Attitudes and interest of pharmacists based on career stage

Pharmacists' attitudes toward independent pharmacy ownership differed by career stage ($F = 3.12$, $df = 2$, $P = 0.047$). Mid-career pharmacists had the most favorable attitude (23.6 ± 27.3), followed by late-career pharmacists (20.8 ± 29.9). Early-career pharmacists held the least favorable attitude (11.05 ± 24.7).

Pharmacists' beliefs about financial risk ($F = 3.01$, $df = 2$, $P = 0.05$), time commitment ($F = 3.47$, $df = 2$, $P = 0.03$), competitive markets ($F = 4.01$, $df = 2$, $P = 0.02$), and business/managerial skills ($F = 3.20$, $df = 2$, $P = 0.04$) were all significantly influenced by career-stage classification.

Late-career pharmacists were less likely to believe that owning an independent pharmacy would increase financial risk (0 ± 5.9) than early-career pharmacists (-2.4 ± 4.9, mean difference = -2.4 [95% CI -0.1 to -4.7]). Mid-career pharmacists were more likely to believe that owning an independent pharmacy would decrease their ability to compete (-0.1 ± 4.5) than early-career pharmacists (-2.6 ± 3.9, mean difference 2.4 [0.4–4.4]). The belief that ownership would require an increase in business/managerial skills was highest in mid-career (3.9 ± 3.8) and late-career (3.5 ± 4.3) pharmacists, compared with early-career pharmacists (1.9 ± 4.5). Time commitment was more burdensome for early-career pharmacists (-1.6 ± 5.8) than for those in the middle (1.1 ± 6.5) or late (1.0 ± 6.6) stages of their careers. However, multivariate results indicated that career stage did not significantly influence attitude when other variables (i.e., age, interest, pharmacy site, gender, and advanced training) were taken into account.

There were no significant differences in interest in pursuing independent pharmacy ownership on the basis of career stage ($F = 0.13$, $df = 2$, $P = 0.88$). Based on the mean values for each of the defined career stages, pharmacists in the early career stage were least likely to pursue independent pharmacy ownership (-2.3 ± 1.6), followed by those in middle (-2.2 ± 1.4) and late (-2.1 ± 1.7) stages.

Discussion

Independent pharmacies represent a significant portion of the pharmacies in the United States.[1] Independent pharmacies have long been identified by their service-oriented environment, and today's independent pharmacies continue that tradition. Pharmacy owners tend to have higher organizational commitment, higher met expectations, and higher job satisfaction than those in other practice environments.[7] Moreover, pharmaceutical care services are frequently developed and implemented first by pharmacists in independent pharmacy environments.[8]

Given the characteristics of today's pharmacists, finding ways of introducing and promoting interest in independent pharmacy practice could be necessary. Sparking new interest in independent pharmacy ownership could be critical to the provision of new and innovative services to patients for generations to come. Attitudes and interest toward independent pharmacy ownership among practicing pharmacists provide insight regarding issues that influence the decision to pursue pharmacy ownership.

Overall, the study showed that although pharmacists practicing in various practice settings held favorable attitudes toward independent pharmacy ownership, they reported a low likelihood of pursuing ownership. This apparent paradox may be explained by examining the relationship between intentions and behaviors.[9,10] For example, the likelihood of performing a behavior considers all issues associated with performing the behavior in addition to attitudes toward the behavior. Thus, the low interest in pursuing pharmacy ownership is likely a reflection of pharmacists' perceived barriers to ownership. Accordingly, identification of helpful resources that provide information and tips on pursuing ownership would aid in minimizing these perceived barriers. Pharmacists identified several sources (e.g., financial advisor, mentor) that they deemed relevant to pursuing independent ownership. Gaither[7] advocated that pharmacists be encouraged to identify mentors or serve as mentors themselves. Such advisement could be critical to the survival of independent pharmacy practice.

Pharmacists' beliefs regarding autonomy and patient loyalty made the largest contributions to their overall attitudes toward ownership. This study showed statistically significant differences in both overall attitudes toward independent ownership and several salient beliefs about ownership based on pharmacists' career stage. However, when other important variables were taken into account, career stage did not significantly influence overall attitudes. Controlling for other important variables, differences in pharmacists' attitudes were significantly explained by their interest in pursuing ownership and whether they had advanced training. More than 40% of pharmacists indicated a need for additional training (continuing education, certification programs) as helpful resources in independent pharmacy ownership. Perhaps these programs can remove or at least minimize barriers so that pharmacists' favorable attitudes will translate to more ownership opportunities.

Interest in pursuing ownership was significantly explained by attitude, geographic location of practice site, ability to obtain financial resources, and involvement in compounding activities. Interest in pursuing ownership did not differ by career stage.

Taken together, these findings suggest that methods of changing attitudes need to be varied and should target those beliefs that are important to the formation of pharmacists' attitudes depending on their pharmacy career stage. Beliefs regarding financial rewards, business/managerial skills, and time commitment were highly associated with interest and should be emphasized when stimulating interest in ownership.

Efforts to encourage independent pharmacy ownership could be focused on all practitioners. However, special focus is needed in early- and mid-career pharmacist populations, as well as in those who practice in urban and suburban settings. Attitudinal change strategies should target early-career pharmacists, particularly regarding their beliefs about financial risk, time commitment, ability to compete, and business/managerial skill requirements associated with ownership. Additionally, providing pharmacists with opportunities for advanced training certification programs could serve to increase favorable attitudes toward ownership. Emphasizing opportunities for meeting the demands of niche markets (e.g., compounding) and offering financial assistance may also stimulate interest in pursuing ownership.

Future studies should determine when and where business management training would be most helpful in stimulating interest in pursuing independent pharmacy ownership (e.g., before, during, or after obtaining one's professional degree). Additionally, studies should address which specific types of continuing education or certification programs are thought to be most helpful (e.g., human resources, tax preparation, privacy and confidentiality training, managing computer software, inventory management). Finally, studies are needed to evaluate perceived barriers of student pharmacists and early-career-stage pharmacists regarding independent pharmacy ownership to provide further insight into how to stimulate interest in ownership in these groups.

Research shows that those interested in pharmacy ownership exhibit an "entrepreneurial spirit."[11] That spirit is reflected in the attitudes of pharmacists in this study, particularly regarding their beliefs about autonomy and patient loyalty. The provision of innovative pharmacy services is the hallmark of present-day pharmacy practice, and continuing education programs and pharmacy schools should offer courses that cultivate future entrepreneurs.

Limitations

The results of this study should be interpreted within some limitations. First, we sampled pharmacists currently licensed and residing in Texas, and findings may not be generalizable to pharmacists in other states. Current owners were removed from the sample, accounting for differences in demographic characteristics with respect to national averages of pharmacists' practice site. Our study consisted of 10.2% of pharmacists who indicated independent community pharmacy as their primary practice site.

Second, differences in attitude and interest accounted for by other characteristics of pharmacists in Texas may not have been identified in this study.

Finally, this cross-sectional study represents one point in time and does not reflect any changes in beliefs, attitudes, and interest in independent pharmacy ownership.

Conclusion

Results of this survey showed that pharmacists practicing in various practice settings held favorable attitudes toward independent pharmacy ownership, but they reported low interest in pursuing ownership. Pharmacists' beliefs about autonomy and patient loyalty made the highest contributions to their overall attitudes toward ownership. Overall attitudes toward independent ownership and several salient beliefs about ownership differed significantly based on pharmacists' career stage. However, when other important variables were taken into account, career stage did not significantly influence overall attitudes. In addition, interest in pursuing ownership did not differ by career stage. Independent pharmacies are identified as a service-oriented environment with many varied opportunities for the practice of pharmaceutical care. Successfully stimulating interest in independent pharmacy ownership is vital to the preservation and growth of patient care services such as disease management in the community setting.

References

1. National Community Pharmacists Association: annual report 2004. In: Preliminary 2004 NCPA–Pfizer Digest. Alexandria, Va.: National Community Pharmacists Association; 2004.

2. Anonymous. Gross margins, net profits up for independents. Drug Store News. 2004;26:30.

3. Mott DA, Doucette WR, Gaither CA. et al. Pharmacists' attitudes toward worklife: results from a national survey of pharmacists. J Am Pharm Assoc. 2004;44:326–36.

4. Fishbein M, Ajzen I. Belief, attitude, intention, and behavior. Englewood Cliffs, N.J.: Prentice Hall; 1980.

5. Guthrie JP, Schwoerer CE. Older dogs and new tricks: career stage and self-assessed need for training. Public Pers Manage. 1996;25:59–72.

6. Reilly NP, Orsak CL. A career stage analysis of career and organizational commitment in nursing. J Vocational Behav. 1991;39:311–30.

7. Gaither CA. Career commitment: a mediator of the effects of job stress on pharmacists' work-related attitudes. J Am Pharm Assoc. 1999;39:353–61.

8. McDermott JH, Christensen DB. Provision of pharmaceutical care services in North Carolina: a 1999 survey. J Am Pharm Assoc. 2002;42:26–35.

9. Sheppard BH, Hartwick J, Warshaw PR. The theory of reasoned action: a meta-analysis of past research with recommendations for modifications and future research. J Consum Res. 1988;15:325–43.

10. Fishbein M, Ajzen I. Formation of intentions. In: Belief, attitude, intention, and behavior: an introduction to theory and research. Reading, Mass.: Addison–Wesley; 1975;288–98.

11. Hermansen-Kobulnicky CJ, Moss CL. Pharmacy student entrepreneurial orientation: a measure to identify potential pharmacist entrepreneurs. Am J Pharm Educ. 2004;68:1–10.

babyboomers

Preparing health care for baby boomers' golden years

U.S. must address looming crisis of an aging population, IOM says

About 60 years ago, Kathleen Casey-Kirschling was born in Philadelphia. Since then, she's been profiled on CNN and in national publications. When she filed for Social Security last year, the Commissioner of the Social Security Administration attended in person. Casey-Kirschling owes this attention to a simple quirk of timing: Born at a second past midnight on January 1, 1946, she is America's first baby boomer.

Casey-Kirschling and her generation represent an impending explosion in the elderly population of the United States. In 2005, 37 million Americans were older than 65 years, making up about 12% of the country's population. By 2030, analysts expect that number to grow to more than 70 million, nearly 20% of the country.

While this dramatic demographic shift has been anticipated for years, a recent report issued by the Institute of Medicine (IOM) points out that "little has been done to prepare the health care workforce" for this rapid growth. "Unless action is taken immediately, the health care workforce will lack the capacity (in both size and ability) to meet the needs of older patients in the future," according to *Retooling for an Aging America: Building the Health Care Workforce.*

The document was produced by the 15-member Committee on the Future Health Care Workforce for Older Americans, chaired by John W. Rowe, MD, Professor, Department of Health Policy and Management, Columbia University Mailman School of Public Health. The committee includes representatives from several fields, including APhA member Miriam A. Mobley Smith, PharmD. They proposed a three-part approach: improve the competence of caregivers, supplement their recruitment and retention, and increase the flexibility of care. "Steps need to be taken immediately to increase overall workforce numbers and to use every worker efficiently," the committee wrote.

Improving and increasing the workforce

The committee considered the "capacity of the health care workforce" the essential issue. In addition to finding the quality of existing education and training "inadequate in both scope and consistency," the committee identified shortages in many geriatric care specialties and emphasized the "need for immediate and dramatic increases in the numbers of workers who care for older patients." Fewer than 1% of pharmacists, physician assistants, and registered nurses are certified or specialize in geriatrics, according to the report.

Caring for older patients requires health professionals, direct-care workers such as nurse aides, informal caregivers, and others. The committee found that "the geriatric competence of virtually all members of the health care workforce needs to be improved" and recommended that hospitals encourage residents to receive training in geriatric care, certifying organizations require competence in the care of older patients, states and the federal government increase minimum training standards for direct-care workers, and public, private, and community organizations fund informal caregiver training.

The committee found that "opportunities for advanced training in geriatrics are scarce or nonexistent and ... very few take advantage of these programs." To address this problem and promote recruitment and retention, they encouraged public and private payers to improve the reimbursement of geriatric specialists and urged states and the federal government to create loan-forgiveness programs, scholarships, and other financial incentives to aid specialists in geriatrics. Because "recruitment and retention are especially dire among direct-care workers," the committee recommended that Medicaid programs increase pay for these caregivers.

Finally, the committee argued that the U.S. health care system has fundamental "deficiencies in quality" with respect to caring for older patients and presented a "vision for the future" incorporating three principles: comprehensive elder care, efficient provision of services, and active participation. However, the committee argued that "there is no single approach or best model that could be broadly adopted for all older patients" and encouraged flexibility. Specific recommendations include payers taking steps to promote proven effective and efficient models of care; Congress and health care foundations promoting relevant research programs; employers, regulators, and other groups expanding the roles of caregivers; and federal agencies supporting new technologies.

To reinforce these recommendations and monitor the industry's progress, the committee also urged Congress to require annual reports from the Bureau of Health Professions to ensure that future problems are reduced or eliminated.

'A sense of urgency'

While 2030 may seem distant, the committee argued that a "sense of urgency" is necessary. "The preparation of a competent health care workforce and widespread diffusion of effective models of care will require many years of effort," they wrote. The year 2030 was chosen as a target to offer enough time to effect meaningful change without risking technological changes that would make the committee's recommendations obsolete.

After an initial review of the document, APhA shares the concerns that the current health care model would be strained by an aging population. APhA is working on initiatives to change the pharmacy practice business model through programs such as medication therapy management (MTM), utilizing the pharmacist's medication use expertise to improve patient outcomes, especially in the vulnerable elderly population. The Association also agrees that financial incentives in the health care system need to better support the level of care articulated in the report.

—**Alex Egervary**

www.pharmacytoday.org

Paving the way for high-quality health care

PQA charts an ambitious course for 2008

Interested in knowing how your pharmacy stacks up against others in your community in quality of asthma services provided? Sometime in the not-too-distant future, you will be able to log on to a Web site created by PQA (a pharmacy quality alliance), enter your ZIP Code, select "asthma services" from the drop-down menu, and, in no time flat, you'll know which pharmacy tops the list.

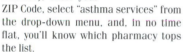

Although the actual launch of such a Web site is still in the planning phase, PQA, in its brief 20-month history, has made considerable progress toward achieving one of its key objectives: providing patients, pharmacists, employers, health insurance plans, and other health care decision makers with the information required to make informed choices. "Here's a huge opportunity for pharmacy to talk about quality—quality of care," said Julie Kuhle, BPharm, of the Iowa Foundation for Medical Care. Kuhle's excitement was shared by many of the approximately 140 other attendees of the November 30 meeting in Washington, D.C.—excitement regarding a paradigm shift that places quality of pharmacist-provided patient care services, not merely cost and convenience, at the forefront of consumers' minds.

Ambitious plans for 2008

Laura Cranston, BPharm, Director of PQA, prioritized PQA's ambitious plan of action for 2008 as follows.

(1) Continue to move PQA's approved quality measures for pharmacy services forward for eventual introduction into the marketplace. Over the past year, 37 proposed quality measures were tested by the National Committee for Quality Assurance (NCQA), and the 14 measures that passed the technical specification and field-testing phases were presented at the meeting (for more information, see www.pharmacist.com/NQFmeasures). Examples of the approved measures include adherence, medication duplication, and high-risk medications in the elderly. Within the next 45 days, the 14 measures discussed at the meeting will be forwarded to the National Quality Forum (NQF) for endorsement. NQF is a private, nonprofit organization that promotes standardization of quality measures and makes comparable data available at a national level. In the PQA-conducted field tests, both pharmacies and drug plans showed enough variation and potential for improvement (e.g., opportunity to improve adherence) that the 14 measures could move forward for endorsement by NQF.

(2) Within the first quarter of 2008, finalize a consumer satisfaction survey for pharmacist/pharmacy services that can be used by pharmacies, drug plans, or employers. The PQA-developed consumer satisfaction survey is undergoing the rigorous process needed to become a survey within the family of assessment tools known as the Consumer Assessment of Healthcare Providers and Systems (CAHPS) instruments. Steven Garfinkel, PhD, of the American Institutes for Research, explained that CAHPS, a program of the Agency for Healthcare Research and Quality (AHRQ), is "arguably the most widely used method to assess quality of care from the patient's perspective" and that CAHPS surveys are recognized as industry standards. In addition to assessing patient-centered care, CAHPS results facilitate consumer choice and, ultimately, improve quality of care. CAHPS surveys promote standardization because users can access the instrument and other related components online and have access to AHRQ-funded technical support. CAHPS surveys are currently available to assess health care provider and facility services such as physicians, dentists, home health, hospitals, and nursing homes.

(3) Refine the concepts needed for conducting demonstration projects and begin the process of rolling out the projects on a limited basis.

(4) Develop educational programs and the speakers for the programs, in order to disseminate PQA's message effectively, with particular focus on identifying potential sites for demonstration projects and educating the projects' caretakers.

(5) Restart the quality metrics effort, define the new cluster groups for 2008, appoint individuals to serve in these various cluster groups, and use input from NCQA and Advanced Pharmacy Concepts (APC) to efficiently develop a second set of measures. Donna Dugan, MS, of NCQA indicated that pilot test results showed promise regarding the readiness of some (e.g., high-risk medication use in the elderly, suboptimal treatment of hypertension in patients with diabetes) but not other (e.g., drug–drug interactions, potentially contraindicated calcium channel blockers in heart failure patients) quality measures. Dugan also indicated that another potential next step is for PQA to consider submitting a subset of measures for inclusion in NCQA's Healthcare Effectiveness Data

pqa

and Information Set (HEDIS), although she said NCQA is "just on the brink of going through our internal committees with the results of the field tests, to make decisions on whether any of the measures make sense on the health plan level."

(6) Continue to develop the template for the above-mentioned pharmacy quality Web site.

Bringing MTM into the fold
In providing CMS's perspective on the use of PQA's starter set of measures for comparing Medicare Part D plans, Jeffrey Kelman, MD, said, "We strongly favor quality assessment, quality feedback, quality transparency, and value-based purchasing. We're interested in expanding the quality measures of Part D plans on an aggressive basis." Kelman also indicated that CMS is interested in "continuing the conversation" regarding medication

therapy management (MTM), a point of considerable interest to Anne Burns, BPharm, APhA Vice President of Professional Affairs, who commended CMS on this stance and highlighted the challenges that PQA has faced in determining the data sources needed to develop quality measures for MTM services.

"Right now, the services are not really being reflected in pharmacy claims data and they're being collected from plans, in our understanding, in a variety of different ways," said Burns. She asked Kelman whether CMS was analyzing how the data for MTM services are being collected at the plan level over and above those measures that are reported to CMS on beneficiary enrollment, cost of drugs, etc.

"We're still working out the best approach to MTM," said Kelman. Kelman indicated that CMS will eventually be able to construct a tool that will capture the

information needed to create a measure centered on quality of MTM services.

Necessary for health care's progress
Former FDA Commissioner and CMS Administrator Mark McClellan, MD, PhD, now affiliated with the Brookings Institution, emphasized the critical importance of effective medication management to a high-value health care system in his lively keynote address. McClellan, whom Cranston cited as instrumental in PQA's launch, told the PQA members, "You have the opportunity in 2008, as you move forward with these measures, to really educate the public about what we need to get high-quality, affordable health care for all Americans, and we're not going to get there unless outfits like yours succeed."

—Joe Sheffer

Medicare Part D update: Additional details
CMS hosted a Pharmacy Open Door Forum in December focused on Medicare Part D preparations of keen interest to pharmacists in 2008. Much of the information presented at the forum was covered in the December issue of *Pharmacy Today* (page 55). Additional relevant details mentioned during the forum are as follows.

■ As of December, nearly 25 million beneficiaries were enrolled in a Part D plan.
■ CMS surveys indicate that about 8 of 10 seniors remain satisfied with their coverage.
■ In 2008, formularies, on average, will cover 2% more distinct drug entities than they did in 2007.
■ More than 90% of beneficiaries in a prescription drug plan (PDP) will have access to at least one plan in 2008 with premiums lower than their 2007 PDP.
■ As of December 31, 2007, the transition phase of Part D vaccine administration cost being covered under Medicare Part B ended. Vaccines covered under Part B—influenza, pneumococcal, and hepatitis B for intermediate- and high-risk beneficiaries—and their associated administration will continue to be covered under Part B in 2008. As of January 1, Part D vaccines and their associated administration fees are covered under Part D. For Part D pharmacies (both in network and out of network) that dispense and administer vaccines, vaccine ingredients and administration fees should be billed under a single claim. Pharmacists should contact their vendor or the National Council for Prescription Drug Programs (NCPDP) for guidance on billing of single claims. A more detailed Medicare Learning Network article on 2008 vaccine administration and claims processing is available at www.cms.hhs.gov/ContractorLearningResources/downloads/JA0727.pdf.
■ CMS enacted measures to ensure that systems have timely, accurate, and complete Part D enrollment

information in 2008. Early processing dates were scheduled for all reassignees and plans were required to submit all billing information for new enrollees into the plans in initial enrollment transactions to CMS. This requirement is expected to result in considerably fewer E1 query responses that do not include accurate enrollment information at the point of sale (POS). CMS believes these enhancements, coupled with the accelerated processing schedules, should result in 2008 information for most reassigned beneficiaries being available in the enhanced E1. (Note: Only pharmacists with the enhanced E1 can query for future enrollment; pharmacists with the original E1 can only query for current-month enrollment.) CMS encourages pharmacists to run an E1 query in January to ensure that dual eligibles or otherwise reassigned individuals have not changed plans subsequent to their reassignment. This will ensure that enrollment information is correct at POS.
■ The toll-free 24/7 pharmacy line remains the same: 866-835-7595. Pharmacists can call this number to find out the name of the plan in which a beneficiary is enrolled, check for Medicare eligibility, obtain limited-income subsidy (LIS) status information, and get assistance on the POS process.
■ CMS's goal is to make POS unnecessary but, while it is being phased out, CMS is attempting to make the POS process as easy as possible for beneficiaries and pharmacists. The agency renewed its contract with WellPoint to conduct POS operations in 2008. The payer sheet, therefore, will not change.
■ For all individuals who qualify for LIS, Part D plans are required to accept and use best available evidence to document beneficiaries' LIS status and to change the beneficiaries' cost-sharing level in the sponsor system.
■ Visit www.cms.hhs.gov/Pharmacy/ for more information.

Glossary

Abstracts:
A short (100–200 words) summary of an article. Abstracts may merely describe the scope of an article, or they may present the key points or data presented in the paper.

Accreditation:
Recognition of a residency or other type of program by comparing it with standards set by the accrediting body. This standard describes the goals or ideals that each program should strive for and sets certain minimum criteria that each should maintain.

Adherence:
The rate at which patients actually take a prescribed treatment. Known formerly as "compliance." A related term, persistence, describes the rate at which patients continue to take their medications over time.

Adulterated:
Products that had been changed or contaminated with impure or foreign substances.

Biopharmaceutics:
The study of a drug's physical and chemical properties as they relate to the effects of the drug on the body (absorption, distribution, and metabolism or elimination).

Certification:
Recognition of an individual for specialized knowledge and/or skills based on demonstration of that knowledge or those skills to the certifying body. The term certification carries the connotation that the certifying body is a nongovernmental entity, and the recognition typically carries no legally defined privileges.

Chronic conditions:
Diseases that last for more than about six months or that have long-term (usually lifelong) effects are referred to as chronic conditions. These include diabetes, hypertension (high blood pressure), and heart conditions. Also, surgery and other therapies may produce a chronic condition. For instance, a colon cancer patient may have all or some of the colon removed, with an ostomy created for the passage of waste. Or a patient whose stomach is removed because of gastric cancer may require special types of enteral nutrition rather than a normal diet of solid foods.

Class of trade:
Customers of a business or industry may be divided into one or more groups based on their purchasing and payment characteristics. Each of these classes of trade is dealt with differently — and may receive different prices or payment policies — because of the interplay between these characteristics and the sellers' goals and objectives relative to that part of the industry.

Closed-shop pharmacies:
A pharmacy not open to the public. It usually provides services to nursing homes or other types of long-term care facilities. These services may be drug dispensing, consulting on patients' drug therapy, or both.

Code blue:
This term refers to the hospital's response when a patient is in cardio-pulmonary arrest (the heart and/or lungs have stopped). Various health care professionals respond to the Code Blue, and the pharmacist attends to help calculate doses and draw up drugs to be administered in this emergency situation. Hospitals differ in what they call the situation; Code Blue is a common term derived from the fact that the patient is turning blue from a lack of oxygen. Other names are Code Red or Code 99.

Compounding:
The preparation of prescriptions specifically for a patient based on an individualized drug order from a prescriber.

Computerized databases:
Used in reference to the literature, this term means computer files containing information from articles that have been published in journals, magazines, and newspapers. These databases are searchable, using either key words from the title or abstract of the article, the authors' names, or the journals' names.

Controlled substances:
Any of several dangerous drugs, such as morphine, cocaine, codeine, diazepam (Valium), and amphetamines, that are handled, dispensed, and recorded specially under federal law. Some controlled substances, such as marijuana and heroin, are completely illegal, since they have no accepted medical use in the United States.

Copayment:
The amount of money a patient must pay when receiving certain types of health care services under insurance programs or prepaid health care plans.

Copyediting:
Correction and preparation of a manuscript for typesetting and printing.

Glossary

Covenant:
A promise or an agreement between two parties in which each provides something of value to the other. In pharmacy, the patient gives money to the pharmacist, who provides a patient-specific pharmaceutical product along with information on the proper use and adverse effects of that product.

Database vendors:
Companies or organizations that obtain several databases and make them available to the public or others. Examples include DIALOG and BRS; bulletin board services such as America Online, CompuServe, and Prodigy also have access to databases.

Decentralized drug distribution:
Systems in hospitals of distributing drugs to patients in which pharmacy services are located in several locations near patient-care areas rather than in one central pharmacy.

Deep discounter:
A type of mercantile outlet that reduces prices far below those of normal retail outlets and relies on volume to make a profit.

Drug information:
A service provided by pharmacists to other health professionals or to the public in which basic or detailed information about drugs is provided.

Drug interactions:
Detrimental (or occasionally positive) effects produced when two or more drugs are used at the same time. By checking the patient profile for interacting drugs, the computer can alert the pharmacist to consider whether both drugs can be safely used together in a patient.

Drug-regimen review:
A clinical pharmacy service provided to residents of nursing homes in which pharmacists review the drug therapy of residents and provide suggestions to physicians about drug selection, duplication, necessity, adverse effects, or monitoring.

Drug-use review:
Review of a prescription, at the time of dispensing (concurrent) or after the fact (retrospective), for appropriateness based on a patient's medical condition, other medications the patient is already receiving, or patient-specific factors that might make the prescribed drug a poor choice. The term can also be applied to retrospective review of large numbers of prescriptions for appropriateness.

Durable medical equipment:
Items such as wheelchairs, walkers, and bedside toilets that patients buy when their health fails or rent during rehabilitative periods after surgery or injury. The term can also include various types of intravenous (also called parenteral) or enteral services that require special catheters or pumps to deliver fluids or nutrition through the patient's veins or the gastrointestinal tract safely.

Efficacy:
The ability of a drug to produce desired therapeutic effects.

Emergency contraceptives:
Also known as "morning-after pills." Medications containing female hormones can be administered within 72 hours of unprotected intercourse, and pregnancy will be averted in more than 90% of women. In Washington State, California, and a few other states, pharmacists can prescribe ECs under physician-approved protocols.

Fellowship:
A postgraduate program, usually research-oriented, often in a narrow field of study that relies on a Socratic teaching method.

Formulary:
A list of drugs that have been selected by the medical staff of a hospital or HMO for use in that institution. Drugs are selected on the basis of efficacy, safety, cost, and quality of life. In recent years, the marketing of many "me-too" drugs by pharmaceutical industry—drugs that have no important advantage over drugs already on the market—has made cost an increasingly important factor in formulary decisions. Another important factor is the number of times per day that a medicine must be given, since in hospitals highly paid personnel must dispense and administer each dose and in HMOs patient compliance is higher with fewer doses.

Galenicals:
Historically used to refer to a class of pharmaceutical products that were compounded through mechanical means.

Galley proofs:
Typeset versions of articles that are provided to editors (and usually to authors) for a final check of spelling, style, and accuracy.

Health care team:
A group of professionals with various skills who work together in providing patient care.

Hypochondriac:
A patient with a psychological disorder in which he or she complains of imagined medical problems.

Indigent:
Unable to pay for certain basic services for oneself, including health care.

Inpatients:
Patients who have been admitted to a hospital or other health care facility and are staying there for treatment. Other patients are called outpatients or, in the community pharmacy setting, ambulatory patients.

Laws:
Acts passed by a legislative body.

License:
A document issued to pharmacists and other citizens that provides special privileges based on specialized knowledge or skills. A drivers' license is one type of such document; it permits the holder to operate motorized vehicles on public roads based on a demonstration to the state of sufficient knowledge. A pharmacy license is similar; it permits the holder to engage in a specialized profession known as pharmacy following demonstration to the state of adequate knowledge. It is a privilege, not a right, and thus the state may withdraw the privilege for various reasons.

Living will:
A legal document that provides guidance to health care professionals about what actions a patient would like taken if he or she is unable to provide an informed decision because of illness or injury. Also known as an advance directive.

Medicaid:
The federal program that reimburses health care providers, including pharmacists, for services provided to the indigent (or poor) patient.

Misbranded:
Drug products that were not properly labeled as to contents and proper use.

Negligence:
Failure of a professional to provide the standard of due care to patients who seek that care.

Nursing homes:
Facilities that provide residential care and health care to residents who live in them. Residents are typically deficient in one or more activities of daily living: ambulating, feeding, bathing, or toileting.

Nutrition support:
For patients whose medical conditions do not permit them to take a normal diet, nutrition support is provided. This may entail oral feedings using liquid foods or intravenous feedings using specialized solutions. The pharmacist is an important member of the nutrition support team because of special expertise in both product preparation and clinical areas.

Objectification:
The viewing of other people in a self-centered way, such as obstacles to one's own goals or a vehicle through which one's owns goals can be realized without regard for the feelings of the other person.

Paradigm:
As used here, paradigm is the typical or standard activities of a pharmacist on a day-to-day basis.

Patient carts:
Hospital pharmacies often use carts with small drawers, one for each patient on a nursing station, to deliver medications from a central or decentral pharmacy to the patient-care floors. Each nursing station cart is exchanged periodically, usually once a day, with a new supply of medications for each patient.

Patient counseling:
Providing the recipient of a prescription medication with oral or written information about the drug product being used.

Patient profiles:
A record, usually computerized, of all medications a patient has received at a given pharmacy. Ideally, the profiles should include both prescription and nonprescription medicines.

Peer review:
Analysis of submitted articles by experts who are not part of the journal's staff.

Pharmacokinetic monitoring:
A part of pharmaceutical care required by patients on certain medications. For some drugs, the difference between a therapeutic blood level and a toxic blood level is very small, and the doses of those drugs need to be calculated carefully and blood levels checked to assure optimal therapy.

Pharmacology:
The study of the action of drugs in biological systems.

Pharmacopeia:
Books listing drugs and other medical devices, including standards for their preparation and analysis, that are recognized by a governmental authority.

Pharmacy benefits managers (PBMs):
Companies that contract with managed-care organizations, insurance companies, or employers to provide prescriptions and pharmaceutical care to a covered population. PBMs often contract with networks of independent or chain pharmacies to provide this care in accordance with guidelines and rules that can reduce the cost of prescriptions.

Pharmacy technician:
A paraprofessional assistant to the pharmacist who helps with the mechanical preparation of medications for dispensing to patients. This person may interpret prescription orders, prepare the medication (including some compounding of medications and preparation of intravenous solutions), and check the work of other technicians in specific situations.

Placebo:
A preparation with no known pharmacologic or medicinal properties. Placebos can sometimes "work" by making the patient believe that a real drug is being given, and placebos are used in some research as a way of identifying the beneficial properties of drugs.

Primary-care providers:
A health care provider to whom patients generally turn first for services.

Product labeling:
The information provided with prescription drugs, including the package insert that lists uses, precautions, adverse effects, and dosages of the drug product. The language in the product labeling must be approved by FDA.

Glossary

Reciprocation:
Once a pharmacist is licensed, he or she can use that license (if in good standing) to practice in other states, after the state board of pharmacy in the new state recognizes the license from the previous state.

Regulations:
Rules promulgated by a part of the executive branch of government, usually based on a law giving the agency statutory authority for the regulation.

Residency:
A postgraduate program of organized training that meets the requirements of a residency-accreditation body.

Rounding:
Once or more often each day in a teaching hospital, members of the health care team gather to conduct "rounds," which usually involve walking to the room of each patient that the team is currently caring for. During rounds, each member of the team has an opportunity to share with the others important information about the patient. Since these are teaching institutions, rounds also serve an important role in imparting knowledge among the members of the team.

Safety:
The ability of a drug not to produce harmful or deleterious side effects or adverse reactions.

Socratic teaching method:
The transfer of knowledge that relies on a person teaching one or a few students in a highly individualized manner. Named after Socrates of ancient Greece.

Style manual:
A book listing preferred ways of stating material in a field or publication.

Terminal position:
A position in a corporate hierarchy from which one has little hope for advancement because of an individual's education and corporate policies.

Tertiary-care institutions:
Hospitals that provide care to patients who could not be treated adequately at the primary (community hospital) or secondary (regional referral hospitals) institutions. Tertiary-care hospitals are often affiliated with medical schools.

Traineeship:
Short-term programs, usually of one week in duration, that provide intensive information and demonstrations about one disease or a small group of similar conditions.

Unit dose packages:
In hospitals and some nursing homes, medications are packaged in strips, with each dose labeled with the brand name, strength, and generic name of the drug. Even though this packaging costs more, it speeds the pharmacy operation and permits return of unused medication to the pharmacy.

Wholesale druggists:
Intermediaries in the mercantile chain between manufacturers and retail outlets such as pharmacies.

Index

Index

Index

Index

Index